Step by Step

Corneal Refractive Surgery

(Techniques and Technology)

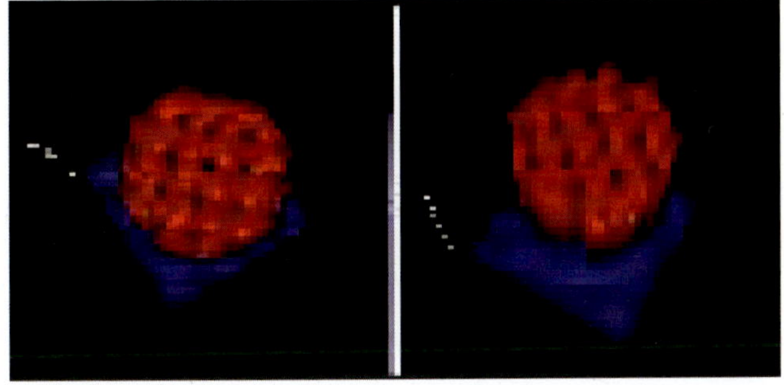

Step by Step

Corneal Refractive Surgery

(Techniques and Technology)

Editors

Ashok Garg
MS PhD FIAO (Bel) FRSM FAIMS
ADM FICA
International and
National Gold Medalist
Medical Director
Garg Eye Institute and Research
Centre
235-Model Town
Dabra Chowk, Hisar-125005 (India)

Dimitrii Dementiev
MD
Chief and Medical Director
Blue Eye Centro di Microchirurgia
Oculare Eye Clinic
Arese 20020 (MI)
Via Campo Gallo 21/10
Milan (Italy)

Ioannis G Pallikaris
MD
Professor and Head
Department of Ophthalmology
University of Crete
VEIC, PO Box 2208
Heraklion 71003
Crete, Greece

Roberto Pinelli
MD
Scientific Director
Instituto Laser Microchirurgia
Oculare
Crystal Palace
Via Cefalonia 70
Brescia-25124 (Italy)

Foreword

Miguel Angelo Padilha

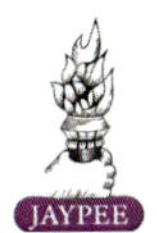

JAYPEE BROTHERS MEDICAL PUBLISHERS

The Health Sciences Publisher

New Delhi | London

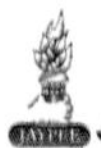

Jaypee Brothers Medical Publishers (P) Ltd

Headquarters
EMCA House
23/23-B, Ansari Road, Daryaganj
New Delhi 110 002, India
Landline: +91-11-23272143, +91-11-23272703
+91-11-23282021, +91-11-23245672
E-mail: jaypee@jaypeebrothers.com

Corporate Office
4838/24, Ansari Road, Daryaganj
New Delhi 110 002, India
Phone: +91-11-43574357
Fax: +91-11-43574314
E-mail: jaypee@jaypeebrothers.com

Overseas Office
J.P. Medical Ltd
83 Victoria Street, London
SW1H 0HW (UK)
Phone: +44 20 3170 8910
E-mail: info@jpmedpub.com

EU GPSR Authorised Representative
Logos Europe, 9 rue Nicolas Poussin
17000, La Rochelle, France
Phone: +33 (0) 6 67 93 73 78
E-mail: contact@logoseurope.eu

Website: www.jaypeebrothers.com
Website: www.jaypeedigital.com

Step by Step Corneal Refractive Surgery (Techniques and Technology)

First Edition: 2006

Reprint: 2026
ISBN: 978-81-8061-746-1

Printed at: Samrat Offset Pvt. Ltd.

To

- My Respected Param Pujya Guru Sant Gurmeet Ram Rahim Singh Ji for his blessings and motivation.
- My Respected Parents, teachers, my wife Dr Aruna Garg, son Abhishek and daughter Anshul for their constant support and patience during all these days of hard work.
- My dear friend Dr Amar Agarwal, a leading International Ophthalmologist from India for his continued support and guidance.

—Ashok Garg

All my colleagues at Vardinoyannion Eye Institute of Crete (Greece).

Ioannis G Pallikaris

My friend and my teacher in Ophthalmology Prof Viktor Zuev, MD.

Dimitrii Dementiev

I dedicate this book to India's Talented ophthalmologists, in the fervent hope that they may become increasingly devoted to refractive surgery.

Roberto Pinelli

Contributors

Amar Agarwal MS FRCS FRC Ophth
Consultant
Dr Agarwal's Eye Hospital
19, Cathedral Road
Chennai-600086
India

AnnMarie Hipsley PT PFS PhD
Director of Research
Global Vision Research Group Ltd
ACE Vision Group
PO Box 328
Blacklick Oh 43004-0328
(USA)

Ariadna Silva-Lepe MD
Terranova No. 676-101
Col. Providencia
Guadalajara, Jal.
Mexico, CP 44630

Ashish Doshi MS
Dr Agarwal's Eye Hospital
19, Cathedral Road
Chennai-600086
India

Ashok Garg MS PhD FIAO (Bel) FRSM FAIMS ADM FICA
Medical Director
Garg Eye Institute and
Research Centre
235-Model Town, Dabra Chowk
Hisar-125005
India

Athiya Agarwal MD DO FRSH
Consultant
Dr Agarwal's Eye Hospital
19, Cathedral Road
Chennai-600086
India

Barbara Kusa MD
Centre Microchirurgia
Ambulatoriale
Via Donizetti, 24 20052 - Monza,
Italy

Carlos Manrique-Lara MD
26, South WillowPoint Circle
The Woodlands
Texas 77382
USA

Charalambos Siganos MD PhD
Department of Ophthalmology
University of Crete
Heraklion, Crete
Greece

Chris P Lohmann MD PhD
Universitats - Augenklinik
Franz - Josef - Strau B-Allee
D-93042, Regensburg
Germany

Cyres K Mehta MS FSVH FAGE
Director and Consultant
Mehta International Eye Institute
Seaside, 147, Colaba Road
Mumbai-400005
India

Dimitrii Dementiev MD
Chief and Medical Director
Blue Eye Centro di
Microchirurgia Oculare Eye Clinic
Arese 20020 (MI)
Via Campo Gallo 21/10
Milan (Italy)

Fabrizio I Camesasca MD
Department of Ophthalmology
Istituto Clinico Humanitas
Rozzano, Milano
Italy

Frederic Hehn MD
Centre de La Vision
Nations - Vision
23, Boulevard de l'europe
54500, Vandoeuvre
France

George D Kymionis MD PhD
Department of Ophthalmology
University of Crete
Heraklion, Crete
Greece

Guillermo Avalos-Urzua MD
Terranova No. 676-101
Col Providencia
Guadalajara, Jal, Mexico
CP 44630

Hetal R Solanki DO
Aditya Jyot Eye Hospital Pvt Ltd
Wadala, Mumbai-400031
India

Hijab Mehta MS DOMS FCPS
Aditya Jyot Eye Hospital Pvt Ltd
Wadala, Mumbai-400031
India

Hitendra Mehta MS
Aditya Jyot Eye Hospital Pvt Ltd
Wadala, Mumbai-400031
India

Ioannis G Pallikaris MD PhD
Prof and Head
Department of Ophthalmology
University of Crete
Heraklion, Crete
Greece

Jaime R Martiz MD
26, South Willow Point Circle
The Woodlands
Texas 77382
USA

Jairo E Hoyos MD PhD
Instituto Oftalmologico Hoyos
Rambla de Sabadell 62 1^0
08201 Sabadell
Barcelona, Spain

Jairo Hoyos-Chacon MD
Instituto Oftalmologico Hoyos
Rambla de Sabadell 62 1^0
08201 Sabadell
Barcelona, Spain

Jean-Marc Legeais MD PhD
Hôtel Dieu de Paris, Service d'
Ophthalmologie, laboratoire
Biotechnologie et oeil 1 Place du
Parvis Notre-Dame
Paris
France 75004

Jes Mortensen MD
The Eye Department
Orebro University Hospital
SE-70185, Orebro
Sweden

Jorge L Alió MD PhD
Instituto Oftalmologico De
Alicante
Avda. Denia 111, 03015
Alicante, Spain

Keiki R Mehta MS DO FIOS
Chairman and Medical Director
Mehta International Eye Institute
147, Shahid Bhagat Singh Road,
Colaba Road, Mumbai-400005
India

Maria C Arbelaez MD
Al Wattiyah, Romaila Building
106, El-Maghraby Eye and
Ear Centre
PO Box 513, PC 112 Rwui
Muscat, Sultanate of Oman

Maria I Kalyvianaki MD
Department of Ophthalmology
University of Crete
Heraklion, Crete
Greece

Matteo Piovella MD
Centro Microchirurgia
Ambulatoriale
Via Donizetti 24
20052, Monza
Italy

Melania Cigales MD
Instituto Oftalmologico Hoyos
Sabadell (Barcelona)
Spain

Michael C Knorz MD
Klinikum Mannheim
Theodor Kutzer Ufer 1-3
Mannheim
Germany

Nilesh Kanjani MS
Consultant
Dr Agarwal's Eye Hospital Pvt Ltd
19, Cathedral Road
Chennai 600086
India

Robert Montés-Micó MD PhD
Instituto Oftalmologico De
Alicante, Avda Denia 111, 03015
Alicante
Spain

Roberto Pinelli MD
Director
Istituto Laser Microchirurgia
Oculare, Crystal Palace
Via Cefalonia, 70
25124 Brescia
Italy

S Natarajan MS
Chairman and Medical Director
Aditya Jyot Eye Hospital Pvt Ltd
Plot No. 153, Road No. 9
Major Parmeshwaran Road
Opp SIWS College, Gate No. 3
Wadala, Mumbai-400031
India

Sanjay Chaudhary MS
Chaudhary Eye Centre and
Laser Vision
4802, Bharat Ram Road
24, Daryaganj
New Delhi-110002
India

Sonika Doshi MS
Dr Agarwal's Eye Hospital Pvt Ltd
19, Cathedral Road
Chennai-600086
India

Soosan Jacob MD DNB FERC
Dr Agarwal's Eye Hospital
19, Cathedral Road
Chennai-600086
India

Sunita Agarwal MS DO PSVH
Dr Agarwal's Eye Hospital
19, Cathedral Road
Chennai-600086, India
15, Eagle Street
Langford Town
Bangalore
India

Tahira Agarwal FORCE DO FICS
Director
Dr Agarwal's Eye Hospital
19, Cathedral Road
Chennai-600086, India

Theokliti G Papadaki MD
Department of Ophthalmology
University of Crete
Heraklion, Crete, Greece

Vikentia J Katsanevaki MD PhD
Vardinoyannion Eye Institute
University of Crete
Greece

FOREWORD

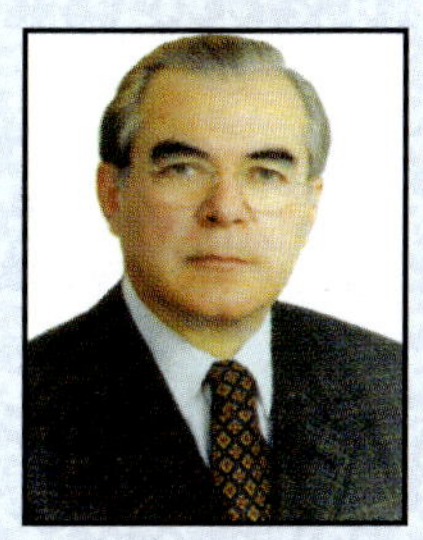

José Barraquer, regarded as the forefather of refractive surgery may not have foreseen in the early sixties that his keratomileusis was the beginning of so long a chain of consequences responsible for the tremendous development of the *armamentarium* of refractive solutions by means of manipulation of the cornea.

Barraquer was followed in continuous movement by Fyodorov's anterior radial keratotomy in 1977 and its introduction into the United States by Leo Bores in 1978, by Kaufman and McDonald's epikeratophakia in 1980, by the advent of Trokel and Seller's excimer laser radiation removing corneal tissues in animal experiments in 1983 and by the introduction of Ruiz's keratomileusis in situ in 1987, all of them fostering the tremendous development in research, technique, methods and management of complications in refractive surgery in the last forty years.

Today, such delicate structure has been unveiled by researchers, who irrepressibly seek ways to reshape it and bring light beams to meet the retina. Such encounter is the perfect conjunction of the external environment with the visual phenomenon which is processed inside, granting the brain with the best vision possible.

The search for refractive surgical solutions is clearly not restricted to the reshaping of the cornea. The other advances are the refractive lensectomy and its replacement by monofocal, bifocal, multifocal or accommodative intraocular lenses and the implantation of IOLs in phakic eyes.

All of these options have advantages and disadvantages, but we know that the unyielding quest for the vision that is as nearly perfect as possible will never cease. As men attempt to achieve immortality and resemblance to their creator, ophthalmologists strive at a breathtaking pace to correct the defects of the visual device, amazed at the power they now bear in their own hands.

Step by Step Book on*Corneal Refractive Surgery* derives from a mighty concentrated effort by Garg, Pallikaris, Dementiev and Pinelli to bring together a select group of exponents in the field of refractive surgery in order to discuss techniques and procedures constantly questioned in contemporary ophthalmology. It is mandatory to speak of contemporaneousness once the evolution of means and methods for the practice of our specialty involves technology in continuous and overwhelming velocity of transformation.

In twenty four chapters, the work exposes the essence of what present-day refractive Surgeons consider important and indicates the direction of their thinking.

Three to two decades ago a skeptic and frightened but also curious and inquisitive ophthalmic community watched the raids of intrepid surgeons on the cornea, cutting it, burning it and excising tissue from its surface with lasers. These are but remote images, now replaced by state-of-the-art technology which provides detailed exams of the corneal structure as well as sophisticated evaluation of aberrations.

Most of us have witnessed already strides in ophthalmology which have perplexed us but the full impact of successful evolution has yet to be realized—the day will come when limitations to visual potentiality will no longer exist.

I heartily congratulate my prestigeous colleagues Dr Ashok Garg, and co-editors **who collaborated in the devising, elaboration and execution of this encompassing work which provides a substantial and opportune update in corneal refractive surgery and grants us the means to meet with the challenge of keeping abreast of the dynamic changes we can already envisage.**

Dr Miguel Angelo Padilha MD FBCS
Professor and Director of the Department of Ophthalmology
Brazilian College of Surgeons
Rua Visconde de Silva, 52/5th Floor
Ed. Colégio Brasileiro de Cirurgiões
Botafogo, 22271-090
Rio de Janeiro, Brazil
tel. (55) 21-2539.2847
fax (55) 21-2527.9994
www.miguelpadilha.com

Preface

Corneal Refractive Surgery has become the state-of-the-art surgery today. Ophthalmologists are able to understand in a better way to modify the corneal surface to suit the patients refractive needs. Wavefront Aberrometry and Biomechanical Customisation have certainly added new dimensions in this field.

This step by step book contains 24 chapters covering all aspects of practical corneal refractive surgery. A number of well-known International Refractive Surgeons have shared their skill and experiences to give you a glimpse of their facts and figures about Corneal Refractive Sugery. A DVD Rom is being given with the book showing latest corneal refractive surgery techniques by International masters of this field.

Our sincere thanks to Shri JP Vij (CMD), Mr Tarun Duneja (General Manager, Publishing) and whole staff of Publishing House for their keen interest and constant support to publish this book in a short time.

We are hopeful this book shall provide useful practical guidance to ophthalmologist doing Refractive Surgery worldwide.

Editors

Contents

DVD Contents

CHAPTER 1

The Evolution of Lamellar Corneal Procedures

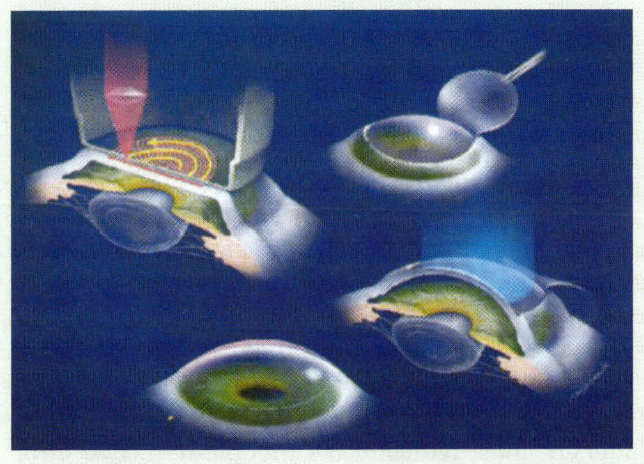

Ioannis G Pallikaris
Theokliti G Papadaki
(Greece)

INTRODUCTION

The roots of lamellar refractive corneal surgery lay in Bogota, Colombia and in the genius, persistent work of Professor Jose Ignacio Barraquer. Based on the fundamental principle that the cornea contributes two-third of the refracting power of the eye, as most light reflection occurs at the air/tear film interface, Barraquer attempted to alter the tear film/anterior cornea interface radius of curvature by adding or removing corneal tissue.[1] Corneal lamellar procedures (Figure 1.1) were developed in an effort to preserve each layer of the cornea. The term *keratomileusis*, which is derived from the Greek roots *keras* (horn-like=cornea) and *smileusis* (carving), was introduced to describe lamellar techniques.[2]

KERATOMILEUSIS *IN SITU*

Keratomileusis *in situ* for myopia, was the first to develop in the late 1940s. The procedure involves raising a corneal cap and removing tissue from the residual stromal bed.

Barraquer's initial technique consisted of performing a free-hand lamellar dissection of the anterior half of the cornea using a Paufique knife or a keratome, to create a corneal cap. Subsequently, the refractive cut was attempted by removing stroma from the bed (*keratomileusis in situ)* with a second pass of the knife or keratome. When the cap was replaced, the anterior corneal curvature was flattened, thus, reducing the myopic refractive error.[3]

The many technical difficulties of keratomileusis *in situ* could not be overcome with the instrumentation available at that time, and the procedure had, therefore, to be temporarily abandoned.[3]

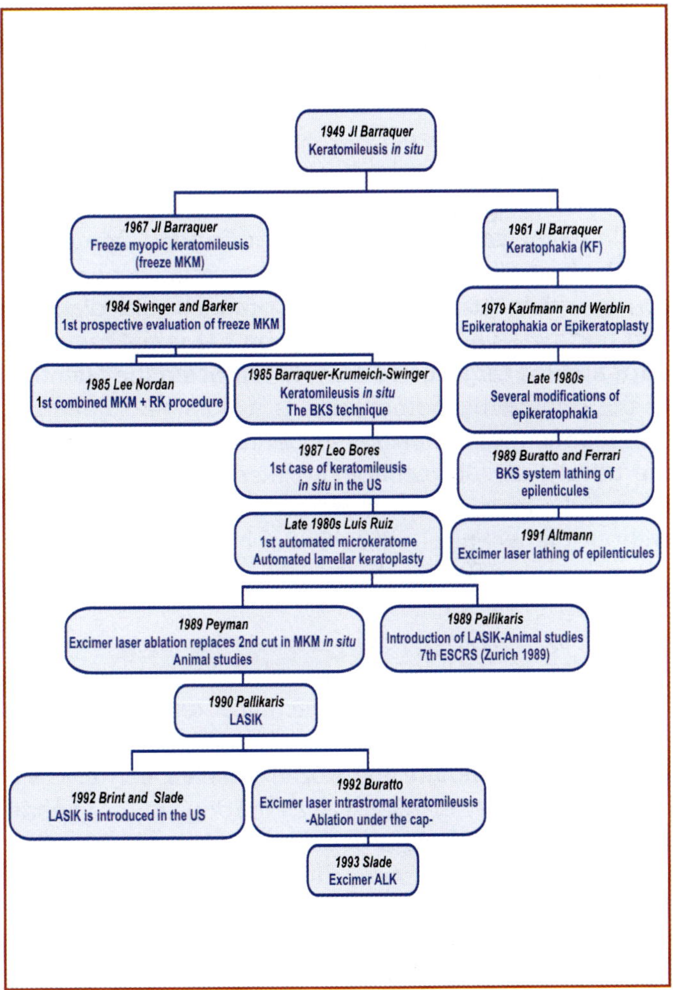

FIGURE 1.1: Evolution of lamellar corneal procedures

KERATOPHAKIA

Barraquer, however, would not abandon the efforts to perfect lamellar techniques. His ingenuity and persistence led to the development of keratophakia (KF), which was first introduced in 1961.[4] KF involves steepening of the central corneal curvature by placing a disk of tissue under the lamellar cap. At that time, the added tissue was invariably an alloplastic stromal disk harvested from a donor cornea with the use of a microkeratome. The disk diameter and thickness varied, depending on the initial refractive error and the target correction. KF attracted the attention of the ophthalmic community as a possible solution in the treatment of aphakia after cataract extraction.[5] With the advent of IOL technology, interest in KF subsided, since IOLs featured the more accurate refractive results without the technical difficulties of harvesting the donor tissue and performing the lamellar cut.

FREEZE MYOPIC KERATOMILEUSIS

In an effort to overcome the technical difficulties of the manual cut, Barraquer was the first to use the contact lens lathe to sculpture the frozen lamellar corneal cap, and so freeze keratomileusis was introduced.[4-7] Theoretically, this new technique could be used to achieve either myopic or hyperopic corrections. However, Barraquer found myopic corrections more successful, thus, he focused his research on refining the freeze myopic keratomileusis (MKM) technique. Barraquer recognized that the cutting speed as well as the relation between IOP and the diameter of the resection, were factors directly affecting the quality and depth of the cut.[3] His efforts for more predictable, reproducible and accurate cuts, led to the development of applanator lenses, suction rings of various diameters and various heights of microkeratome tracks.[6] This work constituted the basis for future microkeratome evolution.

Although first reported results on freeze MKM were encouraging,[3] the technique proved to have two major disadvantages:

- The cryolathe was too expensive to obtain and too complex to maintain
- The learning curve was too steep, involving high rate of complications such as irregular astigmatism or corneal scarring.[7]

At the same time, other techniques were introduced for the correction of refractive errors, such as epikeratophakia,[5,8-13] incisional keratotomy[14-16] and IOL implantation.[17,18]

EPIKERATOPHAKIA (EPIKERATOPLASTY)

Kaufmann and Werblin introduced epikeratophakia or epikeratoplasty in 1979.[8] In an effort to avoid the use of a cryolathe, the innovators attempted to use preprocessed refractive lenticles. A stromal disk was removed from a donor eye with the use of a microkeratome. The disk was frozen and lathed into a concave or convex lens. The lens was then lyophilized and stored for later use. Epikeratophakia was intended for use in the treatment of aphakia, myopia, hyperopia and keratoconus.[11-13] Its major advantages were simplicity and reversibility. Unfortunately, the initial reports showed that the technique was neither predictable nor safe.[18-22] Major problems related to the procedure were poor predictability and complications related to the re-epithelialization of the donor lenticle (persistent epithelial defects, epithelial ingrowth, melting, scarring). Furthermore, it was shown that upon removal of the epilenticle, there remained, occasionally, irreversible changes in the patient's initial refractive error.[23] Several modifications were proposed in an effort to improve epikeratophakia.[29,30] Burrato and Ferrari used the BKS system and Altmann used the excimer laser to shape epilenticles without freezing.[31] However, as the difficulties could not be overcome, epikeratoplasty was withdrawn from the market and research turned once again towards keratomileusis techniques.

BARRAQUER-KRUMEICH-SWINGER (BKS) TECHNIQUE

By that time it was well understood that one of the major problems regarding freezing procedures was that they were often complicated with corneal haze and induced irregular astigmatism.[24-28] Inaccuracy of both epikeratoplasty and freeze MKM was in part attributed to the changes and variables introduced during the excessive processing of the epilenticle button or the corneal cap, respectively.[32,33] Investigations in the direction of developing nonfreezing techniques led to the development of the Barraquer-Krumeich-Swinger (BKS) technique in 1985.[34] This technique included an improved microkeratome (the BKS microkeratome), a set of dyes and a suction stand. The microkeratome was used to perform a total lamellar cap. The cap was then placed epithelial side down, on one of the suction dyes for the microkeratome to perform the second refractive cut at the stromal aspect of the cap. The dye was selected depending on the amount of the attempted correction of myopia or hyperopia. The sculptured lamellar disk was finally sutured back to the bed. Despite their technical difficulty, nonfreezing techniques proved to have a major advantage—the rapid and comfortable recovery of the patients. This was attributed to the preservation of fibroblasts and corneal epithelium. However, significant amounts of irregular astigmatism could not be avoided.[35]

In 1987, Leo Bores performed the first keratomileusis *in situ* in the US.[2] Keratomileusis *in situ* with the use of manual microkeratomes, however, was reported as being not technically safe, precise or predictable and failed to be adopted by a large number of surgeons.[36] Research began in the direction of developing new improved microkeratomes in an effort to improve the reproducibility and accuracy of the *in situ* technique.[37]

AUTOMATED LAMELLAR KERATOPLASTY (ALK)

The development of the automated geared microkeratome by Ruiz in the late 1980s introduced automated lamellar keratoplasty (ALK) in the field of lamellar refractive corneal surgery. The speed of the cut could be controlled by the foot pedal resulting in more even and consistent cuts. The keratome would also automatically reverse at the end of the procedure, without disturbing the lamellar cut. The second, refractive cut was subsequently performed on the bed. The depth of the second cap was adjusted by altering the height of the suction ring.

ALK has been a breakthrough for lamellar surgery. Initially, the corneal cap was sutured back to the stromal bed, but very soon suturing was abandoned as unnecessary. The total operative time was reduced and the procedure could be safely performed under topical anesthesia. Recovery time improved. ALK was greatly popularized as many surgeons who found it difficult to use the manual microkeratomes adopted the new technique.

The first clinical trials on ALK revealed its advantages: (i) ease of use, (ii) rapid recovery and stability of refraction, and (iii) efficacy in the correction of high myopia. Major disadvantages, however, where the relative high rate for irregular astigmatism (2%) and the poor predictability of the procedure (within 2D).[38] The latter was attributed to the imprecision of the depth obtained with the second resected disk. Research now focused on improving the accuracy of the second disk resection. *It was at that time when we thought to combine the precision of photorefractive keratectomy (PRK) with the technique of ALK.*

Trokel et al suggested PRK in 1983.[39] As the use of 193 nm excimer laser in refractive surgery generated, it was revealed that for myopias greater than 6D, PRK resulted in significant central corneal haze, regression of refractive effect and poor predictability.[40]

LASER *IN SITU* KERATOMILEUSIS (LASIK)

Laser in situ keratomileusis (LASIK) was introduced, designed and developed at the University of Crete and the Vardinoyannion Eye Institute of Crete (VEIC) in 1988.[41] The term laser *in situ* keratomileusis (LASIK) was introduced to describe a combination of lamellar refractive corneal surgery and excimer laser photoablation of the cornea under a hinged corneal flap. The idea of raising a corneal flap and removing central tissue from the bed was first described by Pureskin in 1966.[42] He attempted to do the cut manually and cut out the *in situ* part with a trephine.

In LASIK the automated microkeratome is used to create a corneal flap. The refractive second cut is then substituted by the excimer laser submicron accuracy of stromal tissue removal. The initial hypothesis was that a flap would assure better fitting of tissues after removing the intrastromal tissue with laser, and would not affect the anatomic relations of corneal layers mainly by two ways:

i. Preservation of Bowman's layer.
ii. Integrity of the nervous net at the superficial part of the cornea, as the latter follows at a great length its route through the base of the flap.

Other important factors were reduction of maneuvers and total time required for the operation.

The first animal studies to determine wound healing reactions after LASIK, began in 1987, using a Lamda Physik excimer laser and a specially designed microkeratome that was designed to produce a 150-micron flap instead of a total cap. It was suggested that stromal ablation could potentially avoid the regression of effect and stromal haze related to PRK, as the ablated area is hidden from the normal healing process of the eye that takes place at the epithelium/stroma interface.[43,48]

The first papers on LASIK were presented at the Seventh European Congress of the ESCRS in Zurich in

August 1989 and published in 1990.[43] The first LASIK on a blind human eye was performed in June 1989, as a part of an unofficial blind eye protocol.

EXCIMER LASER INTRASTROMAL KERATOMILEUSIS

Later on, in 1992, Lucio Buratto reported on excimer laser intrastromal keratomileusis, a technique where photoablation was performed under a corneal cap. First results on a large series of human eyes proved that this technique was efficient yet not safe. Complication rates were comparable to that of MKM.[44]

Stephen Slade and Brint were the first to perform LASIK in the US in 1992. During the 1993 American Academy of Ophthalmology Meeting, George Waring gave LASIK the temporary names "flap and zap" in order to emphasize the alacrity of the procedure. The major advantages of the procedure, appreciated by patients and surgeons alike include:

- Minimal postoperative discomfort
- Early recovery of visual function
- Lack of adverse healing phenomena such as haze formation
- Increased range of efficacy over PRK in myopia, hyperopia and astigmatism.

To date, there have been published several articles concerning healing of partially sighted eyes,[45,46] results on partially sighted eyes,[47] a comparative study between LASIK and PRK in partially sighted eyes[51] and series of normal sighted eyes with varying follow-up.[49]

Several clinical studies on LASIK since 1995, reveal that refractive results are far from optimum. Accuracy and predictability proves greater with lower diopters of myopia, while certain studies report a high rate of intraoperative complications, comparable to that of other lamellar techniques.[50-72]

LASIK is the most recent step in the evolution of lamellar corneal techniques, initiated by Barraquer 50 years ago. Reports to date are encouraging, although longer follow-up data are expected. Meanwhile, continuous research in the direction of improving microkeratomes and readjusting laser algorithms will hopefully improve the predictability, safety and stability of the procedure.

Reviewing the history of lamellar refractive surgery is essential for better understanding and further refining the currently used techniques. Continuing evolution in all fields of refractive surgery is the only way to approach the ultimate goal, which should be to offer our patients a better vision, both Qualitatively and Quantitatively.

REFERENCES

1. Barraquer JI. Oueratoplastia refractiva. Estudios Inform 1949;10:2-21.
2. Bores L. Lamellar refractive surgery. In Bores L (Ed): Refractive Eye Surgery. Blackwell Scientific Publications: Boston 1993;324-92.
3. Barraquer JI. Keratomileusis. Int Surg 1967;48:103-17.
4. Barraquer JI. Method for cutting lamellar grafts in frozen corneas—new orientations for refractive surgery. Arch Soc Am Ophthalmol 1958;1:237.
5. Kaufmann HE. The correction of aphakia. Am J Ophthalmol 1980;89:1-10.
6. Barraquer JI. Results of myopic keratomileusis. J Refract Surg 1987;3:98-101.

7. Littman H. Optic of Barraquer's keratomileusis. Arch Oftal Optom 1966;6:1.
8. Werblin TP, Klyce SD. Epikeratophakia—the correction of aphakia: I—lathing of corneal tissue. Curr Eye Res 1981; 1:591-97.
9. Barraquer JI. Modification of refraction by means of intracorneal inclusions. Int Ophthalmol Clin 1966;6:53-78.
10. Baumgartner SD, Binder PS, Deg JK, et al. Epikeratophakia—clinical and histopathologic evaluation in non-human primates. Invst Ophthalmol Vis Sci 1983;24:148.
11. Werblin TP, Kaufmann HE, Friedlander MH, et al. A prospective study of the use of hyperopic epikeratophakia grafts for the correction of aphakia in adults. Ophthalmology 1981;88:1137-40.
12. Kaufmann HE, Werblin TP. Epikeratophakia—a form of lamellar keratoplasty for the treatment of keratoconus. Am J Ophthalmol 1982;93:342-47.
13. Werblin TP, Blaydes JE, Kaufmann HE. Epikeratophakia—the correction of astigmatism: Preliminary experimental results. CLAOJ 1983;9:61-63.
14. Bores LD, Myers W, Cowden J. Radial keratotomy—an analysis of the American experience. Ann Ophthalmol 1981;13:941-48.
15. Arrowsmith PN, Sanders DR, Marks RG. Visual, refractive and keratometric results of radial keratotomy. Arch Ophthalmol 1983;101:873-81.
16. Deitz MR, Sanders DR, Marks RG. Radial keratotomy—an overview of the Kansas city study. Ophthalmology 984;91:467-78.
17. Shearing SP. Posterior chamber lens implantation. Int Ophthalmol Clin 1982;22:135-53.
18. McDonald MB, Kaufmann HE, Aquavella JV, et al. The nationwide study of epikeratophakia for aphakia in adults. Am J Ophthalmol 1897;103:350-65.
19. McDonald MB, Kaufmann HE, Aquavella JV, et al. The nationwide study of epikeratophakia for myopia in adults. Am J Ophthalmol 1897;103:375-83.
20. Reidy JJ, McDonald MB, Klyce SD. The corneal topography of epikeratophakia. Refract Corn Surg 1990;6:26-31.

21. Wilson DR, Keeney AH. Corrective measures for myopia. Surv Ophthalmol 1990;34:294-304.
22. Goosey JD, Prager TC, Goosey CB, et al. Stability of refraction during two years after myopic epikeratoplasty. Refract Corneal Surg 1990;6:4-8.
23. Rozakis GW, Slade SG, et al. Refractive Lamellar Keratoplasty Slack: Thorofare 1994.
24. Swinger CA, Barker BA. Prospective evaluation of myopic keratomileusis. Ophthalmology 1984;91:785-92.
25. Nordan LT, Fallor MK. Myopic keratomileusis—74 consecutive non-amblyopic cases with one year follow-up. J Refr Surg 1986;2:124-28.
26. Maquire LJ, Klyce SD, Sawelson H, et al. Visual distortion after myopic keratomileusis—computer analysis of keratoscope photographs. Ophthalmic Surg 1987;18:352-56.
27. Nordan LT. Keratomileusis. Int Ophthalmol Clin 1991;31:7-12.
28. Barraquer C, Guitierrez A, Espinoza A. Myopic keratomileusis—short-term results. Refract Corneal Surg 1989; 5:307-13.
29. Slade SG, Strauss GH. Use of tissue adhesive (Tisseel) in epikeratophakia. Invest Ophthalmol Vis Sci 1990;31:30.
30. Goosey JD, Prager TC, Marvelli TL, et al. Epikeratophakia without annular keratectomy. Ann Ophthalmol 1987;19:388-91.
31. Altmann J, Grabner C, et al. Corneal lathing using the excimer laser and a computer-controlled positioning system: part I—lathing of epikeratoplasty lenticules. Refract Corneal Surg 1991;7:377-84.
32. Friedlander MH, Rich LF, Werblin TP, et al. Keratophakia using preserved lenticles. Ophthalmology 1991;87:687-92.
33. Zavala EY, Krumeich J, Binder PS. Laboratory evaluation of freeze vs no-freeze lamellar refractive keratoplasty. Arch Ophthalmol 1991;105:1125-28.
34. Swinger CA, Krumeich J, Cassiday D. Planar lamellar refractive keratoplasty. I Refract Surg 1986;2:17-24.
35. Colin J, Mimouni F, Robinet A. The surgical treatment of high myopia—comparison of epikeratoplasty, keratomileusis

and minus power anterior chamber lenses. Refract Corneal Surg 1990;6:245-51.

36. Arenas-Archila E, Sanchez-Thorin JC, et al. Myopic keratomileusis *in situ*—a preliminary report. J Cataract Refract Surg 1991;17:424-35.
37. Hofmann RF, Bechara SJ. An independent evaluation of second generation suction microkeratomes. Refract Corneal Surg 1992;8:348-54.
38. Slade SG, Updegraff SA. Complications of automated lamellar keratectomy (comment). Arch Ophthalmol 1995;113 (9):1092-93.
39. Trokel S, Srinivasan R, Braren B. Excimer laser surgery of the cornea. Am J Ophthalmol 1995;94:125.
40. Seiler T, McDonnell PJ. Excimer laser photorefractive keratectomy. Surv Ophthalmol 1995;40(2):89-118.
41. Pallikaris I, Papatzanaki M, Stathi EZ, et al. Laser *in situ* keratomileusis. Laser Surg Med 1990;10:463-68.
42. Pureskin N. Weakening ocular refraction by means of partial stromectomy of the cornea under experimental conditions. Vestn Oftalmol 1967;8:1-7.
43. Pallikaris I, Papatzanaki ME, Georgiadis A, et al. A comparative study of neural regeneration following corneal wounds induced by argon fluoride excimer laser and mechanical methods. Lasers Light Ophthalmol 1990;3:89-95.
44. Buratto L, Ferrari M, Rama P. Excimer laser intrastromal keratomileusis. Am J Ophthalmol 1992;113:291-95.
45. Pallikaris IG, Papatzanaki ME, Siganos DS, et al. A corneal flap technique for laser *in situ* keratomileusis. Arch Ophthalmol 1991;109(12):1699-1702.
46. Pallikaris IG, Papatzanaki ME, Siganos DS, et al. Tecnica de colajo corneal para la queratomileusis *in situ* mediane laser—estudios en humanos. Arch Ophthalmol (Ed Esp) 1992;3(3):127-30.
47. Siganos DS, Pallikaris IG. Laser *in situ* keratomileusis in partially sighted eyes. Invest Ophthalmol Vis Sci 1993;34(4):800.

48. Pallikaris IG, Siganos DS. Excimer laser *in situ* keratomileusis and photorefractive keratectomy for the correction of high myopia. J Refract Corneal Surg 1994;10(15):498-510.
49. Pallikaris IG, Siganos DS. Corneal flap technique for excimer laser *in situ* keratomileusis to correct moderate and high myopia—two year follow-up (best papers of sessions). ASCRS Symposium on Cataract, IOL and Refractive Surgery 1994;9-17.
50. Bas AM, Onnis R. Excimer laser *in situ* keratomileusis for myopia. J Refract Surg 1995;11(suppl): 229-33.
51. Fiander DC, Tayfour F. Excimer laser *in situ* keratomileusis in 124 myopic eyes. J Refract Surg 1995;11(suppl): 234-38.
52. Knorz MC, Liermann A, Steiner H. Laser *in situ* keratomileusis to correct myopia of –6 to –29 diopters. J Refract Surg 1996;12:575-84.
53. Salah T, Waring III GO, El Meghraby A, et al. Excimer Laser *in situ* keratomileusis under a corneal flap for myopia of 2 to 20 diopters. Am J Ophthalmol 1996; 121:143-55.
54. Guell JL, Muller A. Laser *in situ* keratomileusis (LASIK) for myopia ranging from –7 to –18 Diopters. J Refract Surg 1996;12:222-28.
55. Perez-Santonja JJ, Bellot Claramonte P, Ismail MM, et al. Laser *in situ* keratomileusis to correct high myopia. J Cat Refract Surg 1997;23:372-85.
56. El Danasoury MA, Waring GO, El Maghraby A, et al. Excimer laser *in situ* keratomileusis to correct compound myopic astigmatism. J Refract Surg 1997;13:511-21.
57. Marinho A, Pinto MV, Pinto R, et al. LASIK for high myopia—1 year experience. Ophthal Surg Lasers 1997;27: S517-20.
58. Casebeer JC, Kezirian GM. Outcomes of spherocylinder treatments in the comprehensive refractive surgery LASIK study. Semin Ophthalmol 1998;13(2):71-78.
59. Argento CJ, Cosentino MJ. Laser *in situ* keratomileusis for hyperopia. J Cataract Refract Surg 1998;24(8):1050-58.
60. Carr JD, Stulting RD, Sano Y, et al. Prospective comparison of single-zone and multizone laser *in situ* keratomileusis for

the correction of low myopia. Ophthalmology 1998; 105(8):1504-11.
61. Farah SG, Azar DT, Gurdal C, et al. Laser *in situ* keratomileusis—literature review of a developing technique. J Cataract Refract Surg 1998;24(7):989-1006.
62. Knorz MC, Wiesinger B, Liermann A, et al. Laser *in situ* keratomileusis for moderate and high myopia and myopic astigmatism. Ophthalmology 1998;105(5):932-40.
63. Davidorf JM, Zaldivar R, Oscherow S. Results and complications of laser *in situ* keratomileusis by experienced surgeons. J Refract Surg 1998;14(2):114-22.
64. Ibrahim O. Laser *in situ* keratomileusis for hyperopia and hyperopic astigmatism. J Refract Surg 1998;14(2 suppl): 179-82.
65. Lavery F. Laser *in situ* keratomileusis for myopia. J Refract Surg 1998;14(2 suppl):177-78.
66. Chayet AS, Magallanes R, Montes M, et al. Laser *in situ* keratomileusis for simple myopic, mixed and simple hyperopic astigmatism. J Refract Surg 1998;14(2 suppl): 175-76.
67. Maldonado-Bas A, Onnis R. Results of laser *in situ* keratomileusis in different degrees of myopia. Ophthalmology 1998;105(4):606-11.
68. Goker S, Er H, Kahvecioglu C. Laser *in situ* keratomileusis to correct hyperopia from +4.25 to +8.00 diopters. J Refract Surg 1998;14(1):26-30.
69. Zaldivar R, Davidorf JM, Oscherow S. Laser *in situ* keratomileusis for myopia from –5.5 to –11.50 diopters with astigmatism. J Refract Surg 1998;14(1):19-25.
70. Salchow DJ, Zirm ME, Stieldorf C, et al. Laser *in situ* keratomileusis for myopia and myopic astigmatism. J Cataract Refract Surg 1998;24(2):175-82.
71. Lindstrom RL, Hardten DR, Chu YR. Laser *in situ* keratomileusis (LASIK) for the treatment of low moderate, and high myopia. Trans Am Ophthalmol Soc 1998;95:285-96.
72. Waring GO 3rd, Carr JD, Stulting RD, et al. Prospective, randomized comparison of simultaneous and sequential bilateral LASIK for the correction of myopia. Trans Am Ophthalmol Soc 1997;95:271-84.

CHAPTER 2

IntraLase FS Laser to Create Corneal Flaps: All Laser Procedure

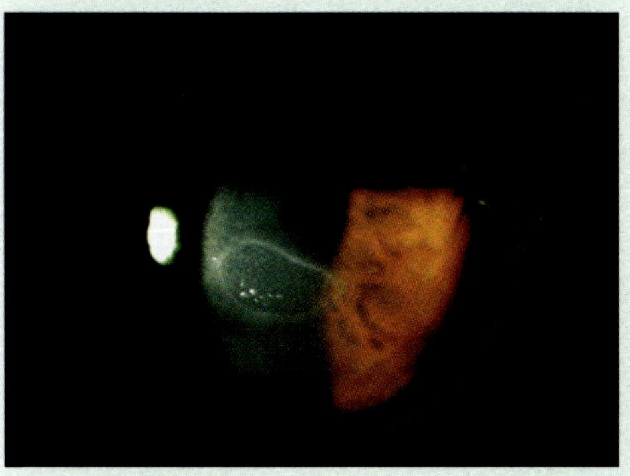

Jaime R Martiz
Carlos Manrique-Lara
(USA)

INTRODUCTION

In conventional laser assisted *in situ* keratomileusis (LASIK), refractive surgeons use a microkeratome with a razor blade to create the flap. Performance of the initial lamellar resection for flap creation remains responsible for a portion of intra and postoperative complications in LASIK.

To date the majority of complications (1 in 1,000 cases) in LASIK are related to mechanical microkeratomes, which use metal blade to create a flap (nicks, irregularities, etc.). The flap depth using standard microkeratomes can vary between eyes depending on blade manufacture, corneal curvature and intraocular pressure of the patients.

The most common intraoperative complication includes "buttonhole", epithelial sloughing, incomplete flaps, thin or thick flaps and free flaps. Complications after LASIK include epithelial in-growth, flap dislocation and diffuse lamellar keratitis. Any of these situations could potentially delay recovery of vision acuity or in a worth case scenario even lead to a permanent vision loss. Using a mechanical keratomes, if the ring that fixates on the eye with suction looses fixation during the creation of the flap, the cap can be cut. The cap is either replaced and the patient has to wait three or more months before a repeat treatment. With the IntraLase FS laser if suction is lost, the laser's focus changes immediately to the surface of the eye (Figure 2.1). There is no laceration of the flap and the surgeon is able to regain suction and begin the case immediately without risk.

The IntraLASIK it used only to create the flap, and then we use an excimer laser to perform the rest of the LASIK procedure (Figure 2.2). The procedure is

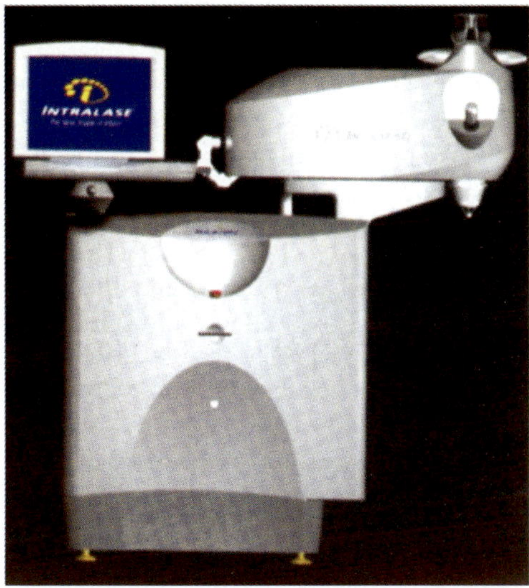

FIGURE 2.1: IntraLase FS pulsion laser

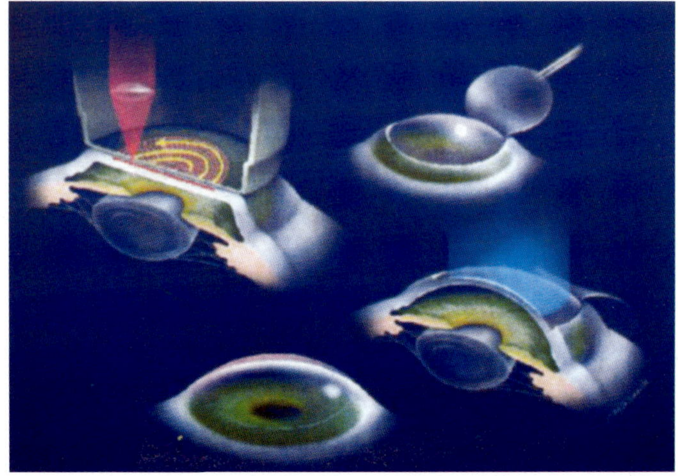

FIGURE 2.2: Resection initiated

distinguished by the speed of the laser pulses, in the femtosecond (one quadrillionth of a second) range. Surgeons have the opportunity to offer their patients a safer, computer controlled alternative for creating the corneal flap and may avoid the complications related to the metal blades from microkeratomes.

THE INTRALASE FS LASER

The laser introduces high precision femtosecond technology; it creates a flap under very low vacuum, delivering the laser energy directly to the corneal stroma through a disposable glass lens (Figure 2.3). The outer surface of the cornea suffers no trauma, and the procedure is painless. The IntraLase FS laser is a solid-state laser that does not rely upon a mixture of gases to generate a beam, as does the excimer laser. It uses a very short pulse with a spot size of 3 microns. This enables the laser to apply

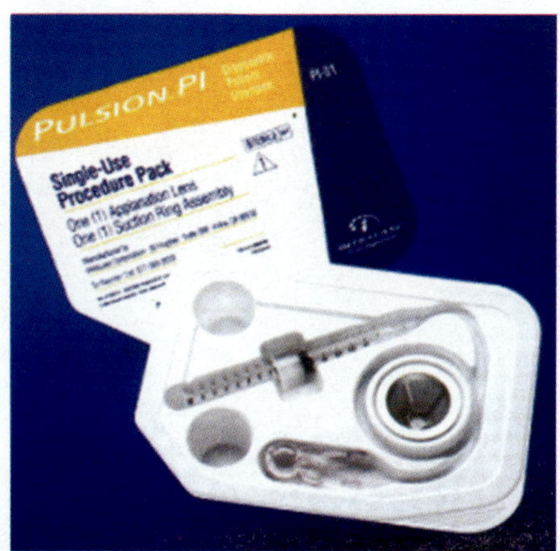

FIGURE 2.3: Suction ring and a flat contact lens

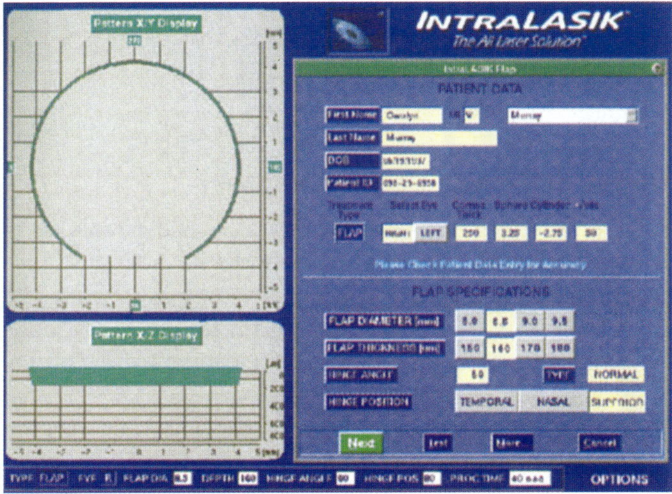

FIGURE 2.4: Computer parameter

less energy to the corneal tissue with micron range accuracy. It use a wavelength of 1053 nm that is not absorbed but instead can pass through the cornea with no effect on the tissue until it reaches the pre-programmed target (Figure 2.4). The beam is optically sharpened into a 3 microns spot size and delivered to the predetermined intracorneal location. The laser pulses are places close together to define precise subsurface areas of photodisruption.

FEMTOSECOND LASER PHOTODISRUPTION PROCESS

The specific features of the process depend for the most part on the pulse duration and focus geometry of a particular system. If the energy is too elevated to start optical breakdown, the resultant shock wave and cavitations bubbles produce significant collateral tissue damage.

Steps of Tissue Photodisruption

1. The femtosecond laser produced optical breakdown.
2. Combination of free electrons and ions that constitutes the plasma state.
3. The optical breakdown created hot plasma expands with supersonic velocity displacing adjacent corneal tissue.
4. Spread of the supersonic displacement front through the corneal tissue as a shock wave.
5. Shock wave loses velocity and energy as it spread out relaxing to a wave that dissolves without risk.
6. Spreading out of the plasma occurs on a time scale that is short in comparison to the local thermal diffusion time constant, thereby confining thermal damage.
7. The cooling plasmas vaporize small volume of corneal tissue, eventually forming a cavitations bubble.
8. The cavitations bubble consists mainly of CO_2, N_2 and H_2O, which can diffuse out from the corneal stroma via normal mechanisms.

INTRALASIK: CREATION OF A FLAP

The localized effects of femtosecond photodisruption allow its use as a high precision cutting device. The laser pulses must be placed contiguously to create a flap within the corneal stroma. This flap can be placed in any orientation: horizontal, vertical or oblique. The only limitation to creating a flap incision is that they must be made from the deepest portion of the cornea to the more superficial. This occurs because, the static gas bubbles that persist in the cornea block the laser if the focus is moved to a plane below the previously produced bubbles. Using a computer controlled scanning optical delivery system and a femtosecond laser; photodisruption can be placed contiguously to create a corneal flap with a high-precision tissue separation.

All corneal procedures with IntraLASIK utilize an applanation system consisting of a suction ring and a flat contact lens located at the tip of the laser delivery system (Figure 2.5). The suction ring fixates the eyes, allowing the contact lens to temporarily flatten the front surface of the cornea. The flat contact lens is securely attached to the suction ring by an internal cylindrical clamp,

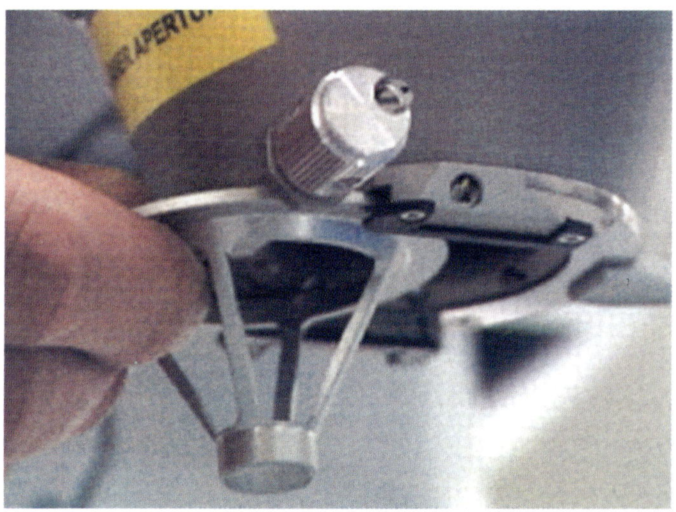

FIGURE 2.5: Cone in laser

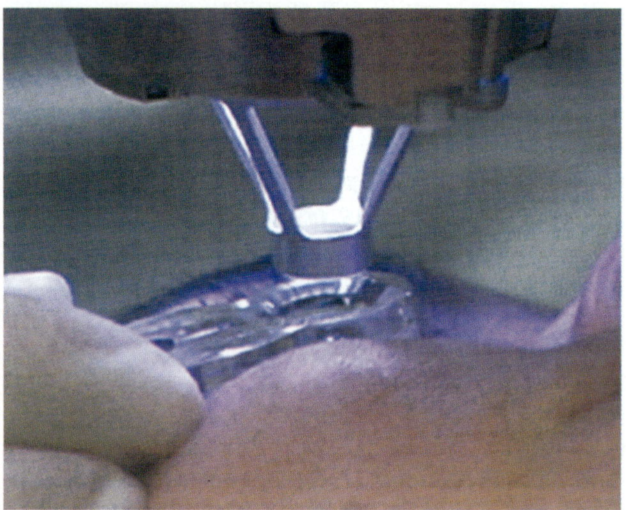

FIGURE 2.6: Applanation cone into eye

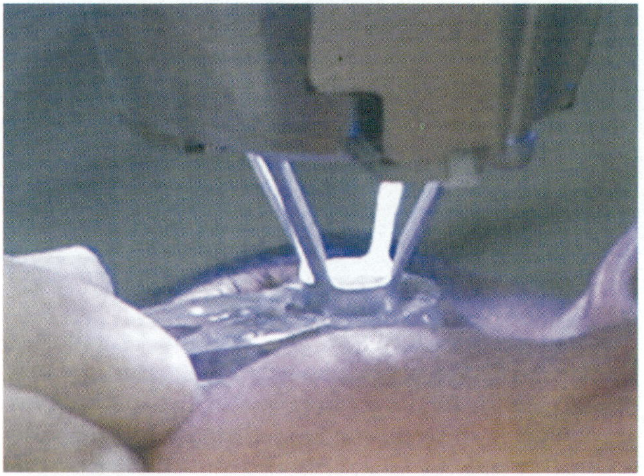

FIGURE 2.7: Applanation cone into eye part 2

mechanically coupling the eye to the beam delivery system (Figures 2.6 and 2.7). This system allows depth precision to be controlled to less than ten microns.

A flap is created by a pattern of laser pulses at the desire depth to create a resection plane parallel to the applanated corneal surface. First a pocket is made, to a gas bubbles to escape, then the resection plane is created in a raster pattern, and finally a side cut is made by advancing the laser towards the surface in a circular pattern (Figures 2.8 to 2.10). The corneal hinge can be placed at any meridian by blocking the beam for a short time during each circle. After the laser reaches the surface gas bubbles escape from the interface and the suction is released. The patient is then placed under the excimer laser and the flap is elevated to ablate the corneal stroma. The flap is repositioned as with standard LASIK.

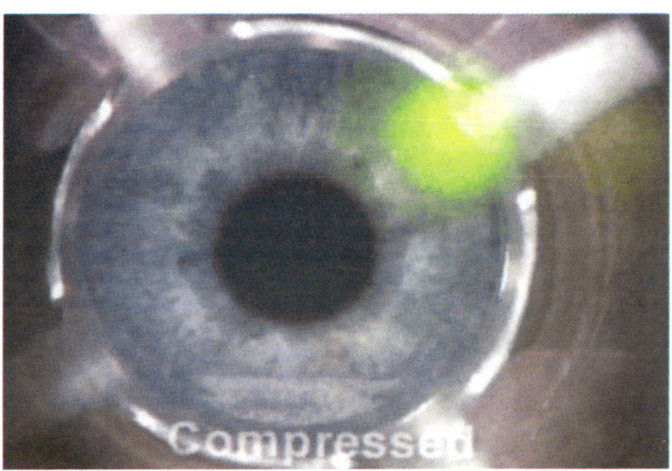

FIGURE 2.8: IntraLASIK pocket

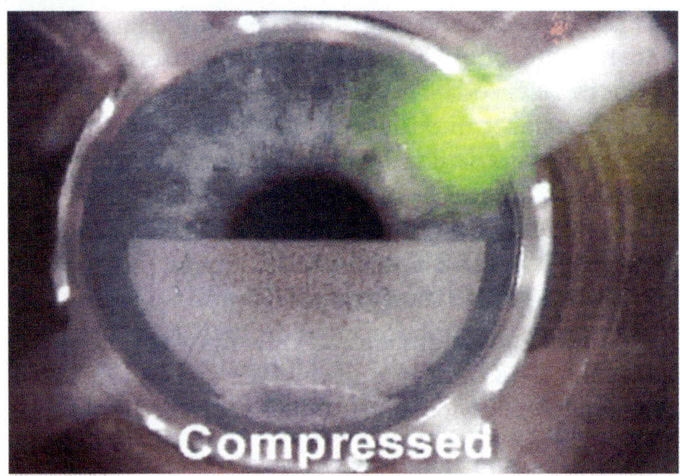

FIGURE 2.9: IntraLASIK created in a raster pattern

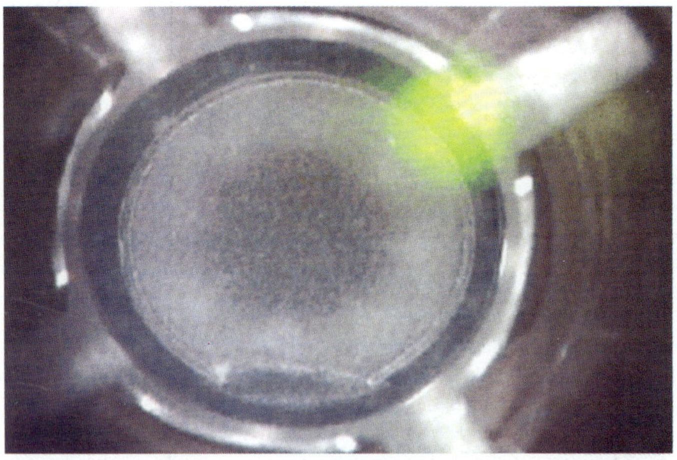

FIGURE 2.10: IntraLASIK side cut

COMPARING INTRALASIK AND LASIK: THE DIFFERENCE IS IN THE CORNEAL FLAP

Some patients not eligible for LASIK may be able to have IntraLASIK. The thickness of the cornea is an important variable in LASIK. Most patients have corneas between 500 and 600 microns thick. Most microkeratomes cut flaps that are between 100 and 200 microns thick. For people with thin corneas, LASIK surgeons tend to move cautiously, balancing the thickness of the cornea against the amount of vision correction needed, and even may decide that the procedure is not recommended in a particular patient.

The IntraLase FS laser can make corneal flaps as thin as 100 microns, which may allow surgeons to perform IntraLASIK in patients with thinner and flatter corneas. It may present fewer complications since the cut follows the curvature of the cornea and produces a flap with vertical edges, unlike the edges left by a microkeratome. This difference in flap architecture may reduce the chance of corneal epithelial ingrowths.

AFTER INTRALASIK

Corneal flaps complete with IntraLASIK appear to adhere more tightly to the corneal bed at the end of the procedure. They demonstrate a more aggressive healing response at the corneal flap edges. Avoid complications such as corneal irregularities and scarring, which can degrade vision, but also offers the potential for better vision after LASIK.

INTRALASIK: DECREASE ENHANCEMENT RATES AND LESS HIGH ORDER ABERRATIONS INDUCED

IntraLASIK could potentially decrease enhancement rate. It provides more precise flaps, better predictability of results and creates more astigmatically neutral flaps than mechanical blade microkeratomes. This is an enormous contribution as we start to perform more custom treatment using wave front technology.

With the microkeratomes, corneal flaps are frequently thicker in the periphery and thinner in the center. In IntraLASIK there is no risk of flap thickness irregularities that can result in induced astigmatism or significant degree of high order aberrations. When the corneal flaps are produced with mechanical blade microkeratomes, crinkles and striaes can occur in the center. In IntraLASIK a planar flap is created, a type of flap that will become more important in the future as we advance into wavefront guided treatments. There is less high order aberrations induced with IntraLASIK because it creates consistent thickness throughout the entire resection.

DISCUSSION

LASIK using a microkeratome to create a corneal flap, has become the most frequently perform surgical procedure worldwide in refractive surgery. Even though LASIK has a high success rate, they're still a percentage of complications including vision loss that still have been reported. The greater parts of these complications are related to microkeratome malfunction. The ability to vary different parameters such a thickness, diameter, hinge location, hinge angle and side cut, side cut angle, pocket side and location can additional offer a superior clinical safety. Precision and control in LASIK surgery have everything to do with accuracy of vision correction, quality of resulting vision and reproducibility among differing patients and surgeons. Replacing the mechanical microkeratome, the source of many LASIK complications, with a computer guided laser may be a significant advantage.

BIBLIOGRAPHY

1. Dastgheib KA, Clinch TE, Manche EE, Hersh P, Ramsey J. Sloughing of corneal epithelium and wound healing complications associated with laser *in situ* keratomileusis in patients with epithelial basement membrane dystrophy. Am J Ophthalmol 2000;130:297-303.
2. Davidorf JM, Zaldivar R, Oscherow S. Results and complications of laser *in situ* keratomileusis by experienced surgeons. J Refract Surg 1998;14(2):114-22.
3. Durairaj VD, Balentine J, Kouyoumdijan G. The predictability of corneal flap thickness and tissue laser ablation in laser *in situ* keratomileusis. Ophthalmology 2000;107:2140-43.
4. Holland SP, Srivannaboon S, Reinstein DZ. Avoiding serious corneal complications of laser assisted *in situ* keratomileusis and photorefractive keratectomy. Ophthalmology 2000;107: 640-52.
5. Jacobs BJ, Deutsch TA, Rubenstein JB. Reproducibility of corneal flap thickness in LASIK. Ophthalmic Surg Lasers 1999;30:350-53.
6. Juhasz T, Kastis GA, Suarez C, et al. Time-resolved observations of shock waves and cavitations bubbles generated by femtosecond laser pulses in corneal tissue and water. Laser Surg Med 1996;19:23-29.

7. Kurtz RM, Horvath C, Liu HH, Krueger R, Juhasz T. Lamellar refractive surgery with scanned picosecond and femtosecond laser pulses. J Refract Surg 1998;14:541-48.
8. Maatz G, Heisterkamp A, Lubatschowski H, et al. Chemical and physical side effects at application of Ultrashort laser pulses for intrastromal refractive surgery. J Opt A Pure Appl Opt 2000;2:59-64.
9. Martiz J. All Laser LASIK with the Pulsion FS Laser: LASIK and Beyond LASIK, Wavefront Analysis and Customized Ablation 2001;8:119-25.
10. Probst LE, Machat JJ. Mathematics of laser *in situ* keratomileusis for high myopia. J Cataract Refract Surg 1998;24(2):190-95.
11. Ratkay I, Juhasz T, Kiss K, Ferencz I, Suarez C, Kurtz R. Ultrashort pulsed laser surgery: Initial Application in LASIK. Ophth Clinics N America 2001;14:347-55.
12. Tham VM, Maloney RK. Microkeratome complications of laser *in situ* keratomileusis. Ophthalmology 2000;107:920-24.

CHAPTER 3

Photorefractive Keratectomy (PRK)

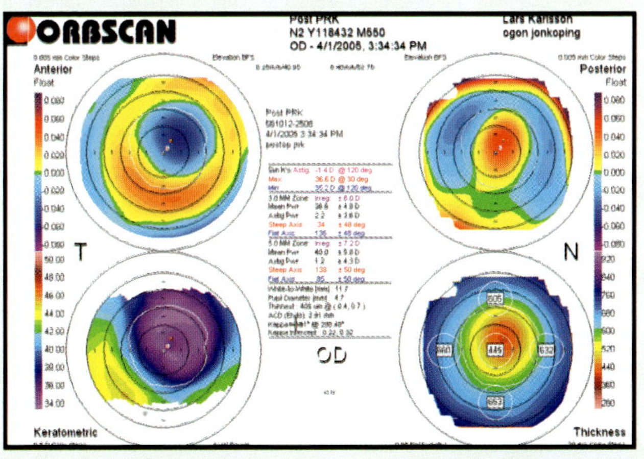

Jes Mortensen (Sweden)

INTRODUCTION

Writing a chapter about PRK is a nostalgic business. PRK disappeared for a while but is now seeing a renaissance as growing concerns about problems in LASIK surgery are becoming more and more evident.

I shall try to cover the subject partly from the literature but mostly from my own experience from excimer laser surgery. To talk about the present and the future you have to first mention the past, the history.

The term excimer is a contraction of excited dimer.

In 1976, Dr. Dave Muller, Ph.D., former President of Summit Technology, Inc., built Cornell University's first Excimer Laser. The excimer laser was initially used for etching silicone computer chips in the 1970s. Excimer laser emission is inherently short pulsed, typically around 10 nsec, with a repetition rate between 1 and 50 Hz.

The ArF excimer laser emission is 193 nm. Research in the early 1980s showed that excimer laser generated UV light can precisely etch a variety of polymers.

Dr. Srinivasan microetched, or photoablated, patterns on human hairs (Figure 3.1). He was impressed as to how sharply defined the edges were and how the microetched hair retained its cylindrical shape. This information was also published, and in 1983, Dr. Steve Trokel, M.D., saw the picture of the microetched hair and visited Dr. Srinivasan at his IBM laboratory in July 1983.

Drs. Srinivasin and Leigh observed that the irradiated substrate is broken into small fragments that are ejected into the surrounding atmosphere. They called the process "ablative photodecomposition". The term preferred today is photoablation. Dr. Srinivasin noticed that you could

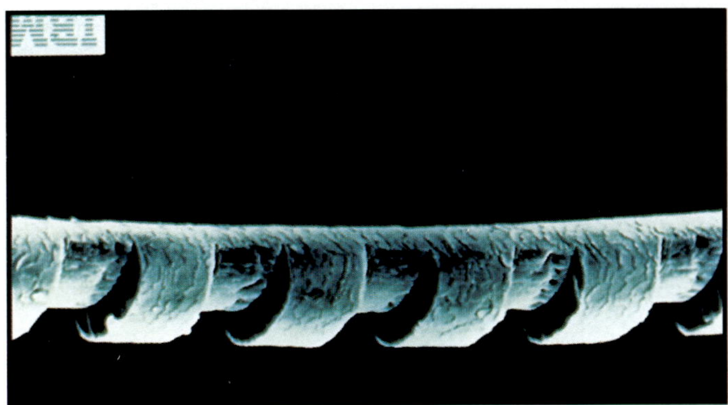

FIGURE 3.1: Microetched human hair

remove tissue with the laser without causing any harm to the neighboring material due to heating.

At 193 nm, a single UV photon has energy of 6.4 eV, which exceeds the covalent bond strength of many molecules. After bond breakage occurs, intense local pressure in a confined volume ejects the molecular fragments into the surrounding atmosphere. Corneal tissue effectively absorbs laser energy at 193 nanometres.

The high photon energy may result in a purely photochemical process. The temperature is only increased by 5° Celsius. Extremely short laser pulses help to limit local heating. Photochemical and photothermal effects of the excimer laser wavelengths on the cornea are due to absorption by solid elements. The excimer laser does not cut like a knife, rather it removes tissue by ablation sending the material ablated up in the air as a plume. That caused the problems of the early broad beam excimer lasers, as the plume shadowed the central part of the ablation zone causing the central island.

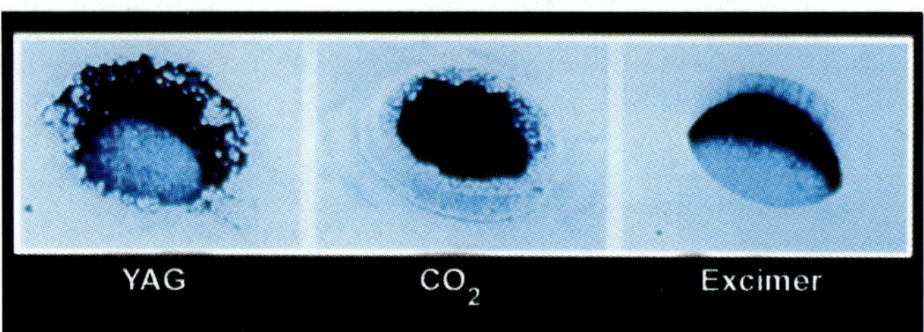

FIGURE 3.2: The precise and controlled etching of the cornea

Mutagenesis and carcinogenesis are always concerns with UV radiation. However in several studies no mutagenic or carcinogenic cellular events[9,10] were seen to be caused by 193 nm irradiation.

In 1983, professor Stephen Trokel and co-workers first reported the precise and controlled etching of the cornea by an argon-fluorine (ArF) excimer laser (Figure 3.2). An excellent preservation of normal corneal stromal microstructure near to the ablation zone was found. In 1996 the first Excimer laser for refractive use in the USA was approved by the FDA.

In 1983 Dr. Munnerly refined the use of excimer lasers to alter the refractive power of the cornea. He presented a mathematical formula to calculate the depth of ablation, diameter and edge angles of the treatment.

The Munnerly's PRK formula:

$$T=S/3\ (D)^2$$

where T is thickness of the removed tissue (microns), S is refractive change diopters and D is diameter of the ablated zone.

The first approaches to excimer laser refractive surgery attempted to build on the strategies developed for radial keratotomy. Growing concerns about the width of the linear incisions that would be expected to fill with an epithelial plug that might persist for months to years turned the investigators to direct ablation of the superficial central cornea.

In 1984, Dr. Marguerite MacDonald from LSU started doing animal research with the Excimer Laser.

From that point on, research and development groups began to spring up all over the world, especially in Western nations. The early pioneers include: Dr. Steve Trokel, M.D., USA; Dr. Francis L'Esperance, M.D., USA; Prof. John Marshall, Ph.D., England; Dr. Malcolm Ker-Muir, M.D., England; Dr. Theo Seiler, M.D., Ph.D., Germany; Dr. Olivia Serdarevic, M.D., USA; Dr. Carmen Puliafito, M.D., USA; Dr. Roger Steinert, M.D., USA; Dr. Marguerite MacDonald, M.D., USA; Dr. Charles Munnerlyn, USA; and others.

In July 1988, Dr. Marguerite MacDonald, M.D., performed Excimer Laser PRK on the first sighted eye thus giving with the longest follow-up in the world. In 1989, in Germany, Dr. Theo Seiler did the first bilateral Excimer Laser PRK for myopia

To induce corneal flattening, the most tissue must be removed centrally, with progressively less removed toward the periphery. Several laser delivery systems accomplish that goal.

Perhaps the most precise term for this approach is laser anterior keratomileusis. More commonly, it is known by the less specific term photorefractive keratectomy; abbreviated (PRK).

The first laser systems were: A scanning beam in conjunction with a diaphragm (Meditec, Novatec), and laser systems (Summith, VISX 20/20) with a laser beam with a diameter of 4 to 6 mm. A diaphragm system places a moveable circular aperture in the path of the laser beam. The aperture can either expand or contract during the exposure. In either case, the central cornea will be exposed to each laser pulse, and the more peripheral cornea will be exposed to fewer pulses. The modern scanning laser systems we see today have a scanning beam with a point size of 1 to 2 mm; the laser beam is steered by a computer system. Modern excimer laser systems have a pulse frequency of 50 to 200 Hz.

The excimer laser removes 0.22 to 0.25 microns of the corneal tissue per pulse.

The larger the diameter of the ablation zone the deeper the ablation. A scanning laser cuts deeper than the old broad beam lasers, which prompted VISX to offer a combination of the two techniques. That even made the ablation faster.

The diameter of the ablation zone was initially 4.0 mm (Summit), but it was soon realized that many patients had problems with glare and halo, disturbing the vision especially during night driving. Eyes with wider ablation zones were much more unlikely to develop such problems. I have never used an excimer laser system with less than a 6 mm zone, so I have not seen a lot of patients with problems from small ablation zones. Most problems disappeared after 6 to 12 months. Today we know that the retina is able to adapt to the smaller ablation zone at least if it is not less than 6 mm.

Another method of reducing the depth of ablation was to use multiple zones in treating moderate and highly myopic eyes.

There were considerable problems with central islands in the beginning, up to 26 percent had that problem. The patients were unhappy, as the UCVA was low. In most cases the central island would disappear without further treatment, but not always.

Different approaches were developed. Multipass multizone technique and multizone ablation in a single pass were superior to the old single ablation zone.[8]

Treating astigmatism was also of concern in the early days. To treat astigmatism you have to accomplish a toric contour of the corneal surface. Two basic strategies were pursued. In the first, the laser beam was directed through a moving aperture of parallel slit blades that progressively closed during the ablation. The ablation could be performed with this aperture alone, or secondly in combination with the moving round diaphragm that was used in spherical myopic PRK.

Today the scanning laser has solved the problem, but pronounced astigmatism is still of some concern; it is possible to treat but there is a problem with regression. In my experience LASIK is superior to PRK in the treatment of severe astigmatism.

CLINICAL RESULTS

The first clinical studies were done outside the USA. It was first in 1996 that the FDA approved PRK. Most studies have focused on the correction of myopia in the range of –1.5 to –6.0 diopters.[11-13] Two studies under the Food and Drug Administration's (FDA)investigational protocols, generated 2-year follow-up results on 500 to 700 patients. Most ablations have been performed with 5 mm optical zones, and patients have been treated postoperatively with moderately intense doses of steroids; gradually, the dose was tapered over 4 to 6 months. With this approach, uncorrected visual acuity at 6 months was 20/40 or better in approximately 93 percent of patients in both trials. Six-month accuracy within ± 1.00 D of emmetropia was achieved in 75 percent of patients with preoperative myopia ranging from –1.5 to –6.00 D. Other investigations have looked into the use of the excimer laser for the correction of higher myopia[14] and astigmatism;[15-18] these studies were performed multinationally.

In 1994 professor Björn Tengroth and co-workers from Sweden published a study with 495 patients followed for 24 months.[19] Preoperative refraction ranged from –1.25 to –7.50 Diopters:

The PRK procedures was performed by the Summit laser (ExciMed UV/200LA excimer laser).

Mean refraction after 24 months was –0.27 ± 0.74 diopters. The correction was stable first after 18 months. Subgroup analysis showed that the patients with low to moderate myopia (up to –3.90 diopters) had a significantly better refractive outcome than those with high myopia. 91 percent of the eyes had an uncorrected visual acuity of ar least 20/40, and 81.5 percent of at least 20/30. 87.5 percent were within ±1 diopter of emmetropia.

The first patient was treated at our clinic in Jonkoping in February 1992. So far 6000 patients have been treated, 1000 with PTK. Our first excimer laser was a VISX Twenty-Twenty B laser. In 1995 we upgraded to a VISX Star, which served us until 2000 when we changed to a scanning laser, Chiron 217 c. Today we have the Chiron 217 Z and use the Zywave technology.

In the early days we scraped off the epithelium with a knife, then we used an automatic brush (we liked it, the patients did not) today we use LASEK (20% alcohol for 20 seconds, roll off the epithelium from the ablation zone, after the excimer laser ablation, carefully roll back the epithelium and put on a contact lens). Until we changed to the Chiron excimer laser we had no Eye Tracker, so free fixation was used. Postoperatively dexametason or prednisone was used topically. Astigmatism > 0.75 D was corrected.

The results I shall present are all from before 1996. The first reports tell about a hyperopic shift the first months; we did not see that with our VISX Twenty-Twenty B laser.

The first group (89 patients, average age 27 years) 118 eyes preoperative refraction –1.0 diopters to –9.75 diopters. Six months follow up: 80 percent achieved refraction between ±1.0 diopter. Fourteen patients had traces of haze.

10 percent had retreatment due to regression.Visual acuity for the whole group, 72 percent ≥ 20/30, and 81 percent ≥ 20/40. In the –1.0 to –4.0 group, 92 percent were better than 20/40.

Before treatment 30 eyes had no astigmatism, 52 eyes between –0.25 to –0.75 diopters, and 36 eyes –1.0 to –6.0 diopters. After treatment 73 eyes had no astigmatism, 27 eyes between –0.25 to –0.75 diopters, 18 eyes between –1.0 to –2.0 diopters.

We achieved an appropriate reduction of the astigmatism especially the high astigmatism group. Unfortunately we also saw induction of astigmatism, particularly in cases with high myopia. Our experience was that astigmatism correction is somewhat difficult to predict. We have tended to under-correct it. The problem with astigmatism is hitting the right axis; 5 degrees off the axis reduces the power of the correction by 20 percent.

If you are 30 degrees from the correct axis you get no correction of the astigmatism at all.

The second group consisted of high myopics (23 patients, average 35 years), 30 eyes between –10.00 and –25,00 diopters. All were treated in three zones; 4.5, 5.0 and 6.0 mm, and in one session. Astigmatism was also treated if present.

The average spherical equivalent before treatment was: –13.44 diopters and after –1.88 diopters. We did not go for full correction in all cases. The follow up was 6 months. Every eye in this group showed a tendency to regression. At least 5 eyes have been retreated. Happily there were very little problems with haze; 7 eyes showed haze +1, and 1 patient +2. A change in best-corrected visual acuity was seen: 11 unchanged, 10 better and 9 worse. One eye lost 3 lines.

Increase of IOP was seen by 10 percent in the low myopic group; and by almost 20 percent in the highly myopic group.

As mentioned this material is from 1992 to 1995. I shall now show you results from a group of high myopics with 12 to 13 years follow-up. That might give some indications of the safety of the excimer laser procedure.

Performing reoperations we have seen that the pattern etched into the cornea is unchanged even after 13 years (Figure 3.3).

I have three patients (6 eyes) with 13 years follow up and 2 patients (4 eyes) with 12 years follow up. Presented as the following cases:

All eyes were treated with the VISX Twenty-Twenty B laser, epithelium was scraped off with a scalpel. Dexametason was given locally for at least 4 months postoperatvely, if regression or haze was seen a longer period of treatment was prescribed.

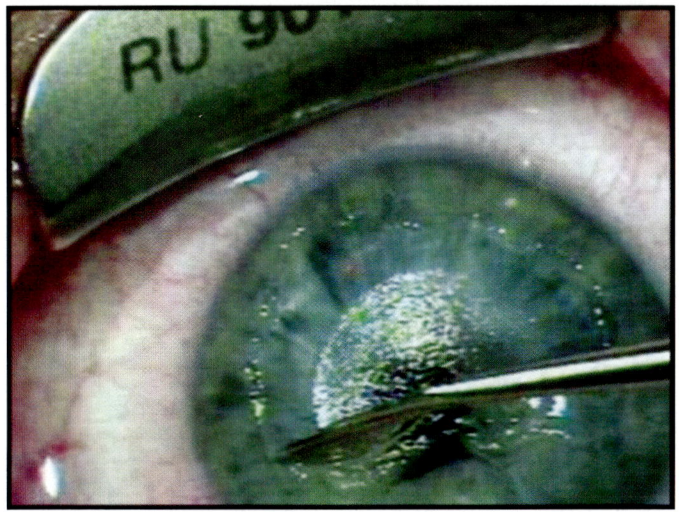

FIGURE 3.3: Retreatment after ten years

1. Woman now 48 years of age. PRK performed May 1992. Refraction left eye: –15.75/–2.25 × 152°. Visual acuity 20/60. PRK ablation: –13.25/ –2.25 × 152°. In August 1992 the right eye was treated. Refraction right eye: –17.75/–1.75 × 49°. Visual acuity 20/40. PRK ablation, full treatment. No retreatment was needed only traces of haze were seen. Last visit, April 2005. Right eye 20/100 without correction, and 20/ 50 with –2,75/–1,0 × 113°. Left eye 20/150 without correction, and 20/30 with –5 spherical. The corneas were clear no trace of haze was seen. Observe the videokeratographies. Posterior ectasia, but no sign of anterior ectasia (Figures 3.4 and 3.5).
2. Woman now 55 years of age. 1992 full treatment left eye: –12.0 Diopters. Visual acuity left eye: 20/50. 1994

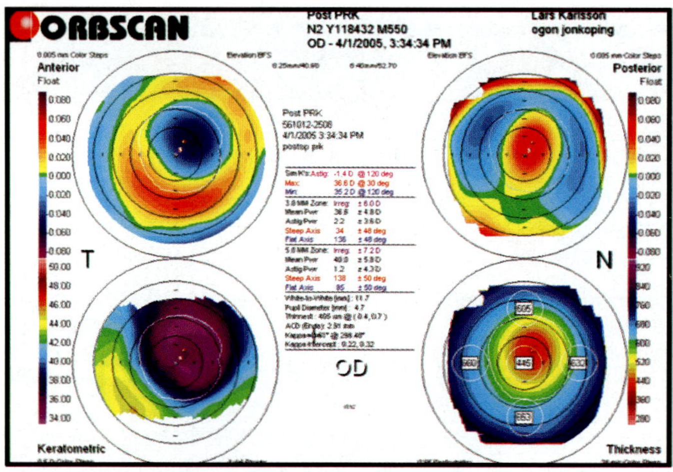

FIGURE 3.4

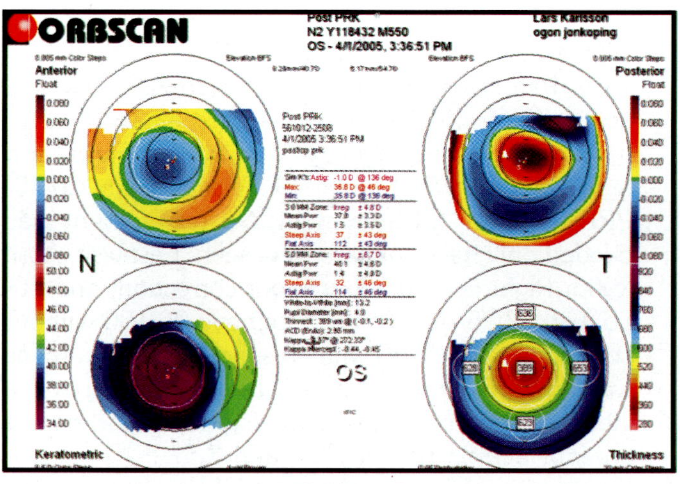

FIGURE 3.5

Full treatment right eye: –8.75/–0.75 × 114°. Visual acuity right eye: 20/20.

December 2001 reoperation left eye: –1.5/–3.0 × 98°. Reoperation due to regression, haze +1.0.

April 2005 right eye: 20/25, refraction –0.75/–0.75 × 65°. Left eye: 20/50, refraction –2.75/-3,75 × 117°. Left eye had macular degeneration. The corneas were clear, no trace of haze. Observe the videokeratographies (Figures 3.6 and 3.7). Left eye posterior ectasia, but no sign of anterior ectasia.

3. Man 45 years of age. Amblyopic due to severe myopia and astigmatism.

May 1992 full treatment: Right eye: 20/60, refraction –14.0/–5.0 × 167°. Left eye full treatment August 1992. Left eye: 20/80, refraction –15.0/–5.0 × 1°.

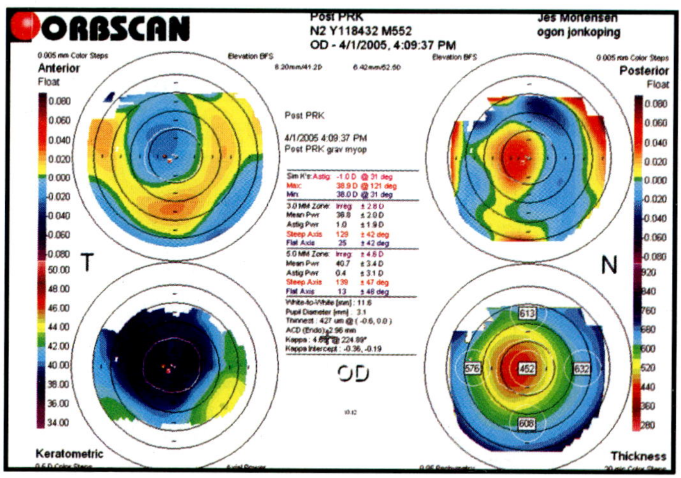

FIGURE 3.6

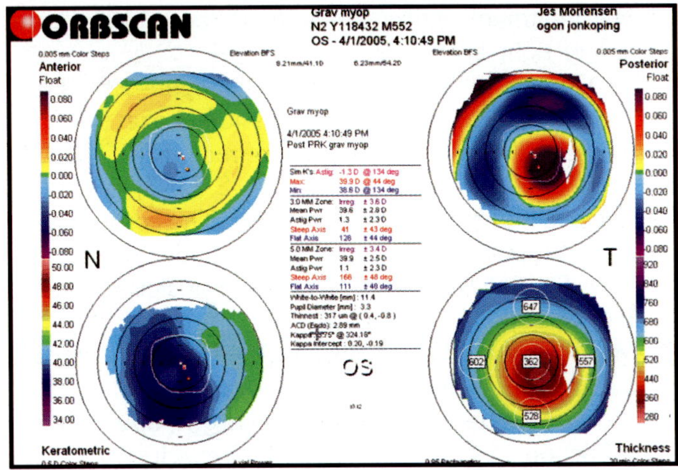

FIGURE 3.7

Due to regression retreatment right eye August 1993: –6.0 sphere. Visual acuity: 20/60

Last visit December 2004. Right eye: 20/60, refraction –5.5/–2.5 × 155°. Left eye: 20/125, refraction –5.5/–5.0 × 170°. Clear corneas no haze. Videokeratographies (Figures 3.8 and 3.9). Posterior ectasia, but no sign of anterior ectasia.

4. Woman now 41 years of age. Both eyes poor vision due to nystagmus, amblyopia; left eye excentric fixation.

   June 1993 left eye full treatment. Left eye: 20/150, refraction –10.0/–1.5 × 0°. November 1993 full treatment right eye. Right eye: 20/60, refraction –4.0/–1.5 × 25°. Last visit Mars 2005. Right eye: 20/50 without correction, emmetropia. Left eye: 20/125 without refraction, 20/50 with –2.0/–4.0 × 145°.

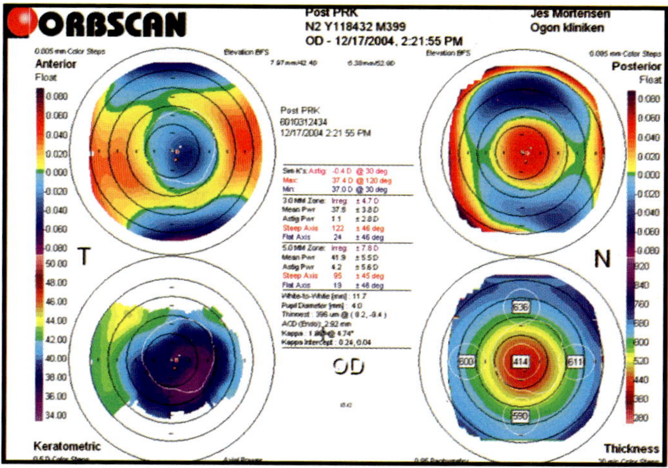

FIGURE 3.8

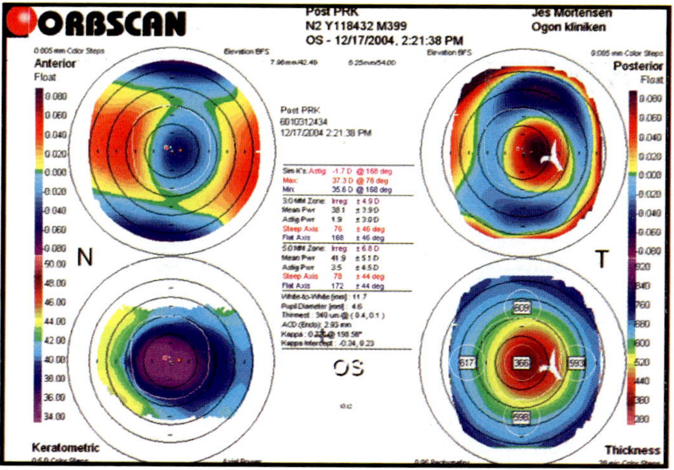

FIGURE 3.9

Videokeratographies show excentric ablation zone left eye, surely caused by the left eyes inborn excentric fixation, the patient does not complain of any problems with halo or glare. She does not wear any correction. Videokeratographies (Figures 3.10 and 3.11).

Mars 2005 OD: 20/50 SC OS: 20/150 SC 20/50 (–2.0/ –4.0 × 145°).

5. Man now 54 years of age. April 1993 right eye treated –11.0/–2.0 × 5°. Right eye: 20/50, refraction –12.0/ –2.25 × 5°. November 1993 left eye full treatment. Left eye: 20/60, refraction –12.25/–4.0 × 168°.

   Last visit March 2005. Right eye: 20/60, refraction –4.5/–1.0 × 100°. Left eye: 20/80, refraction –5.0/ –1.25 × 75°. Videokeratographies (Figures 3.12 and 3.13). Rather nice videokeratographies. No haze was seen. Again posterior ectasia, but no sign of anterior ectasia.

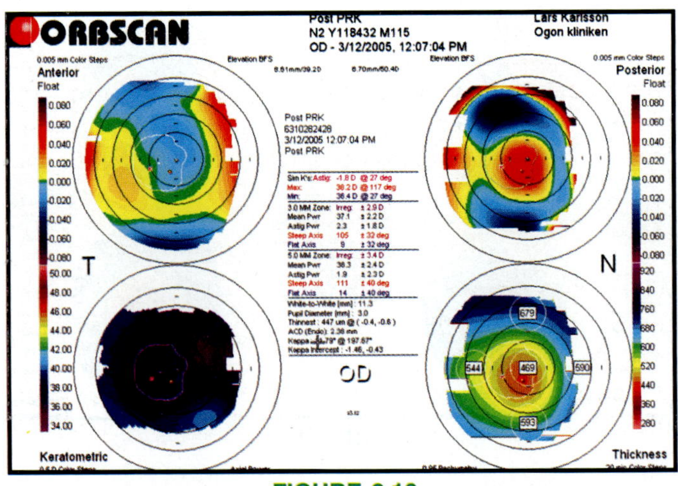

FIGURE 3.10

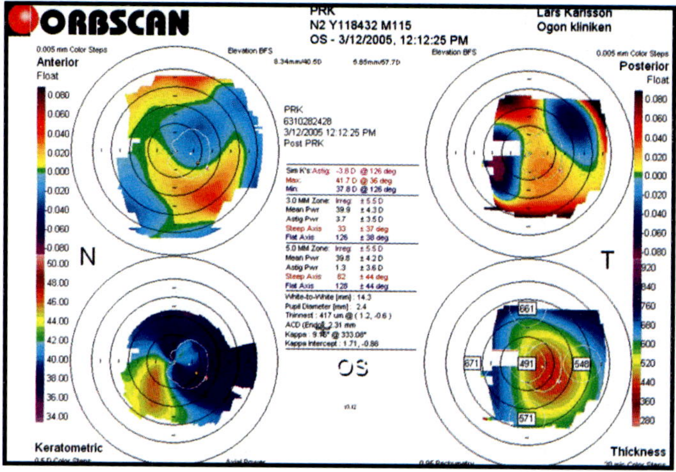

FIGURE 3.11

What we can learn from these cases is that it is possible to treat very high myopia without getting an anterior ectasia. The cornea is clear and regular. Regression was seen in all cases; in spite of that the patients were very satisfied with the reduction of the very high myopia they had from the beginning, none regretted the treatment.

COMPLICATIONS

Where the complications that we saw the same as the complications that we had feared? We were interested in: healing, haze, size of the ablation zone, regression, hyperopic shift, irregularity, keratoconus, postoperative infection and pain during the 2 to 3 first postoperative days.

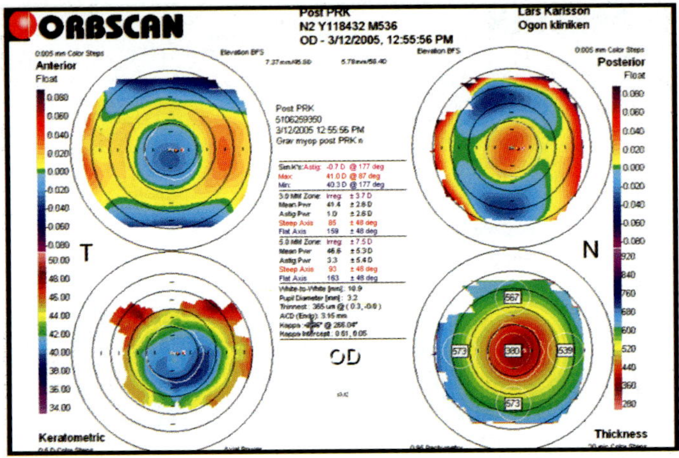

FIGURE 3.12

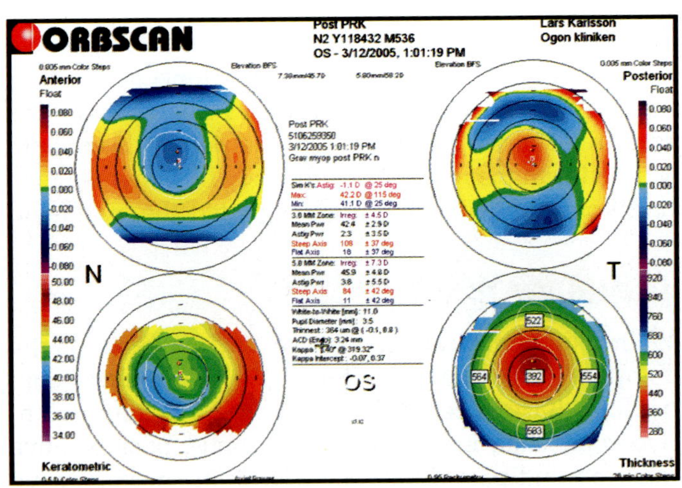

FIGURE 3.13

The worst complication I have seen was a melting of the cornea. The history: Woman early twenties underwent PRK for myopia of –8 diopters one year earlier. She suffered a regression of one diopter; we had read a paper that suggested the removal of the epithelium without further keratectomy would suffice. This was performed and the patient was prescribed diclophenac (Voltaren) eye drops 4 times a day as a painkiller. She experienced severe pain and administrated drops every half to one hour for three days, when she was re-examined as she complained of extremely bad vision in her treated eye. The slit lamp examination revealed a cornea that had almost melted down with only a few microns left of the tissue centrally. She underwent PK the next day and regained good vision but the refraction ended at –8 diopters, no one ever tried to treat this.

Healing was a concern in the very beginning. The first eyes to be treated were from the rabbit. All treated eyes developed severe scarring. When the monkey was used, a more controlled healing was seen.[20, 21] Reepithelialization was seen within 24 to 48 hours. Stromal reorganization was accompanied by an initial phase of vacuolation and invasion by keratocytes. By 6 months a return to normal was seen.

Haze is a part of the healing response. The deeper you ablate the larger the risk of getting haze. The smoother the surface after the ablation the less risk for haze. Professor Theo Seiler et al. concluded in an article 1994, that except for corrections greater than 6 diopters, complications after PRK were rare.[22]

Haze is a kind of scarring taking place during the healing process. Regression will also occur as a part of the haze process. Steroids were suggested to ameliorate the haze and regression.[27] Some investigators however found that steroids were not necessary.[28, 29]

We have had very few problems with haze after PRK with the VISX excimer lasers. Today we use the LASEK method and in treating higher myopes always use mitomycin C 0.02 percent after the ablation. The whole process is described in an article by McCorbett et al.[23] They conclude that Epithelial and keratocyte disturbances only transiently affect visual function. The subepithelial deposits are more persistent and can have lasting effect on the visual performance. Another concern was that a recurrent erosion would occur. The opposite was seen; we actually use the excimer laser ablation to cure recurrent erosions. Phototherapeutic keratectomy is our first choice with recurrent erosions seen after trauma or with various types of anterior corneal dystrophies.

The size of the ablation zone is still a big issue even with LASIK. Today we use the aberrometer (Zywave) to estimate the size of the pupil under scotopic conditions using that as the size for the ablation zone. Not everyone agrees with this. As mentioned we have had very little complaints after using the 6.0 mm zone in all treatments during our VISX period. A certain retinal adaptation takes place. If you have a decentred zone you might get into trouble. Decentration was a problem treating the highly myopic eyes, as you could get a drifting of fixation during the relatively long time the operation took. Today we have a high speed eye tracker, which solves the problem. Reoperating decentration is not an easy task, but the Zywave technology has helped us to reoperate older cases. (Figures 3.15 and 3.16).

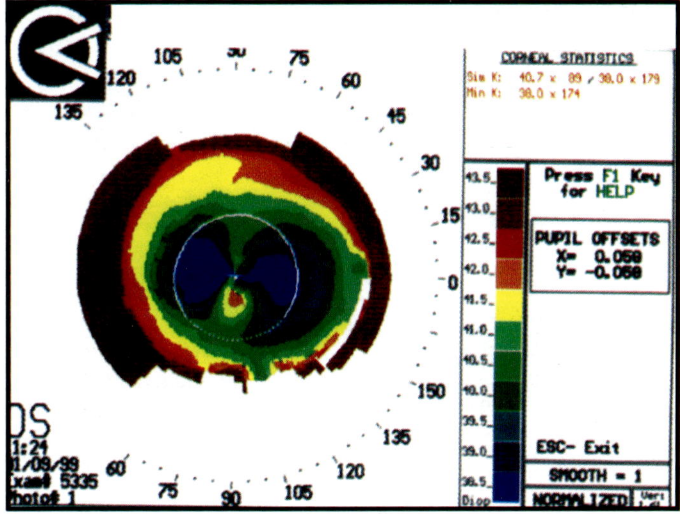

FIGURE 3.14

Regression was a problem especially in cases with haze. Dr. Ca Gauthier et al concluded that that both subepithelial and epithelial layers contribute to regression in the Summit treated eyes.[24] Treating regression after PRK we always use mitomycin C 0.02 percent after the ablation. There are many reports in the litterature confirming this.[25,26]

After the experience from the RK procedure a progressive hyperopic shift was feared. Hyperopic shift is seen after the PRK procedure, but disappears after 3 to 6 months.

Irregularity of the ablated zone is caused by the healing response. If we get haze and regression leading to an irregular surface with inferior visual acuity, we always wait until we are sure that the healing is complete. It is not

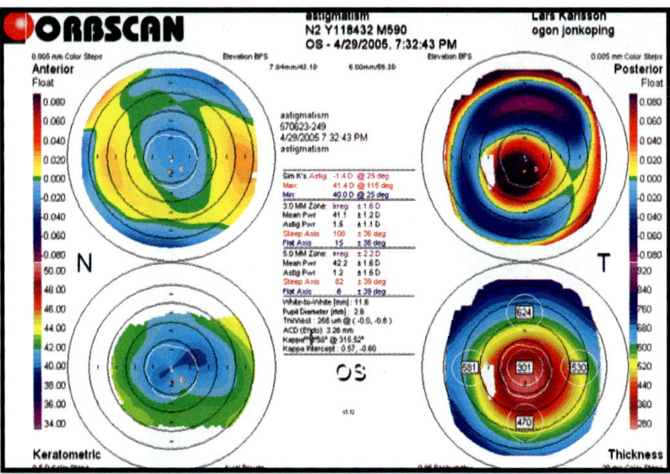

FIGURE 3.15

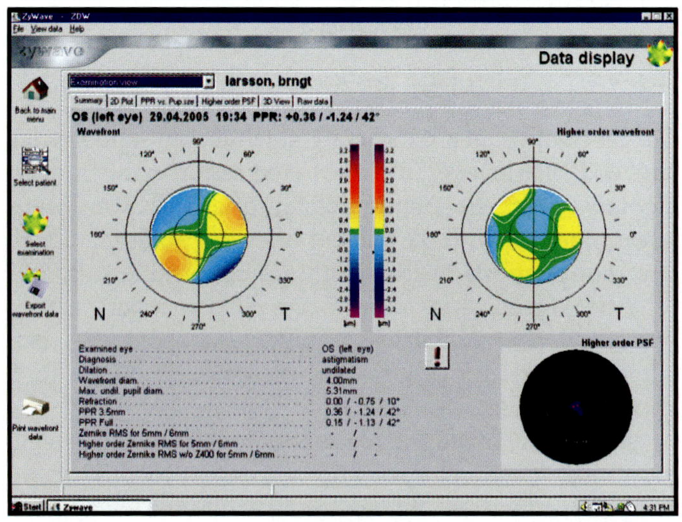

FIGURE 3.16

always easy to convince the disappointed patient that you have to wait perhaps for 1 to 2 years before retreatment can take place. We give the patient a contact lens, which often helps. We do not use steroids for a long time as we find that the potential complications are more threatening than taking your time with the patient and convincing him/her that we will find a solution in the end.

A patient with primary keratoconus is not regarded as a suitable patient for PRK by most surgeons. We treated 24 eyes of 23 patients with primary keratoconus; all eyes were scheduled for penetrating keratoplasty. We concluded that: no increased risk was associated with treating primary keratoconus with excimer laser PRK. We found that excimer laser surgery could improve vision and the ability to wear contact lenses, and it did not interfere with subsequent corneal transplantation surgery.[30] Do we still treat primary keratoconus? Yes but not as often. If we find that the odds for postponing the PK operation are good we consider treatment if the patient agrees. Today we operate the young people with keratoconus with lamellar keratoplasty.

We are starting to treate the lamellae with the excimer laser, especially after lamellar keratoplasty for post LASIK ectasia. We hope that it will be possible to restore a normal vision to the patient. The first patient is scheduled for operation autumn 2005.

To illustrate what has been said I will tell the story about my patient BL born 1957. August 1996 he underwent PRK left eye –6.50/–1.75 × 145°. Visual acuity (VA) was preoperatively 20/20. Haze developed, and regression followed. February 1997 VA left eye: 20/25, refraction left eye –1.5/–1.0 × 145°. August 1997 regression had continued refraction left eye –2.5/–1.5 × 180°. October 1997 retreated –2.5/–1.5x 180°. All went well until new haze was followed by further regression. January 1999 refraction left eye was –0.25/–1.5 × 179°. Full retreatment was done. Haze and new regression retreatment number 3 was performed. April 2002 +1.75/–2.25 × 155°. After that treatment his VA without correction was 20/25 and 20/20 with 0/–1.25 × 140°. But the patient was still not satisfied with the quality of his vision. Last treatment was done with the help of the Zywave aberrometer and as you can see his PSF is very good and the patient is now very satisfied. Visual acuity is 20/20 without correction and 20/16 with 0/–0.75 × 10° (Figures 3.15 and 3.16).

What we learned from this is you should never give up and never abandon the patient. The modern aberrometers can be very helpful.

LASER EPITHELIAL KERATOMILEUSIS (LASEK)

I started this chapter with the statement that ´PRK disappered for a while but is now seeing a renaissance as growing concerns about problems in LASIK surgery are becoming more and more evident‘. During the autumn of 1999 we started performing LASIK at my clinic. After half a year almost every procedure was LASIK. We even successfully reoperated some difficult cases with regression after PRK with the LASIK procedure. However we stopped treating eyes with very high myopia; the limit was set to –10 to –12 diopters. We had very few problems with the flaps using the Hansatom. Then 2 years ago I saw my first case with post-LASIK ectasia. I studied all the available material I could find about this subject. We use the Orbscan videokeratograph and the Zywave aberrometer. We look especially for eyes with forme fruste keratoconus and of course with pachymetry less than 500 microns.

This experience caused a revival of the older PRK technique which was modified (LASEK). The advantage of LASIK over PRK (LASEK) is the absence of pain in the post-operative period, rapid visual recovery and very little response in the wound healing, minimising haze. The problems are well known: Flap problems and risk of developing ectasia. To the associated flap problems I would even add the impact of higher order aberrations. This potential problem could even become the major cause of the revival of the surface ablation techniques. With the new technology of treating higher order aberrations you cannot perhaps give the patient " the vision of an eagle", but restore the same quality of vision as the patient had before the operation; however postoperative problems with contrast sensitivity and night vision are still a concern.

In three articles about Laser-assisted subepithelial keratectomy (LASEK) vs PRK, a reduction in postoperative pain, significantly quicker visual recovery and reduced haze in the eyes with low to moderate myopia was seen.[31-33] In a two year follow up study by Autrata et al 92 patients were operated. LASEK was performed in one eye and the fellow eye had PRK. Preoperative mean spherical equivalent (MSE) was –4.65 diopters (range –1.75 to –7.50 D) after two years the MSE in the PRK group was –0.18 ±0.53 D, in the LASEK group –0.33 ± 0.46. No LASEK eye lost a line of BSCVA.[31]

We often find that the eyes in the high myope group are candidates for LASEK . We use mitomycin C

0.02 percent and after we started with this we have not seen any problems with haze.

Another sign of this shift to the surface ablation techniques is that the inventor of LASIK, professor I Palikaris, is now promoting the EPI LASIK technique, which involves the mechanical removal of the epithelium from Bowman´s membrane. The advantage vs LASEK is that you have not killed the epithelium with the alcohol, so the epithelium you put back after ablation of the surface is still alive. The advantages of the method over LASEK is still to be determined.

SUMMARY

Dr. Steve Trokel, M.D., saw the picture of microetched hair in July 1983, and visited Dr. Srinivasan at his IBM laboratory; that was the start of the whole era of photorefractive keratectomy. Never before has a new surgical technique been brought to the benefit of patients so quickly. The dream of changing the refraction of the eye is very old; different techniques have been tested. Radial keratotomy (RK) was developed by the famous Russian eye surgeon, Professor Fydorov; the RK was the leading technique until the excimer laser came onto the market -today it has disappeared.

In two decades millions of patients have undergone surgery with excimer laser keratectomy all over the world. The results are very good; but no one should forget that it is a surgical method; you can never promise the patient that complications will not happen. This is even more important to bear in mind as excimer keratectomy today in many countries is marketed as a procedure without any risks. The many scientific articles written, and still being produced, on this subject are the best guarantee that the evolution of excimer keratectomy will continue.

REFERENCES

1. Srinivasan R, Leigh WJ. Ablative photodecompensation on poly(ethylene terephthalate) films. J Am Chem Soc 1982;104:6784.
2. Srinivasan R, Mayne-Bayton V. Self-developing photoetching of poly(ethylene terephthalatate) films by far-ultraviolet excimer laser radiation. Appl Phys Lett 1983;41:576-578.
3. Burlamacchi P. Laser Sources. In: Hillenkamp F, Pratesi R, Sacchi CA, ed. Lasers in Biology and Medicine. New York: Plenum, 1980: 1-16.
4. Puliafito CA, Stern D, Krueger RR, Mandel ER. High-speed photography of excimer laser ablation of the human cornea. Arch Ophthalmol 1987;105:1255.
5. Kahle G, Stadter H, Seiler T, Wollensak J. Gas chromatograph/mass spectrometer analysis of excimer and erbium-YAG laser ablated human corneas. Invest Ophthalmol Vis Sci 1992;33(7):2180-2184.
6. Trokel SL, Srinivasan R, Braren B. Excimer laser surgery of the cornea. Am J Ophthalmol 1983;96:710.
7. Seiler T, Wollensack J. Ophthalmology. 1991 Aug;98(8): 1156-63. Myopic photorefractive keratectomy with the excimer laser. One-year follow-up.
8. Carones F, et al. Ophthalmic Surg Lasers. 1996 May;27(5 Suppl):S458-65
9. Kremer F, Blumenthal M. Myopic keratomileusis in situ combined with VISX 20/20 photorefractive keratectomy. J Cataract Refract Surg. 1995;21:508-11.
10. Pallikaris IG, Siganos DS. Excimer laser in situ keratomileusis and photorefractive keratectomy for correction of high myopia. J Refract Corneal Surg 1994;10:498-510.
11. Maguen E, Salz JJ, Nesburn AB, et al. Results of excimer laser photorefractive keratectomy for the correction of myopia. Ophthalmology 1994;101(9):1548-56.

12. Talley AR, Hardten DR, Sher NA, et al. Results one year after using the 193-nm excimer laser for photorefractive keratectomy in mild to moderate myopia. Am J Ophthalmol 1994;118(3):304-11.
13. Dutt S, Steinert RF, Raizman MB, Puliafito CA. One year results of excimer laser photorefractive keratectomy for low to moderate myopia. Arch Ophthalmol 1994;112:1427-1436.
14. Sher NA, Hardten DR, Fundingsland B, et al. 193-nm excimer photorefractive keratectomy in high myopia. Ophthalmology 1994;101(9):1575-82.
15. Hersh PS, Patel R. Correction of myopia and astigmatism using an ablatable mask. J Refract Corneal Surg 1994;10 Supplemental:250-254.
16. Cherry PM, Tutton MK, Bell A, Neave C, Fichte C. Treatment of myopic astigmatism with photorefractive keratectomy using an erodible mask. J Refract Corneal Surg 1994;10(2 Suppl):S239-245.
17. Taylor HR, Kelly P, Alpins N. Excimer laser correction of myopic astigmatism. J Cataract Refract Surg 1994;20(Suppl):S243-251
18. Pender PM. Photorefractive keratectomy for myopic astigmatism: phase IIA of the Federal Drug Administration study (12 to 18 months follow-up). Excimer Laser Study Group. J Cataract Refract Surg 1994;20(Suppl):S262-264.
19. Epstein D, Fagerholm P, Hamberg-Nystrom H, Tengroth B. Twenty-four-month follow-up of excimer laser photorefractive keratectomy for myopia. Refractive and visual acuity results. Ophthalmology. 1994 Sep;101(9):1558-63;discussion 1563-4
20. Marshall J, Trokel SL, Rothery S, Krueger RR. Long.term healing of the central cornea after photorefractive keratectomy using an excimer laser. Ophthalmolohy. 1988 Oct;95(10):1411-21.
21. Fagerholm P, Hamberg NH, Tengroth B. Wound healing and myopic regression following photorefractive keratectomy. Acta Ophthalmol (Copenh) 1994;72(2):229-34.

22. Seiler T, Holschbach A, Derse M, Jean B, Genth U. Complications of myopic photorefractive keratectomy with the excimer laser. Ophthalmology. 1994 Jan;101(1):153-60.
23. Corbett MC, Prydal JL, Verma S, Oliver KM, Pande M, Marshall J. An in vivo investigation of the structures responsible for corneal haze after photorefractive keratectomy and their effect on visual function. Ophthalmology. 1996 Sep;103(9):1366-80.
24. Ca Gauthier, Ba Holden, D Epstein, B Tengroth, P Fagerholm, , H Hamberg.Nystrom. Role of epithelial hyperplasia in regression following photorefractive keratectomy. British Journal of Ophthalmology, 1996, Vol 80, 545-548.
25. Porges Y, Ben-haim O, Hirsch A, Levinger S. Phototherapeutic keratectomy with mitomycin C for corneal haze following photorefractive keratectomy for myopia. J Refract Surg. 2003 Jan-Feb;19(1):40-3.
26. Vigo L, Scandola, Carones F. Scraping and mitomycin C to treat haze and regression after photorefractive keratectomy for myopia. J Refractive Surg. 2003 Jul-Aug;19(4):449-54.
27. Fagerholm P, Hamberg NH, Tengroth B, Epstein D. Effect of postoperative steroids on the refractive outcome of photorefractive keratectomy for myopia with the Summit excimer laser. J Cataract Refract Surg 1994;20(Suppl):212-215.
28. Gartry D, Kerr Muir M, Lohmann CP, Marshall J. The effect of topical corticosteroids on refractive outcome and corneal haze after photorefractive keratectomy: a prospective, randomized, double-blind trial. Arch Ophthalmol 1992;110:944-952.
29. O'Brart DP, Lohmann CP, Klonos G, et al. The effects of topical corticosteroids and plasmin inhibitors on refractive outcome, haze, and visual performance after photorefractive keratectomy. A prospective, randomized, observer-masked study. Ophthalmology 1994;101(9):1565-74.
30. Jes Mortensen, MD, Kent Carlsson, MD, Arne Öhrström, MD, PhD. Excimer laser surgery for keratoconus. J Cataract Refract Surg 1998; 24:893-898.

31. Autrata R, Rhurek J. Laser-assisted subepithelial keratectomy for myopia:two-year follow-up. J Catarct Refract Surg. 2003 Apr;29(4):661-8.
32. Lee JB, Seong GJ, Lee JH, Seo KY, Lee YG, Kim EK. Comparison of laser epithelial keratomileusis and photorefractive keratectomy for low to moderate myopia. J Cataract Refract Surg. 2001 Apr;27(4):565-70.
33. Anderson NJ, Beran RF, Schneider TL. J Catract Refract Surg. 2002 Aug; 28(8): 1343-7.

CHAPTER 4

LASIK: Indications and Surgical Procedures

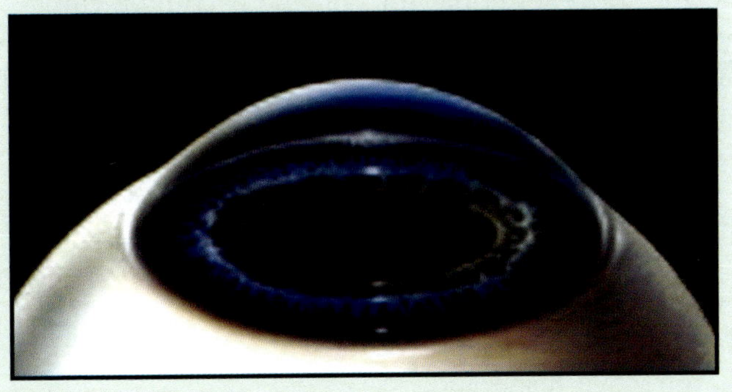

Hijab Mehta
S Natarajan
Hitendra Mehta
Hetal R Solanki

(India)

LASER IN SITU KERATOMILEUSIS (LASIK)

The term *keratomileusis* comes from the Greek words for "cornea" and "to carve." Laser *in situ* keratomileusis, which combines keratomileusis with excimer laser stromal ablation, has become the most popular refractive procedure performed today because of its safety, efficacy, quick visual recovery, and minimal patient discomfort.

BACKGROUND

Barraquer first described corneal lamellar surgery for the correction of refractive error in 1949. The microkeratomes in use today employ many of the same general principles as ***Barraquer's*** original design of a manually advancing electric microkeratome for creating a corneal cap.

A number of innovations occurred over the next few decades till ***Pallikaris*** in 1990 performed the first LASIK procedure using excimer laser for removal of tissue to induce the refractive change.

The excimer laser produced better optical results for three reasons:

1. The excimer laser ablates tissue with submicron accuracy.
2. The laser does not deform the tissue during the refractive reshaping.
3. Larger optical zones are achieved.

Modification in the microkeratome to stop the pass just short of creating a full free cap further improved results. By leaving a narrow hinge of tissue, the outer cornea becomes a flap which is reflected out of the way during the laser exposure. After it is returned to its original position, natural corneal dehydration causes the flap to adhere to the underlying stromal bed. Repositioning of the flap in its original position avoids the distortion induced by sutures and reduces irregular astigmatism.

PATIENT EVALUATION

A thorough preoperative patient evaluation is of critical importance in achieving a successful outcome following refractive surgery. It is during this encounter that the physician begins to develop an impression as to whether the patient is or is not a good candidate for refractive surgery.

Preoperative Evaluation

Important parts of the preoperative evaluation include an assessment of the patient's expectations, the history, the manifest and cycloplegic refractions, a complete ophthalmologic evaluation including slit-lamp and fundus examinations, and ancillary testing. If the patient is a good candidate for surgery, the appropriate refractive surgery procedures, benefits, and risks need to be discussed, and informed consent must be obtained.

Patient Expectations

One of the most important aspects of the entire evaluation is assessing the patient's expectations. The surgeon should explore expectations relating to both the refractive result (e.g. uncorrected visual acuity) and the emotional result (e.g. improved self-esteem). Patients need to understand that they should not expect refractive surgery to improve their best-corrected visual acuity. In addition, refractive surgery will not prevent possible future ocular problems such as cataract, glaucoma, or retinal detachment. If the patient has obviously unrealistic desires, such as a guarantee of 20/20 uncorrected visual acuity, or perfect uncorrected reading and distance vision even though he or she is presbyopic, the patient may need to be told that refractive surgery cannot currently fulfill his or her needs. The refractive surgeon should exclude patients with unrealistic expectations.

HISTORY TAKING

Social History

The social history and medical history can identify the visual requirements of the patient's profession. Certain jobs require that best vision be at a specific distance. For example, a surface laser procedure may be preferable to a lamellar procedure for a patient who wrestles, boxes, or rides horses and is at high risk of ocular trauma. A highly myopic stamp collector or jeweler, who is used to examining objects without glasses a few inches from the eyes, may not be happy with postoperative emmetropia.

Medical History

The medical history should include systemic conditions, prior surgeries, and current and prior medications. Certain systemic conditions, such as connective tissue disorders, can lead to poor healing after refractive surgery. An immunocompromised state, for example from cancer or HIV/AIDS, may increase the risk of infection after refractive surgery. Medications that affect healing or the ability to fight infection, such as systemic corticosteroids or chemotherapeutic agents, should be specifically noted. The use of corticosteroids, and some diseases such as diabetes, increases the risk of cataract development, which could compromise the long-term postoperative visual outcome.

Caution should be taken in performing any excimer laser surgery in patients with cardiac pacemakers and implanted defibrillators, due to the unknown effects of the laser's electromagnetic emissions. Refractive surgery is also generally contraindicated in pregnant and nursing women, due to possible changes in refraction and corneal hydration status. Many surgeons recommend waiting at least 3 months after delivery and cessation of nursing before performing refractive surgery.

Pertinent Ocular History

The ocular history should focus on previous and current eye problems such as dry eye symptoms, blepharitis, recurrent erosions, and retinal tears or detachments. Ocular medications should be noted. A history of previous methods of optical correction, such as glasses and contact lenses, should be taken. The stability of the current refraction is very important. Have the glasses or the contact lens prescription changed significantly in the past few years? A significant change is generally thought to be greater than 0.5 D in either sphere or cylinder over the past year. A contact lens history should be taken. Important information includes the type of lens (e.g. soft, rigid gas-permeable, PMMA); the wearing schedule (e.g. daily wear disposable, daily wear frequent replacement, overnight wear indicating number of nights worn in a row); the type of cleaning, disinfection, and enzyming; and how old the lenses are. Occasionally, a patient may have been happy with contact lens wear and only needs a change in lens material or wearing schedule to eliminate the recent onset of discomfort symptoms.

Because contact lens wear can change the shape of the cornea (corneal warpage), discontinuing contact lens wear is recommended prior to the refractive surgery evaluation and also prior to the surgery. The exact amount of time the patient should be out of contact lenses has not been established. Current clinical practice typically involves discontinuing soft contact lenses for at least 3 days to 2 weeks and rigid contact lenses for at least 2 to 3 weeks. Patients with irregular or unstable corneas should discontinue their contact lenses longer and then be re-refracted every few weeks until the refraction is stable before being considered for refractive surgery.

Patient Age, Presbyopia and Monovision

The age of the patient is very important in predicting postoperative patient satisfaction. The loss of near vision with aging should be discussed with all patients. Prior to age 40 years, emmetropic patients generally do not require reading adds to see a near target. After this age patients need to understand that if they are made emmetropic refractive surgery, they will require reading glasses for near vision. This point cannot be overemphasized for myopes who are approaching age 40. These patients can read well with and without their glasses. Some may even read well with their contact lenses. If they are emmetropic after surgery, many of these patients will not read well with glasses. The patient needs to understand this phenomenon and must be willing to accept this result, prior to undergoing any refractive surgery that aims for emmetropia. A trail with contact lenses will approximate the patient's reading ability after surgery.

A discussion of monovision (one eye corrected for distance and the other eye for near) often fits well in the evaluation at this point. The alternative of monovision correction should be discussed with all patients in the prepresbyopic and presbyopic groups. Generally the dominant eye is corrected for distance and the nondominant eye is corrected to approximately –1.50 to –1.75 D. Such refraction allows good uncorrected distance and near vision without intolerable anisometropia for most patients. Some surgeons prefer a "mini-monovision" procedure, where the near-vision is corrected to approximately –0.75 D, allowing some near vision with better distance vision and less anisometropia. The exact amount of monovision depends on the desires of the patient. Higher amounts of monovision (up to –2.50 D) can be used successfully in selected patients who desire excellent postoperative near vision. While improving the near vision, loss of depth perception and anisometropia may be unwanted from the higher add in some patients.

Many patients have successfully used monovision in contact lenses and want it after refractive surgery. Others have never tried it but would like to, and still others have no interest. If a patient has not used monovision before but is interested, the attempted result should be demonstrated to them in glasses at near and distance. It is often best to try it in contact lenses prior to refractive surgery to make sure the patient is happy with the refractive goal. Although typically the nondominant eye is corrected for near, some patients prefer the dominant eye corrected for near. There are several methods to test ocular dominance. One of the simplest is to have the patient point to a distant object, such as a small letter on the eye chart, and then close each eye to determine which eye he or she was using to point, which is the dominant eye, or to have a patient make an "okay sign" with one hand and look at the examiner through the opening.

EXAMINATION

Uncorrected Visual Acuity and Manifest and Cycloplegic Refraction Acuity

The refractive elements of the preoperative examination are critically important because they directly determine the amount of surgery that is performed. Uncorrected visual acuity at distance and near should be measured. The current glasses prescription and vision with those glasses should also be measured. The manifest refraction should then be performed. The sharpest visual acuity with the least amount of minus should be the final endpoint. The Duochrome test should not be used as the final end-point because it tends to overminus patients. Document the best visual acuity obtainable, even if it is better than 20/20. After the patient's eyes are dilated, a cycloplegic refraction is also necessary. Appropriate cycloplegic drops and enough waiting time between the drops and the cycloplegic refraction are required. Tropicamide 1 percent or cyclopentolate 1 percent is generally used. Waiting at least 30 or 60 minutes, respectively, for full cycloplegia is recommended. The cycloplegic refraction should refine the sphere and not the cylinder from the manifest refraction. For eyes with greater than 5 D of refractive error, a vertex distance measurement should be performed to obtain the most accurate refraction. When there is a large difference between the manifest and cycloplegic refractions (e.g. >0.75 D), a postcycloplegic refraction should be performed to recheck the manifest refraction. In myopes, this is often caused by an overminused manifest refraction. In hyperopes, there may be significant latent hyperopia, and in such cases the surgeon and patient need to decide on exactly how much hyperopia to treat. If there is significant latent hyperopia, a pushed plus spectacle or contact lens correction can be worn for several weeks preoperatively to lessen the postoperative adjustment of treating the true refraction.

Pupillary Examination

After the manifest refraction (but before placing dilating drops) the external and anterior segment examinations are performed. Specific attention should be given to the pupillary examination, evaluating the pupil size in bright room light and dim illumination and looking for an afferent pupillary defect. There are a variety of techniques to measure pupil size in dim illumination, including a near card with pupil sizes on the edge (with the patient fixating at distance), a light amplification pupillometer, or an infrared pupillometer. The actual amount of light entering the eye during the dim light measurement should closely approximate normal night-time activities, such as night driving, and not necessarily complete darkness.

Large pupil size may be one of the risk factors for postoperative glare and halo symptoms after refractive surgery. Another risk factor for postoperative glare includes a higher degree of myopia or astigmatism. As a general rule, pupil size greater than the effective optical zone (usually 6 to 8 mm) increases the risk of glare, but large pupil size is certainly not the only determinant of glare. When asked, patients often have glare under dim light conditions even before refractive surgery. It is important to make patients aware of their glare and halo symptoms preoperatively, as this may minimize postoperative complaints.

Measuring the low-light pupil diameter preoperatively and using the measurement to direct surgery remains controversial. Conventional wisdom suggests that the optical zone should be larger than the pupil diameter to minimize visual disturbances such as glare and haloes. However, it is not clear that pupil size can be used to predict which patients are more likely to have symptoms. It is possible that the size of the effective optical zone, which is related to the ablation profile and the level of refractive error, is more important in minimizing visual side effects than the low-light pupil diameter.

Ocular Motility, Confrontation Fields and Ocular Anatomy

Ocular motility should also be evaluated. Patients with an asymptomatic tropia or phoria may develop symptoms after refractive surgery if the change in refraction causes the motility status to breakdown. If there is a history of strabismus or there is a concern regarding ocular alignment postoperatively, a trial with contact lenses before surgery should be considered. An orthoptic evaluation can be obtained preoperatively if strabismus is an issue. Confrontation fields should be performed in all patients. The general anatomy of the orbits should also be assessed.

Patients with small palpebral fissures and/or large brows may not be ideal candidates for LASIK because there may be inadequate exposure and difficulty in achieving suction with the microkeratome.

Intraocular Pressure

The IOP should be checked after performing the manifest refraction and corneal topography measurements. Patients with glaucoma should be aware that certain refractive surgery procedures elevate the IOP dramatically during the procedure, potentially aggravating optic nerve damage. Also, topical corticosteroids are used after most refractive surgery procedures and may be used for months after PRK or LASEK. Long-term topical corticosteroids may cause marked elevation of IOP in corticosteroid responders. Laser refractive surgery procedures such as PRK and LASIK thin the cornea and typically cause a falsely low measurement of IOP postoperatively. Patients and surgeons need to be aware of this issue, especially if the patient has glaucoma or is a glaucoma suspect.

Slit-lamp Examination

A complete slit-lamp examination of the eyelids and anterior segment should be performed. The eyelids should be checked for significant blepharitis and meibomitis. The tear lake should be assessed for aqueous tear deficiency. The conjunctiva should be examined, looking specifically for conjunctival scarring which may cause problems with microkeratome suction. The cornea should be evaluated for surface abnormalities such as decreased tear break-up time and punctate epithelial erosions. Significant blepharitis, meibomitis, and dry eye syndrome should be addressed prior to refractive surgery, as they are associated with increased postoperative discomfort and decreased vision. A careful examination for epithelial basement membrane dystrophy is required, because its presence increases the risk of flap complications during LASIK. Patients with epithelial basement membrane dystrophy are not good candidates for LASIK; they may be better candidates for PRK. Signs of keratoconus, such as corneal thinning and steepening, may also be found. Keratoconus is typically an absolute contraindication to refractive surgery. The endothelium should be examined carefully, looking for signs of cornea guttata and Fuchs and other dystrophies. Corneal edema is generally considered a contraindication to refractive surgery.

Careful undilated and dilated evaluation of the crystalline lens for clarity is essential especially in patients over age 50. Patients with mild lens changes that are visually insignificant should be informed of these findings and of the fact that the changes may become more significant in the future, independent of refractive surgery. In patients with moderate lens opacities, cataract extraction may be the best form of refractive surgery. Patients should be informed that if they do not undergo refractive surgery at this time, significant refractive error could be addressed at the time of future cataract surgery. Some surgeons give patients a record of their preoperative refractions and keratometry measurements along with the amount of laser ablation performed and the postoperative refraction. This information should help improve the accuracy of the IOL calculation should cataract surgery be required at some future date.

Patient Selection

Many reports indicate that postoperative dry eye is more common with LASIK than PRK. Preoperative evaluation for dry eyes is preformed by assessment of history, the tear meniscus, rose bengal staining, and/or Schirmer testing. Dry eyes should be treated preoperatively with artificial tear supplementation, topical anti-inflammatory medications (corticosteroids or cyclosporine), and/or punctual occlusion, in order to limit keratopathy that can lead to postoperative flap irregularity.

When evaluating the cornea prior to LASIK, it is of particular importance to look for signs of a basement membrane dystrophy that could predispose the patient to epithelial defects with the microkeratome pass. These patients are usually best served by having PRK, if their refractive error permits.

Dilated Fundus Examination

A dilated fundus examination is also important prior to refractive surgery to be certain the posterior segment is normal. Special attention should be given to the optic nerve (glaucoma, optic nerve drusen) and peripheral retina (retinal breaks, detachment). Patients and surgeons should realize that highly myopic eyes are at increased risk for retinal detachment, even after the refractive error has been corrected.

ANCILLARY TESTS

Corneal Topography

An evaluation of corneal curvature is necessary. While manual keratometry readings can be quite informative, they have largely been replaced by computerized videokeratographic analyses. There are several different methods with which to analyze the corneal curvature, including Placido disk systems and scanning slit-beam methods. These techniques image the cornea and provide color maps representing corneal power and/or elevation. This analysis gives a "simulated keratometry" reading and an overall evaluation of the corneal curvature. Eyes with visually significant irregular astigmatism are generally not good candidates for corneal refractive surgery. The curvature analysis should reveal a spherical cornea or regular astigmatism. Early keratoconus, pellucid marginal degeneration, or contact lens warpage should be considered as causes in eyes with visually significant irregular astigmatism. Irregular astigmatism secondary to contact lens warpage usually reverses over time, although it may take months; serial corneal topography should be performed to document the disappearance of visually significant irregular astigmatism prior to any refractive surgery.

Unusually steep or unusually flat corneas can increase the risk of poor flap creation with the microkeratome. Flat corneas (flatter than 40 D) increase the risk of small flaps and free caps and steep corneas (steeper than 48 D) increase the risk of buttonhole flaps. Femtosecond laser (e.g. IntraLase) flap creation theoretically may avoid these risks. These issues may be reduced or eliminated by the use of a smaller flap diameter, slower passage of the microkeratome, higher suction levels and higher IOP, use of a microkeratome head designed to create thicker flaps. Excessive corneal flattening and steepening after refractive surgery may increase the risk of poor quality of vision. Patients with corneas flatter than approximately 34 D or steeper than approximately 50 D postoperatively may be at risk for this complication. Postoperative keratometry for myopes is estimated by subtracting approximately 80 percent of the refractive correction from the average preoperative keratometry reading. For example, if the preoperative keratometry reading is 42 D and 5 D of myopia is being corrected, an estimated postoperative keratometry reading would be 42 D – (0.8 × 5 D) = 38 D. Postoperative keratometry for hyperopes is estimated by adding 100 percent of the refractive correction to the average preoperative keratometry reading. For example, if the preoperative keratometry reading is 42 D and 3 D of hyperopia is being corrected, the estimated postoperative keratometry reading would be 42 D + (1 × 3 D) = 45 D.

When keratometric or corneal topographic measurements reveal an amount or an axis of astigmatism significantly different from the refraction, the refraction should be rechecked for accuracy. Lenticular astigmatism or posterior corneal curvature may account for the difference between refractive and keratometric/ topographic astigmatism.

Pachymetry

A measurement of corneal thickness should be done to determine whether the cornea is of adequate thickness for keratorefractive surgery. This procedure is usually performed with ultrasound pachymetry; however, certain corneal topography systems (e.g. scanning slit-beam, such as OrbScan) can also be used. This latter system can provide a map representing the relative thickness of the cornea at various locations. The accuracy of the pachymetry measurements of scanning slit-beam systems decreases markedly after keratorefractive surgery is performed. Because the thinnest part of the cornea is typically located centrally, a central measurement should always be performed. Unusually thin corneas may reveal early keratoconus. Some surgeons also check the midperipheral corneal thickness for inferior thinning, which may suggest early keratoconus. Unusually thick corneas may suggest mild Fuchs dystrophy. The thickness of the cornea is an important factor in determining whether the patient is a candidate for refractive surgery and which procedure may be best. Most refractive surgeons will not consider LASIK below a certain lower limit of corneal thickness. We do not perform LASIK if the corneal thickness is less than 480 μ. If LASIK is performed and results in a relatively thin residual stromal bed, for example around 250 μm, future enhancement surgery that further thins the stromal bed may not be possible. If there is a question of endothelial integrity causing an abnormally thick cornea, specular microscopy may be helpful to assess the health of the endothelium.

Wavefront Analysis

Wavefront analysis is a relatively new technique that can provide an objective refraction measurement. Certain excimer lasers can use this wavefront analysis information directly to perform the ablation, a procedure called wavefront-guided or "custom" ablation. Some surgeons are using wavefront analysis to document levels of preoperative higher-order aberrations. Refraction data from the wavefront analysis unit can also be used to refine the manifest refraction.

Calculation of Residual Stromal Bed Thickness After LASIK

A lamellar laser refractive procedure such as LASIK involves creation of a corneal flap, ablation of the stromal bed, and replacement of the flap. The strength and integrity of the cornea postoperatively depends on the thickness of the residual stromal bed. Stromal bed thickness is calculated by taking the preoperative central corneal thickness and subtracting the flap thickness and the calculated laser ablation depth for the particular refraction. For example, if the central corneal thickness is 550 µm, the flap thickness is estimated to be 160 µm, and the ablation depth for the patient's refraction is 50 µm, the residual stromal bed thickness would be 550µm - (160 µm + 50 µm) = 340 µm.

Exactly how thick the residual stromal bed needs to be is unclear. However, most surgeons believe that it should be at least 250 µm thick, and many surgeons believe it should be even thicker, in the 275 to 300 µm range. If the calculation reveals a residual stromal bed thickness that is thinner than desired, LASIK may not be the best surgical option. In these cases, a surface laser procedure such as PRK or epithelial-sparing PRK (LASEK) may be a better option because no stromal flap is required.

Refractive Errors Amenable for Treatment with LASIK

The improvement of visual results with the evolution of laser technology has been substantial. A 1999 clinical trial using a conventional laser for myopic astigmatic LASIK yielded postoperative UCVA of 20/20 in 47 percent of eyes. The more recent 2003 clinical trials of wavefront-guided ablation for myopic astigmatic LASIK achieved UCVA of 20/20 in 79 percent to 98 percent of eyes. The following section describes LASIK outcomes using results from FDA clinical trials and publications.

Low Myopia

Series of eyes treated with conventional (non-wavefront-guided) LASIK for low myopia (less than 6.0 D) in FDA clinical trials report that 67 percent to 86 percent of eyes achieved UCVA of 20/20 or better, 93 percent to 100 percent achieved 20/40 or better.

Moderate Myopia

In patients with moderate myopia (approximately –6.0 to –12.0 D), results from large published series and FDA clinical trials report that 26 percent to 71 percent of eyes achieved an UCVA of 20/20 or better, 55 percent to 100 percent reached at least 20/40, and 41 percent percent to 96 percent were within 1.0 D of intended correction.

High Myopia

High myopia is most often defined as myopia greater than –12.0 D, with several studies reporting treatment results in patients with up to –29.0 D. In this range, the predictability of the procedure is markedly reduced, with 26 percent to 65 percent of eyes achieving at least 20/40 UCVA and 32 percent to 65 percent attaining a postoperative refraction within 1.0 D of the intended correction. In addition, when treating such high amounts of myopia, there was a higher incidence of loss of BCVA than in the correction of lower levels of myopia. However, patients with high myopia often gain BCVA after LASIK, probably due to decreased image minification compared with preoperative spectacles.

As experience with LASIK has accumulated, an increasing number of surgeons choose to rarely, if ever, perform LASIK or PRK for corrections above –12.0 D. The required ablation depths for high corrections may leave an inadequate stromal bed (less than 250 μm at a minimum) for long-term structural stability of the cornea.

Myopia with Astigmatism

Overall, the results for toric LASIK ablations are not as predictable as for spherical LASIK ablations. Most often, the procedure undercorrects the cylinder, which may simply indicate the need for improved nomograms or may indicate an inaccuracy of the axis ablated. Often it is difficult to determine the outcome of treatment for myopic astigmatism when reviewing large series of patients. Some clinical trials summarize the final outcome for all patients and do not distinguish between results for myopia and for myopic astigmatism.

In FDA clinical trials, including patients undergoing LASIK for myopic astigmatism, 43 percent to 87 percent of eyes achieved UCVA of 20/20 or better and 84 percent to 99 percent achieved UCVA of 20/40 or better, with 82 percent to 92 percent within ±1.0 D of the intended refraction.

Hyperopia

In contrast to a myopic ablation, where the central cornea is ablated and flattened, a hyperopic ablation steepens the central cornea by ablating a doughnut-shaped area in the midperiphery. With enlargement of both, the optical zone and the peripheral blend zone, as well as improved centration with the assistance of tracking devices, studies of hyperopic LASIK with longer follow-up periods have shown improved outcomes.

In FDA clinical trials of LASIK for hyperopia up to 6.0 D, 49 percent to 59 percent of eyes achieved postoperative UCVA of 20/20 or better, 93 percent to 96 percent achieved postoperative UCVA of 20/40 or better, 86 percent to 87 percent were within 1.0 D of emmetropia postoperatively.

Studies have demonstrated good results for refractive errors up to +4.0 to +5.0 D, but predictability and stability are markedly reduced with hyperopic treatments above this level.

Hyperopic Astigmatism

In several FDA clinical trials of hyperopic astigmatic correction, 37 percent to 65 percent of eyes achieved postoperative UCVA of 20/20 or better, 91 percent to 99 percent had UCVA of 20/40, 87 percent to 91 percent were within 1.0 D of emmetropia. Efficacy was decreased with higher refractive errors

Mixed Astigmatism

LASIK has been approved by the FDA for mixed astigmatism of up to 6.0 D of sphere and cylinder. The outcomes of LASIK for mixed astigmatism are similar to the results for hyperopia and hyperopic astigmatism. From 46 percent to 62 percent of eyes had UCVA of 20/20 or better, 93 percent to 99 percent had postoperative UCVA of 20/40 or better, 88 percent to 96 percent were within 1.0 D of emmetropia.

SURGICAL TECHNIQUE

Preoperative Preparation of the Patient

A mild sedative, such as oral diazepam 5 to 10 mg, may be administered to the patient approximately 30 minutes prior to the procedure. Topical anesthetic drops are instilled and the skin is usually prepped with povidone-iodine or another skin antiseptic. Preoperative topical antibiotic may be used.

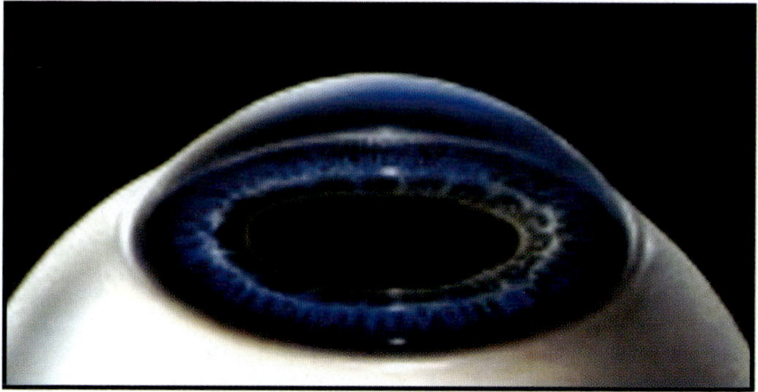

FIGURE 4.1A: Normal cornea

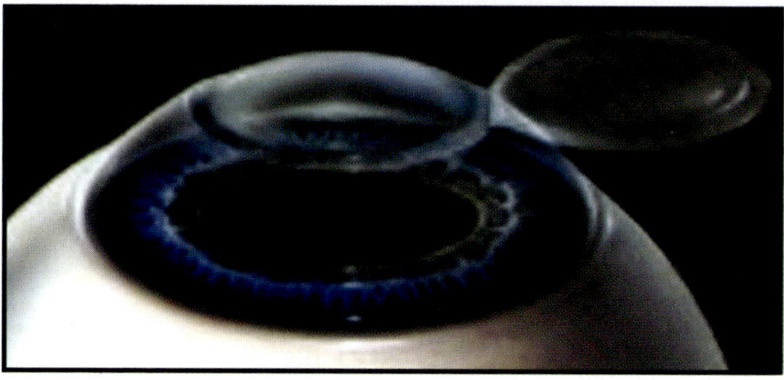

FIGURE 4.1B: Creation of corneal flap

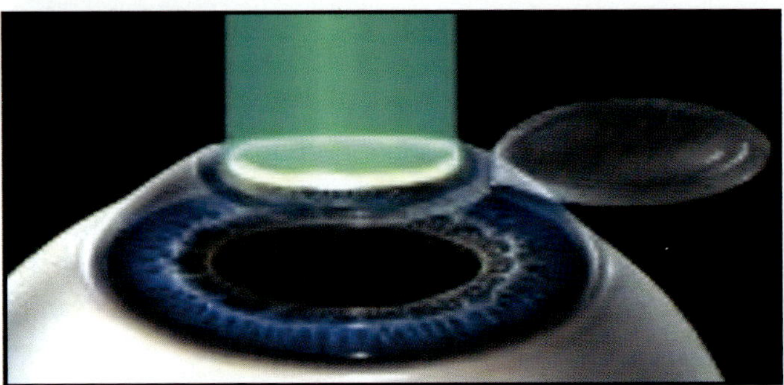

FIGURE 4.1C: Laser ablation

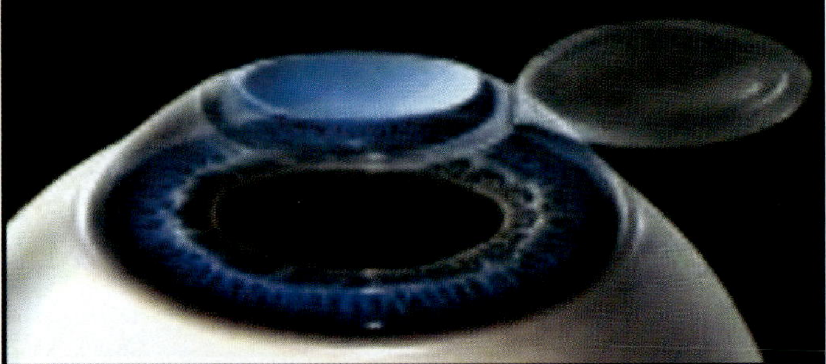

FIGURE 4.1D: Appearance following laser ablation

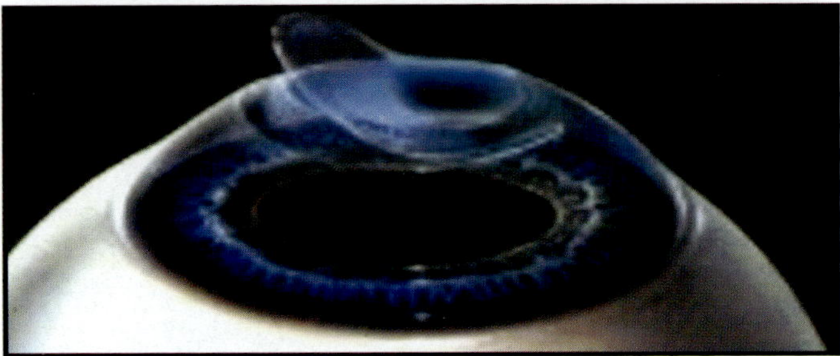

FIGURE 4.1E: Repositioning of corneal flap

FIGURES 4.1A to E: Diagrammatic representation of the LASIK procedure

Many surgeons drape the skin or eyelashes with a plastic drape or with Steri-Strips, while others consider this unnecessary and a potential source of material that might jam the microkeratome. An eyelid speculum is placed that has a configuration to accommodate the suction device and the path of the microkeratome. The cornea may be marked with an optical zone marker to assist in proper centration of the suction ring, and one or more pararadial lines are usually placed to ensure proper realignment of the flap.

Programming the Laser

The actual treatment value programmed into the laser is typically an adjustment of the final refractive goal, derived from each surgeon's individual nomogram as developed by monitoring outcomes. Major variables that some but not all surgeons find to be important include: specific laser, individual surgeon, amount of correction, gender, and age. In addition, the size of the ablation zone and whether to include a blend will be determined by the patient's refractive error, the calculated residual stromal bed, and the pupillary diameter.

Creation of the Flap by the Microkeratome

The diameter of the flap is determined by the surgeon based on such variables as the type of refractive error to be treated (hyperopic corrections and wavefront-guided treatments require a larger flap because of the larger ablation diameter), the corneal curvature and microkeratome suction ring dimensions (flatter corneas result in a smaller flap for the same size ring), the patient's anatomy (peripheral corneal blood vessels and corneal diameter), and the surgeon's preference. Depending on the manufacturer, the suction ring is usually centered over the entrance pupil, but if a suction ring is being used that creates a flap less than 9.5 mm in diameter, some surgeons prefer to skew it toward the hinge to ensure that the hinge will not be located within the laser optical zone.

Thinner flaps leave more stromal bed thickness for the ablation and possible enhancements. However, thicker flaps have a lower risk of unexpected buttonholes and flap folds and may be more stable. Each type of microkeratome characteristically creates a flap with a range of thickness that the surgeon must know and include in the surgical plan to make sure there is an adequate residual stromal bed.

Once the ring is properly positioned, suction is activated. The IOP should be assessed at this point, because low IOP can result in a poor-quality, thin, or incomplete flap. It is essential to have both excellent exposure of the eye, allowing free movement of the microkeratome, and proper suction ring fixation. Inadequate suction may result from blockage of the suction ports from eyelashes under the suction ring or from redundant or scarred conjunctiva. To avoid the possibility of pseudosuction, the surgeon can confirm that true suction is present by observing that the eye moves when the suction ring is gently moved and that the patient can no longer see the fixation light. Methods employed to assess whether the IOP is adequately elevated include use of the Barraquer plastic applanator, use of a pneumotonometer, or palpation of the eye by the surgeon. Beginning surgeons are advised to use an objective rather than a subjective method.

Prior to making the lamellar cut, the surface of the cornea is moistened with proparacaine containing glycerin or with nonpreserved artificial tears. Balanced salt solution is avoided at this point due to the possibility of creating mineral deposits within the microkeratome that can interfere with its proper function. The microkeratome is placed on the suction ring and its path is checked to make sure it is free of obstacles such as the eyelid speculum, drape, or overhanging eyelid. The microkeratome is then activated, passed over the cornea until halted by the hinge-creating stopper, and then reversed off the cornea. With some models, some surgeons feel that epithelial defects may be reduced by lowering the vacuum or discontinuing the suction during the reversal; other models require the vacuum to remain at full pressure during reversal. Improvements in microkeratomes have decreased the incidence of epithelial defects. If a patient develops an epithelial defect in one eye during a microkeratome pass, an epithelial defect will usually develop when the second eye is treated regardless of alterations in the microkeratome vacuum level. This implies that there may be a subclinical epitheliopathy such as epithelial basement membrane disease that is made manifest by the microkeratome pass.

The Ablation

The excimer laser system is then focused and centered over the pupil and the patient is asked to look at the fixation light. The flap is reflected and the patient is asked to continue to fixate. The lights in the room and laser may need to be adjusted to allow the patient to be able to continue to visualize the fixation light through the irregular stromal surface after the flap has been lifted. If excess

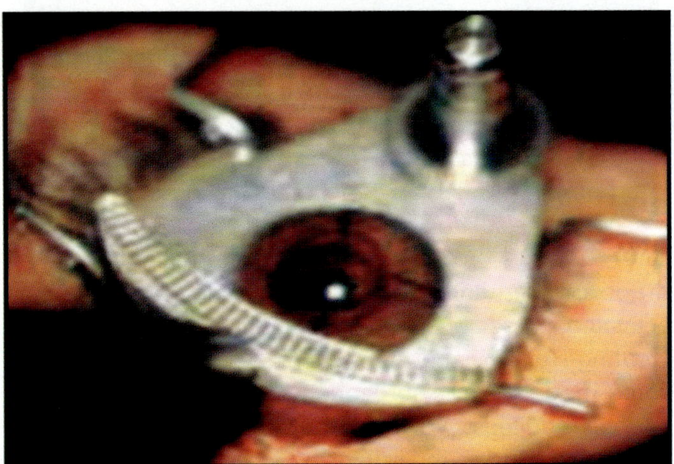

FIGURE 4.2: The suction ring of the Chiron Microkeratome in place also shown are the corneal markings

moisture is noted, the stromal bed is dried with a microsurgical debris-free sponge. The laser is refocused on the stromal bed and centered, most commonly on the pupil. A tracking system, if present, is activated. Once the patient confirms that the fixation light of the excimer laser is still visible and that the patient is looking directly at it, ablation is begun. With or without a tracking device, the surgeon must monitor the patient to make sure that the patient's fixation is maintained throughout the laser exposure. It is important to initiate the stromal ablation promptly, before excessive stromal dehydration has taken place. If centration is lost, however, the ablation should be halted immediately, and fixation regained prior to finishing the treatment. During larger-diameter ablations, a flap protector may be needed to shield the underside of the flap near the hinge from the laser pulses.

Replacing the Flap

After the ablation is completed, the flap is replaced onto the stromal bed. The interface is irrigated until any interface debris is eliminated (which is better visualized with oblique rather than coaxial illumination). The surface of the flap is stroked with a smooth instrument, such as the irrigation cannula or a moistened microsurgical spear sponge, from the hinge to the periphery to ensure that wrinkles are eliminated and that the flap settles back into its original position, as indicated by the radial marks made earlier. The physiologic dehydration of the stroma by the endothelial pump will begin to secure the flap in position within several minutes. If a significant epithelial defect is present, a bandage contact lens should be placed. Once the flap is adherent, the eyelid speculum is carefully removed (taking care not to move the flap). Most surgeons place a drop of antibiotic and corticosteroid over the eye at the conclusion of the procedure. The flap is usually rechecked at the slit-lamp before the patient leaves to make sure it has remained in proper alignment. A clear shield or protective goggles are often placed to guard against accidental trauma that could displace the flap.

Many surgeons instruct their patients to use topical antibiotics and corticosteroids postoperatively for 5 to 7 days. In addition, it is very important to keep the surface of the flap well lubricated in the early postoperative period. Patients may be told to use the protective shield when they shower or sleep for 1 day to 1 week and to avoid swimming or hot tubs for 2 weeks. The patient is examined 1 day after surgery to make sure that the flap has remained in proper alignment and that there is no evidence of infection or excessive inflammation. In the absence of complications, the next examinations are typically at approximately 3 weeks, 1 month, 3 months, 6 months, and 12 months postoperatively.

CONCLUSION

LASIK studies vary considerably in the techniques employed, the degree of refractive error treated, the postoperative follow-up, and the variables analyzed. Consequently, it is often difficult to compare outcomes of different studies. However, LASIK is the most predictable, safe and effective refractive surgery procedure and will also remain the most popular for some time to come.

BIBLIOGRAPHY

1. Basic and Clinical Science Course – Refractive Surgery; American Academy of Ophthalmology. Section 14; 2004-2005.
2. Boxer Wachler BS. Effect of pupil size on visual function under monocular and binocular conditions in LASIK and non-LASIK patients. J Cataract Refract Surg 2003;29:275-8.
3. Casebeer JC, Kezerian Gm. Outcomes of spherocylinder treatments in the comprehensive refractive surgery LASIK study. Sem Ophthalmol 1998;13:71-8.
4. Davidorf JM, Eghbali F, Onclinx T, et al. Effect of varying the optical zone diameter on the results of hyperopic laser *in situ* keratomileusis. Ophthalmology 2001;108:1261-5.
5. El Danasoury MA, El-Maghraby A, Klyce SD, et al. Comparison of photorefractive keratectomy with excimer laser *in situ* keratomileusis in correcting low myopia (from –2.00 to –5.50 diopters): a randomized study. Ophthalmology. 1999;106:411-20.

6. El-Maghraby A, Salah T, Waring III GO, et al. Randomized bilateral comparison of excimer laser *in situ* keratomileusis and photorefractive keratectomy for 2.50 to 8.00 diopters of myopia. Ophthalmology 1999;106:447-57.
7. Fernandez AP, Jaramillo I, Jaramillo M. Comparison of photorefractive keratectomy and laser *in situ* keratomileusis for myopia of –6 D or less using the Nidek EC-5000 laser. J Refract Surg 2000;16:711-5.
8. Hersh PS, Brint SF, Malonery RK, et al. Photorefractive keratectomy versus laser *in situ* keratomileusis for moderate to high myopia: A randomized prospective study. Ophthalmology 1998;105:1512-22.
9. Kawesh GM, Kezerian GM. Laser *in situ* keratomileusis for high myopia with the VISX Star laser. Ophthalmology 2000; 107:653-61.
10. Lui MM, Silas MA, Fugishima J. Complications of photorefractive keratectomy and laser *in situ* keratomileusis. J Refract Surg 2003;19:S247-49.
11. McDonald MB, Carr ID, Frantz JM, et al. Laser *in situ* keratomileusis for myopia up to –11 diopters with up to – 5 diopters of astigmatism with the Summit Autonomous LADAR-Vision excimer laser system. Ophthalmology 2001;108:309-16.
12. Mutyala S, McDonald MB, Scheinblurn KA, et al. Contrast sensitivity evaluation after laser *in situ* keratomileusis. Ophthalmology 2000;107:1864-7.
13. Pallikaris IG, Siganos DS. Excimer laser *in situ* keratomileusis and photorefractive keratectomy for correction of high myopia. J Refract Surg 1994;10:498-510.
14. Pop M, Payette Y. Photorefractive keratectomy versus laser *in situ* keratomileusis: A control-matched study. Ophthalmology 2000;107:251-7.
15. Price FW Jr, Koller DL, Price MO. Central corneal pachymetry in patients undergoing laser *in situ* keratomileusis. Ophthalmology 1999;106:2216-20.
16. Price FW. LASIK. In Focal Points: Clinical Modules for Ophthalmologist. San Francisco: American Academy of Ophthalmology 2000;18(3).

17. Randleman JB, Russell B, Ward MA, et al. Risk factors and prognosis for corneal ectasia after LASIK. Ophthalmology 2003;110:267-75.
18. Reviglio VE, Bossana EL, Luna ID, et al. Laser *in situ* keratomileusis for myopia and hyperopia using the Lasersight 200 laser in 300 consecutive cases. J Refract Surg 2000;16:716-23.
19. Salz JJ, Stevens CA, and the LADARVision LASIK Hyperopia Study Group. LASIK correction of spherical hyperopia, hyperopic astigmatism, and mixed astigmatism with the LADARVision excimer laser system. Ophthalmology 2002;109:1647-56.
20. Tabbara KF, El-Sheikh HF, Islam SM. Laser *in situ* keratomileusis for the correction of hyperopia from +0.50 to +11.50 diopters with the Keracor 117C laser. J Refract Surg 2001;17:123-8.
21. Tole DM, McCarty DJ, Couper T, et al. Comparison of laser *in situ* keratomileusis and photorefractive keratectomy for the correction of myopia of –6 diopters or less. Melbourne Excimer Laser Group. J Refract Surg 2001;17:46-54.

CHAPTER 5

Topography-assisted LASIK

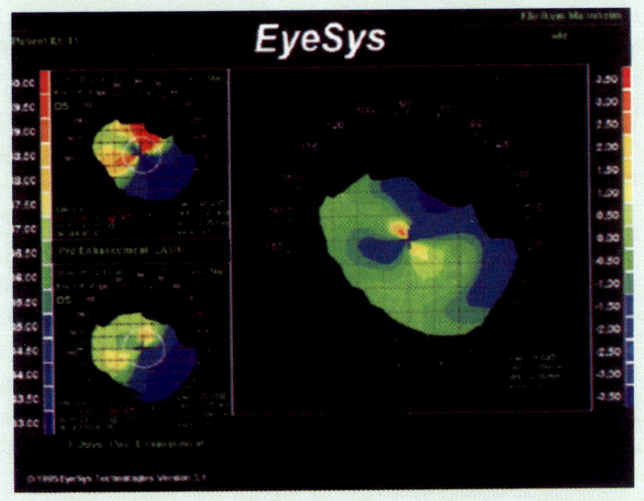

Michael C Knorz (Germany)
Maria C Arbelaez (Sultanate of Oman)

INTRODUCTION

The invention of excimer lasers led to a tremendous improvement in the predictability of refractive surgical procedures. By moving the ablation inside the cornea, the introduction of laser *in situ* keratomileusis (LASIK) virtually eliminated scarring and regression, making it possible to treat high myopia as well as hyperopia. By adding LASIK to their spectrum, refractive surgeons were able to treat almost any refractive error.

Besides myopia, hyperopia, and astigmatism, we all know the rare cases with grossly irregular patterns following, e.g. penetrating corneal grafts, penetrating injuries, or peripheral corneal scars that cause irregularity. All these eyes could be treated rather unsuccessfully to date. In these eyes, we wished we had a software to custom-tailor the ablation and that is exactly what topography-assisted LASIK, (TA-LASIK) is about.

A custom-tailored ablation is also extremely useful and ultimately even more important in slight corneal asymmetries. Today, we use standardized and symmetrical ablation pattern, which is similar to buying a suit "off-the-rack". The individual corneas of our patients, however, show a lot of asymmetry. As many as 40 percent of eyes show some degree of asymmetry, and all these eyes would be far better off with a customized laser ablation. TA-LASIK is the ideal tool to create a perfect cornea as it allows us to reshape the cornea in any pattern we may decide. All that is required is corneal topography (Technomed C-Scan or EyeSys), the proprietary software, a Hansatome microkeratome (Bausch and Lomb Surgical), and a Keracor 117C or 217 excimer laser from Bausch and Lomb Surgical.

HOW DOES TA-LASIK WORK?

As in all refractive procedures, the first requirement to be met is stability of the cornea. It does not make sense to operate as long as the shape of the cornea is still changing. There should be a time interval of at least one year following penetrating grafts or large penetrating injuries. In small scars, of course, the interval could be shorter. Whenever uncertain, the surgeon should wait for three months and reexamine the patient. Now, as soon as the cornea is stable, a corneal topography is taken in the routine fashion. This topographic map should be of as high a quality as possible because it is used as the basis of the ablation. This means that the lids are wide open, that the tear film is regular, that there are no "dark spots" on the map, that the picture is well-centered and well-focused, and that the entrance pupil is visible on the map. All these requirements are easy to meet for experienced observers in normal corneas, but sometimes quite difficult in abnormal ones, which are the corneas we will treat with TA-LASIK. If it is not possible to obtain a good picture, the examination should be repeated at a later date. It is also a good idea to perform topography prior to any other examinations. In addition, we learned from mistakes in the beginning and now require a set of three topographic maps taken at the same day to calculate the ablation.

Assuming perfect maps were obtained, the respective data files are exported onto a disk which is either physically or electronically transferred to Bausch and Lomb Surgical Technolas, Munich, Germany. This procedure is state-of-the-art even today. Later on, the required software will definitely be available either on the laser or on the topography unit. The respective software then converts measurements of radii of curvature to true height values. Based on the height, the ablation is calculated by a proprietary algorithm. All we have to do is to tell the software which K-value it should target. This is another tricky issue in very irregular corneas, but only the correct K-value will create an emmetropic eye and therefore an extremely happy patient. Should the K-value not be accurate, however, this will result in some spherical deviations from emmetropia which is still much better than an irregular cornea. To establish the actual K-value of a specific cornea, we used topographic maps (normalized scale) and subjectively estimated the average refractive power of the part of the cornea overlying the entrance pupil. In irregular corneas, this requires some guessing.

In addition to the K-value, we must provide the diameter of the desired ablation zone and, of course, pachymetry of the central cornea. Pachymetry is especially important in repair procedures following previous refractive surgery, e.g. PRK (photorefractive keratectomy) or LASIK. The cornea is thinner after PRK or LASIK, which leaves less space for further ablations. Therefore, it is very important to measure corneal thickness in these cases.

After all parameters are set, the computer will calculate a treatment based on the corneal topography of the individual eye.

CASE REPORTS

PATIENT CW: IRREGULAR ASTIGMATISM AFTER PENETRATING INJURY

This 6-year-old patient had suffered a penetrating injury in her left eye. A light bulb exploded, and glass fragments penetrated her eye, causing corneal lacerations extending from 10 to 12 O'clock peripherally. One year after the initial repair, scar formation caused significant irregular astigmatism. Uncorrected visual acuity (UCVA) was 20/200. With a correction of +0.5 sphere –5.0 cyl axis 170°, an acuity of 20/100 was achieved. Contact lenses were tried but not tolerated by the patient. Corneal topography showed marked irregular astigmatism. Therefore, the authors discussed treatment options with the parents of this child. As contact lenses were not tolerated, surgery seemed to be the only option to prevent amblyopia. We considered T-cuts, corneal grafts and TA-LASIK. LASIK was selected as the least invasive and most predictable option. Surgery was performed under general anesthesia. Figure 5.1 shows the topographic work place on which the ablation is planned. The preoperative topographic map (scale in diopters) is on the upper left, and the ablation profile suggested by the TA-LASIK software (scale in mm) is on the upper right. On the lower left, the surgeon can add individual fudge factors, and the expected result is displayed on the lower right hand side. Comparing maps, we can see that the flat area at the lower right (blue colors) of the preoperative topography map is steepened by the ablation (red color at the lower right of the ablation map). Superposing the two maps in the upper row, the resulting map, which is displayed at the lower right, should be a perfect sphere, at least theoretically.

Figure 5.2 shows the results of the calculated ablation we just described. The preoperative topographic map and the topographic map one day after surgery are shown in Figure 5.2. The color scale is the same in both maps, which can therefore directly be compared. As clearly

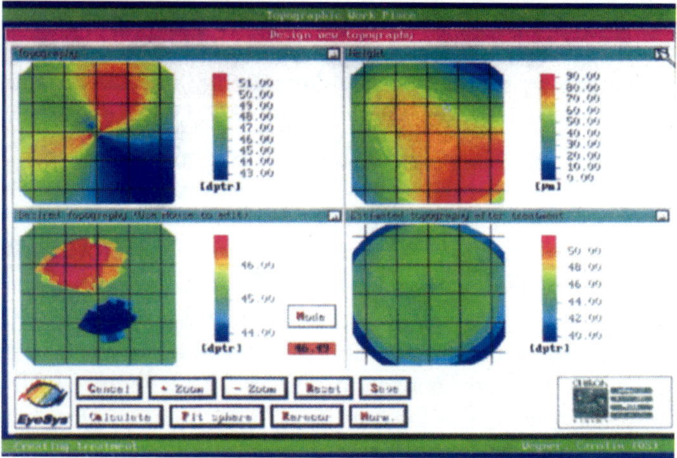

FIGURE 5.1: Topographic workplace used to design the ablation of patient CW. The preoperative topographic map (scale in diopters) is on the upper left, and the ablation profile suggested by the TA-LASIK software (scale in µm) on the upper right. On the lower left, the surgeon can add individual fudge factors, and the expected result is displayed on the lower right hand side

visible, the steep area on the upper left is considerably flatter, and visual acuity without correction improved to 20/60 on day one. Figure 5.2 also shows the differential map. The change map, which visualizes the ablation that was performed, closely resembles the planned ablation (Figure 5.1, upper right, for comparison). One year after surgery, visual acuity without correction was 20/80, and with correction of –2 cyl axis 140° acuity was 20/60. To prevent amblyopia, the right eye was occluded 4 hours a day. Corneal topography at one year shows considerable regression of effect. The cornea was still more regular than

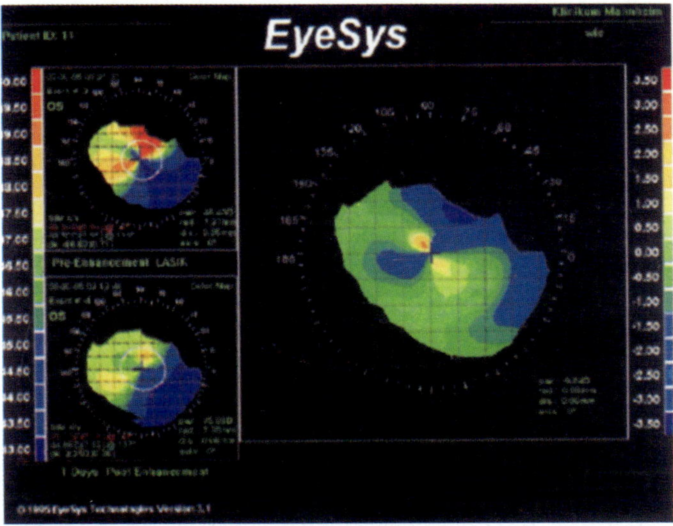

FIGURE 5.2: Pre- and postoperative topographic maps and differential map of patient CW (penetrating injury with irregular astigmatism)

preoperatively, but most of the effect had regressed. We considered a retreatment and calculated an ablation of 50 m. Preoperatively, corneal thickness was 587 μ. Flap thickness was 160 μ, and ablation depth during the first TA-LASIK procedure was 86 μ. Central corneal thickness after the first procedure was 430 μ. We therefore decided against a retreatment to avoid possible late keratectasia due to corneal thinning.

PATIENT AT: DECENTERED ABLATION AFTER PRK

Mr AT is a 40-year-old patient who had PRK in his right eye in July 1994 (Meditec MEL 60 excimer laser). His

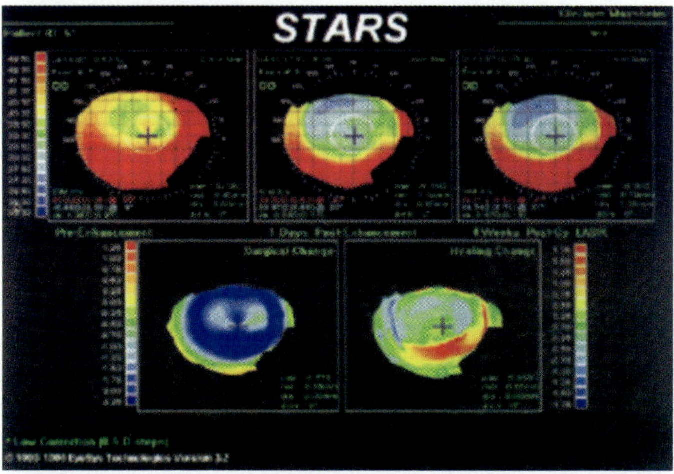

FIGURE 5.3: STARS display of patient AT (decentered ablation after PRK). The preoperative map is shown on the upper left, the map on day 1 in the center, and the map at 1 month on the upper right. The differential map on the lower left (surgical change) shows that the ablation zone was enlarged and the central astigmatism was removed. The map on the lower right (healing change) shows some regression of effect, indicated by the steepening (red colors) around the edge of the ablation zone

preoperative refraction was –8 D in his right eye. After PRK, he complained about halos and double vision, most pronounced in dim light and at night, and had refused PRK in his second eye because of these problems. He was referred to us for possible retreatment. Corneal topography revealed a small ablation zone which was also decentered superotemporally (Figure 5.3, upper left). The average refractive power of the cornea overlaying the entrance pupil was estimated to be 41 D. UCVA was 20/

30, spectacle-corrected visual acuity (SCVA) was 20/20 (–1.0 sphere –1.5 cyl axis 160°). Central corneal thickness was 469 μ. We decided to perform TA-LASIK. Considering a corneal refraction of, on average, 41 D and a manifest spherical equivalent (SE) of –1.75 D, we aimed for a target K-value (corneal refraction) of 39 D. Optical zone size was 6 mm, ablation depth 95 μ. As a flap thickness of 160 μ was used, this left a stromal bed of roughly 200 μ which we consider to be the minimum in order to avoid possible late ectasia. Corneal topography at day 1 shows a much larger ablation zone (Figure 5.3, center). Visual acuity was 20/20 without correction on day one, and the halos had disappeared. Visual acuity and refraction remained stable throughout the postoperative follow-up which is now 6 months. Corneal topography is shown in Figure 5.3. The STARS display allows for evaluation of both the surgical change and the healing change, or regression. The differential map on the lower left (surgical change) shows that the ablation zone was enlarged and the central astigmatism was removed. The map on the lower right shows some regression of effect, indicated by the steepening (red colors) around the edge of the ablation zone.

PATIENT DK: IRREGULAR ASTIGMATISMAFTER PKP AND RK

The patient, a judge at a local court, had had a penetrating corneal graft because of recurrent stromal herpetic keratitis in 1992. He was first referred in 1993. Manifest refraction was +0.25 sphere –6 cyl axis 135°. Corneal astigmatism was –8 D axis 135° and slightly asymmetric. Initially, astigmatic keratotomy was performed in 1994. After AK, manifest refraction was –2.5 sphere –4 cyl axis 165°. UCVA was 20/400 and best-corrected visual acuity (BCVA) was 20/60. Corneal topography showed marked irregularity and axis shift (Figure 5.4, upper left). We therefore decided to perform TA-LASIK. Average refractive power of the cornea overlaying the entrance pupil was estimated to be 45 D. Spherical equivalent of manifest refraction was –4.5 D. We therefore selected a target K-value of 40.5 D. A 5.4 mm optical zone was used, and ablation depth was 150 μ. Corneal thickness was 610 μ centrally, and both the internal and external margins of the graft were well aligned with the host cornea. It is very important to check alignment prior to the lamellar cut. In poor alignment or localized ectasia at the edge, corneal thickness might be reduced, and the keratome cut may cause further weakening of the cornea, inducing more ectasia, or even a penetration of the anterior chamber. In this patient, alignment was perfect, and the LASIK procedure performed in July 1997 was uneventful. A 160 μ flap was used. One day after TA-LASIK, UCVA had improved to 20/30, and BCVA was 20/25 (correction: +0.75 sphere). After 4 months, UCVA was 20/30 and BCVA 20/25, but manifest refraction had changed slightly to +1 sphere – 2.0 cyl axis 10°. Corneal topography 4 months after TA-LASIK showed marked improvement of the irregularity (Figure 5.4). Some residual with-the-rule (WTR) astigmatism was still present, but the irregular astigmatism which was present preoperatively had virtually disappeared as shown by the differential map (Figure 5.4).

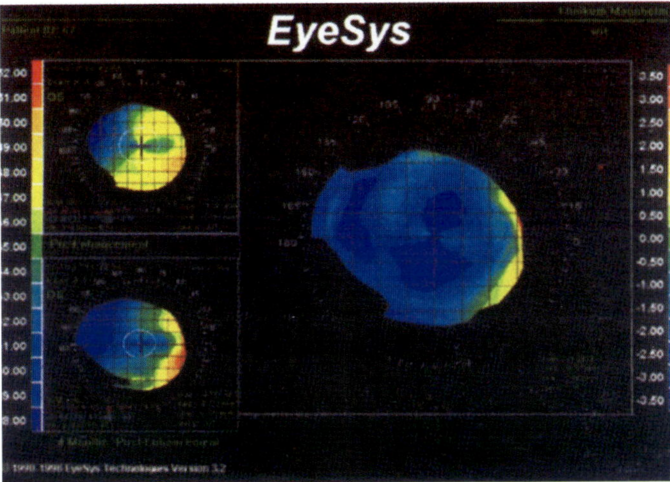

FIGURE 5.4: Pre- and postoperative topographic maps and differential map of patient DK (irregular astigmatism after PKP and RK)

PATIENT ASJ: ASYMMETRIC WTR-ASTIGMATISM

This patient is an excellent example for the use of TA-LASIK in a cornea with "just" some asymmetric astigmatism. Remember, as many as 40 percent of human corneas show some asymmetries like the one shown here ! This 29-year-old lady had a refraction of –7 sphere –1.25 cyl axis 170° in her right eye. SCVA was 20/20. Corneal topography showed asymmetric WTR-astigmatism, with the lower half-meridian being steeper than the upper half-meridian (Figure 5.5, upper left). A symmetrical ablation pattern would have left part of the astigmatism in the lower half-meridian. We therefore decided to perform TA-LASIK

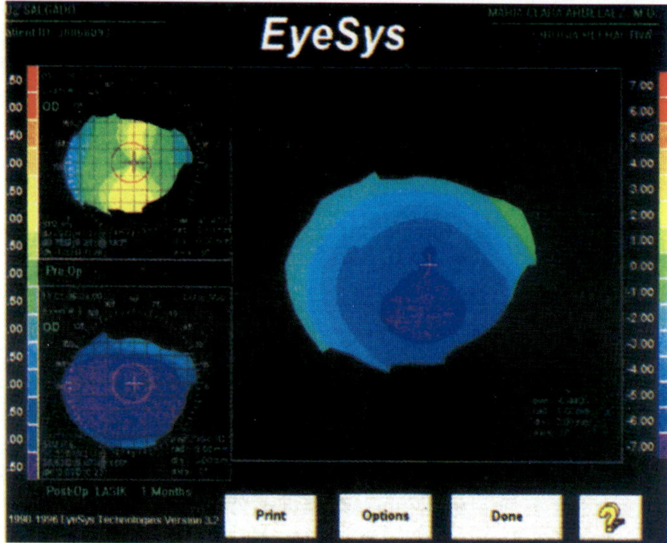

FIGURE 5.5: Pre- and postoperative topographic maps and differential map of patient ASJ (asymmetric WTR-astigmatism)

in this patient. Preoperative pachymetry was 579 μ. An optical zone size of 5 mm was used. Flap thickness was 160 μ, and ablation depth was 109 μ.

On day 1, UCVA was 20/30 and BCVA (+1.25) was 20/20. At 1 month.

UCVA was 20/20, and results remained stable throughout the follow-up period of 6 months. Corneal topography showed a spherical surface after the ablation (Figure 5.5, lower left). The differential maps nicely demonstrates the asymmetric ablation performed—flattening was greater in the lower half-meridian than in the upper half-meridian, as clearly visible by the asymmetric blue bow-tie pattern (Figure 5.5).

PATIENTS AND RESULTS

In a prospective, noncomparative case series, we operated 29 consecutive eyes of 27 patients between July 1996 and July 1997. All eyes have one year follow-up, and the data were presented at the annual meeting of the American Academy of Ophthalmology in New Orleans in 1998. Results were evaluated in four groups:

Group 1 (post-keratoplasty group) consisted of six eyes (five patients) with irregular corneal astigmatism after penetrating keratoplasty. All grafts were performed more than 2 years ago.

Group 2 (post-trauma group) consisted of six eyes (six patients) with irregular corneal astigmatism after corneal trauma. The trauma dated back more than 2 years in all eyes.

Group 3 (decentered/small optical zones group) consisted of 11 eyes (10 patients) with irregular corneal astigmatism after PRK (one eye) or LASIK (10 eyes) due to decentered or small optical zones. All patients complained about halos and image distortion even during the day.

Group 4 (central islands group) consisted of six eyes (six patients) with irregular astigmatism after PRK (two eyes) or LASIK (four eyes) due to central islands or keyhole patterns. All patients complained about blurred vision or image distortion even during the day.

Corneal topography was performed using the corneal analysis system (EyeSys System 2000, Software Version 3.10 and 3.20, EyeSys Premier, Irvine, CA) and more recently the Technomed C-Scan (Technomed Co., Baesweiler, Germany). The topographic changes from the preoperative examination to the postoperative examination at 12 months were subjectively graded as follows—planned correction fully achieved (irregularity less than 1 D and optical zone size as predicted), attempted correction partially achieved (decrease of irregularity of more than 1 D on the differential map and/or increase of optical zone size by at least 1 mm), flattening or steepening of the corneal contour level only, no change of irregularity (change 1 D or less on differential map), no change at all. The term "topographic success rate" (Table 5.1) was introduced and defined to include eyes in which the planned correction was fully achieved and eyes in which the planned correction was partially achieved. In addition, a short questionnaire was completed 12 months after surgery by all patients. Patients were asked to rate their satisfaction with the result of the surgery (high, moderate, not satisfied).

The results of all groups are given in Table 5.1. In the postkeratoplasty group, corrective cylinder was significantly reduced as compared to the preoperative value, and UCVA improved significantly. In the post-trauma group, corrective cylinder was also significantly reduced, and UCVA improved significantly. In the decentered/small optical zones group, both corrective cylinder and SE were reduced, and UCVA improved accordingly, but differences were not statistically significant.

In the central islands group, both corrective cylinder and SE were reduced, and UCVA improved accordingly, but the difference of corrective cylinders was statistically significant only.

Comparing the groups, UCVA improved most in the postkeratoplasty and the post-trauma groups. Results were worst in the central island group, with 33 percent loosing two or more lines of UCVA.

TABLE 5.1: Refraction, visual acuity, corneal topography, and patient satisfaction12 months after topographically-guided LASIK

	Group 1 Postkeratoplasty	*Group 2 Post-trauma*	*Group 3 Decentered/small*	*Group 4 Central islands*
No. of eyes	n = 6	n = 6	n = 11	n = 6
Cylinder preoperatively	5.83 +/– 1.25 D (4.00 to 8.00 D)	2.21 +/– 1.35 D (1.00 to 5.00 D)	0.73 +/– 0.71 D (0 to 2.00 D)	1.42 +/– 1.13 D (0 to 3.50 D)
Cylinder at 12 months	2.96 +/– 1.23 D* (1.50 to 4.50 D)	0.50 +/– 0.84 D** (0 to 2.5 D)	0.36 +/– 1.05 D (0 to 3.5 D)	0.50 +/– 0.84 D* (0 to 2.00 D)
UCVA improved 2 or more lines	83%	83%	55%	50%
UCVA +/–1 line	17%	17%	36%	17%
UCVA lost 2 or more lines	0%	0%	9%	33%
Topographic success rate	66% (n = 4)	83% (n = 5)	91% (n = 10)	50% (n = 3)
Patient response: "Very satisfied"	66% (n = 4)	66% (n = 4)	18% (n = 2)	34% (n = 2)
Patient response: "Moderately satisfied"	17% (n = 1)	0%	46% (n = 5)	0%
Patient response: "Not satisfied"	17% (n = 1)	34% (n = 2)	36% (n = 4)	66% (n = 4)
Reoperation rate	50% (n = 3)	50% (n = 3)	36% (n = 4)	50% (n = 3)

SE—spherical equivalent of manifest refraction, UCVA—uncorrected visual acuity, * p—0.01; ** p—0.001

Results of corneal topography were best in the decentered/small optical zones group, with a success rate, defined as the percentage of eye with the planned result and the percentage of eyes that improved, of 91 percent, followed by the post-trauma group with a success rate of 83 percent. The lowest success rate was observed in the central island group, being 50 percent only (Table 5.1).

SUMMARY

We observed a significant improvement of UCVA, a significant reduction of corrective cylinder, and a more regular corneal topography in all but one of the treatment groups. However, results were poor in one group (central islands group). Our results confirm that topographically-guided LASIK works clinically, and that it is clearly indicated in decentered or small optical zones and useful in postkeratoplasty and post-trauma irregularities. Following refinement of targeting, ablation algorithms, and corneal topography systems, topographically-guided LASIK will in the near future be a tool to create hard-contact lens vision in patients with irregular or asymmetric corneas. Topography-assisted LASIK will take refractive surgery to new limits by ultimately providing a quality of vision which is better than ever before in those 40 percent of patients with corneal irregularities.

CHAPTER 6

Zyoptix

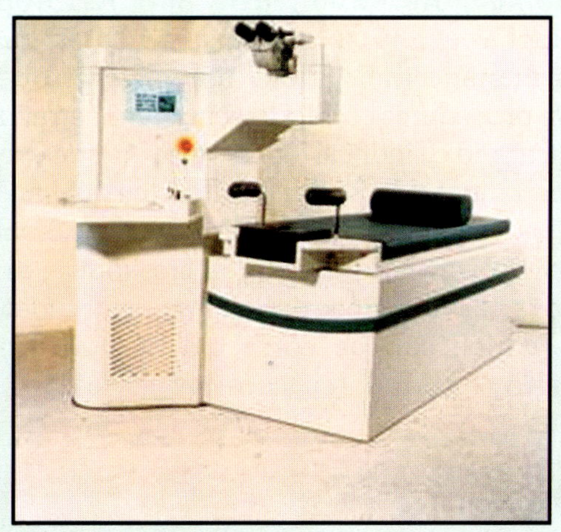

Amar Agarwal
Ashish Doshi
Sonika Doshi
Nilesh Kanjani
Sunita Agarwal
Athiya Agarwal
Ashok Garg

(India)

INTRODUCTION

Since as early as middle of 19th century it has been known that the optical quality of human eye suffers from ocular errors (aberrations) besides the commonly known image errors such as myopia, hyperopia and asigmatism.[1] In early 1970's Fyodorov introduced the anterior radial incisions to flatten the central cornea to correct myopia.[2] Astigmatic keratotomy[3], Keratomileusis and Keratophakia, Epikeratophakia[4] and currently Excimer Laser[5] have been used to manage the various refractive errors. These refractive procedures correct lower order aberrations such as spherical and cylindrical refractive errors however higher order aberrations persist, which affect the quality of vision but may not significantly affect the Snellen visual acuity. Refractive corrective procedures are known to induce aberrations.[6] It is the subtle deviations from the ideal optical system, which can be corrected by wavefront and topography guided (customized ablation) LASIK procedures.[7]

ABERRATIONS

Optical aberration customization can be corneal topography guided which measures the ocular aberrations detected by corneal topography and treats the irregularities as an integrated part of the laser treatment plan. The second method of optical aberration customization measures the wavefront errors of the entire eye and treats based on these measurements.[7] Wavefront analysis can be done either using Howland's aberroscope[8] or a Hartmann Shack wavefront sensor.[9] These techniques measure all the eye's aberrations including second-order (sphere and cylindrical), third-order (coma–like), fourth-order (spherical), and higher order wavefront aberrations. Based on this information an ideal ablation plan can be formulated which treats lower order as well as higher order aberrations.

ZYOPTIX LASER

Zyoptix TM (Bausch and Lomb) is a system for Personalized Vision Solutions, which incorporates Zywave TM Hartmann Shack aberrometer coupled with Orbscan TM II z multi-dimensional device, which generates the individual ablation profiles to be used with the Technolas® 217 Excimer Laser system. Thus this system utilizes combination of wavefront analysis and corneal topography for optical aberration customization.

ORBSCAN

The Orbscan (BAUSCH & LOMB) corneal topography system (Figure 6.1) uses a scanning optical slit scan that is fundamentally different than the corneal topography that analyses the reflected images from the anterior corneal surface. The high-resolution video camera captures 40 light slits at 45 degrees angle projected through the cornea similarly as seen during slit lamp examination. The slits are projected on to the anterior segment of the eye: the anterior cornea, the posterior cornea, the anterior iris and anterior lens. The data collected from these four surfaces are used to create a topographic map. This technique provides more information about anterior segment of the eye, such as anterior and posterior corneal curvature and

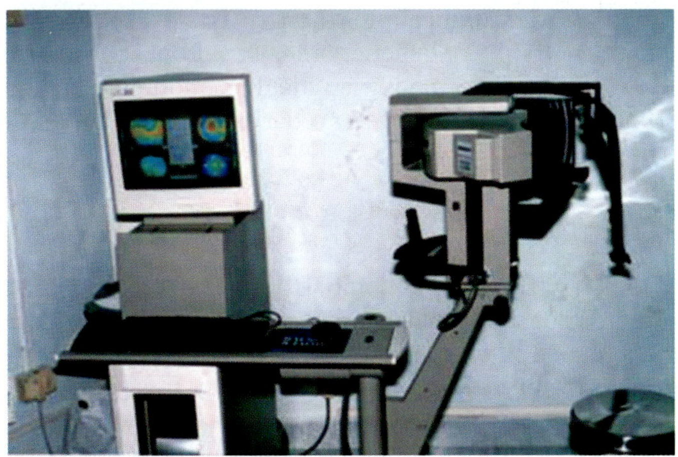

FIGURE 6.1: Orbscan

corneal thickness.[10] It improves the diagnostic accuracy and it has passive eye-tracker from frame to frame, 43 frames are taken to ensure accuracy. It is easy to interpret and has good repeatability. Three different maps are taken, and the one featuring the least eye movements is used. The maximum movements considered acceptable are 200μ.

ABERROMETER

Zywave™ is based on Hartmann–Shack aberrometry (Figure 6.2) in which a laser diode (780 nm) generates a laser beam that is focused on the retina of the patient's eye (Figure 6.3). An adjustable collimation system compensates for the spherical portion of the refractive error of the eye. Laser diode is turned on for approximately 100 milliseconds. The light reflected from the focal

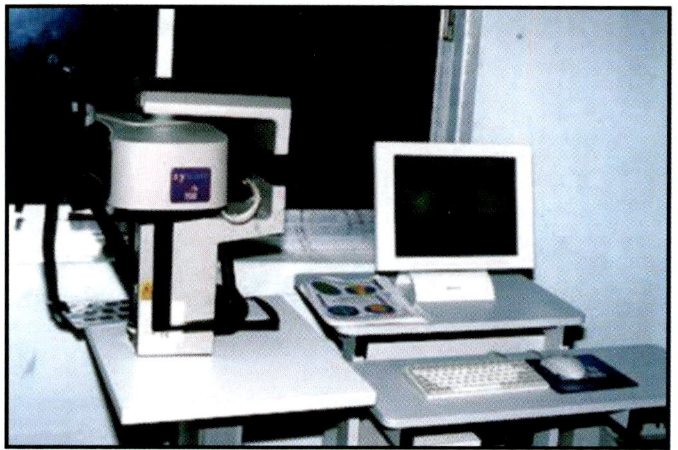

FIGURE 6.2: Hartmann Shack aberrometer

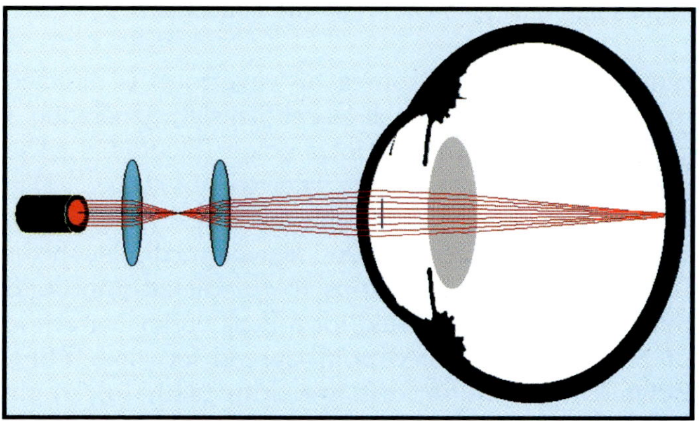

FIGURE 6.3: Zywave projects low-intensity HeNe infrared light into the eye and use the diffuse reflection from the retina

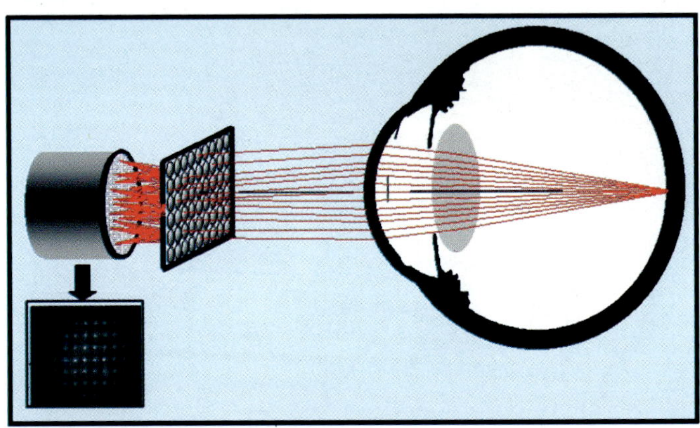

FIGURE 6.4: Schematic illustration of the Bausch & Lomb Zywave aberrometer. A low-intensity HeNe infrared light is shone into the eye; the reflected light is focused by a number of small lenses (lenslet-array), and pictured by a CCD-camera. The capture image is shown on the bottom left.

point on the retina (source of wavefront) is directed through an array of small lenses (lenslet) generating a grid like pattern (array) of focal points (Figure 6.4). The position of the focal points are detected by Zywave™ .Due to deviation of the points from their ideal position, the wavefront can be reconstructed. Wavefront display shows (a) higher order aberrations (b) predicted phoropter refraction (PPR) calculated for a back vertex correction of 15mm.(c) Simulated point spread function (PSF). Zywave™ examinations are done with (a) single examination with undilated pupil (b) five examinations with dilated pupil (mydriasis) non-cycloplegic, using 5% Phenylephrine drops. One of these five measurements, which matched best with the manifest refraction of the undilated pupil, is chosen for the treatment.

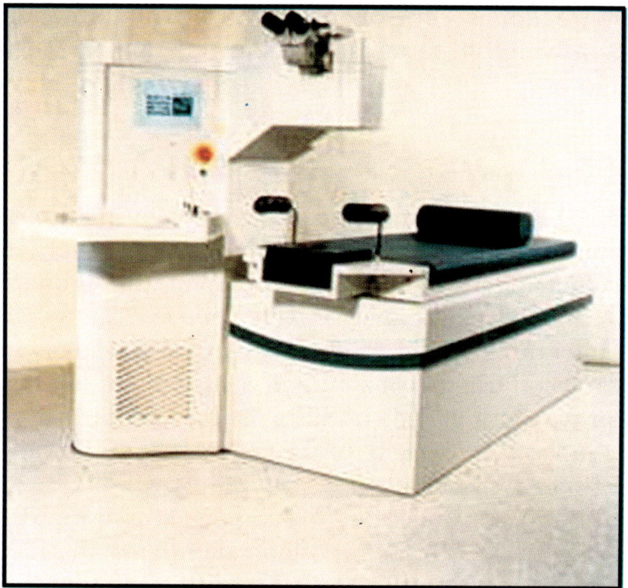

FIGURE 6.5: Technolas 217 z excimer laser system.

ZYLINK

Information gathered from Orbscan and Zywave are then translated into treatment plan using Zylink™ software and copied to a floppy disc. The floppy disc is then inserted into the Technolas 217 system (Figure 6.5), fluence test carried out and a Zyopitx treatment card was inserted. A standard LASIK procedure is then performed with a superiorly hinged flap. A Hansatome™ microkeratome is used to create a flap. Flap thickness varied from 160 μm to 200 μm. A residual stromal bed of 250 μm or more is left in all eyes. Optical zone varied from 6 mm to 7 mm depending upon the pupil size and ablation required.

Eye tracker is kept on during laser ablation. Postoperatively all patients are followed up for at least 6 months.

RESULTS

We did a study comprising 150 eyes with myopia and compound myopic astigmatism. Preoperatively, the patients underwent corneal topography with Orbscan II z ™ and wavefront analysis with Zywave ™ in addition to the routine pre-LASIK work up. The results were assimilated using Zylink ™ and a customized treatment plan was formulated. LASIK was then performed with Technolas® 217 system. All the patients were followed up for at least six months.

Mean preoperative BCVA (in decimal) was 0.83 ± 0.18 (Range 0.33- 1.00). Mean postoperative (6 months) BCVA was 1.00 ± 0.23 (Range 0.33-1.50). Difference was statistically significant (p=0.0003). Out of 150 eyes that underwent customized ablation, 3 eyes (2%) lost two or more lines of best spectacle corrected visual acuity (BSCVA).

Safety Index = Mean postoperative BSCVA / Mean preoperative BSCVA = 1.20 (Figure 6.6). Mean preoperative UCVA was 0.06 ± 0.02 (Range 0.01-0.50). Mean postoperative UCVA was 0.88 ± 0.36 (Range 0.08 – 1.50). Difference was statistically significant (p =0.0001). Efficacy index = Mean postoperative UCVA / Mean preoperative UCVA = 14.66 (Figure 6.7). Preoperatively, none of the eyes had UCVA of 6\6 or more and one eye (0.66%) had UCVA of 6/12 or more. At 6 months post-operatively, 105 eyes (69.93%) had UCVA of 6\6

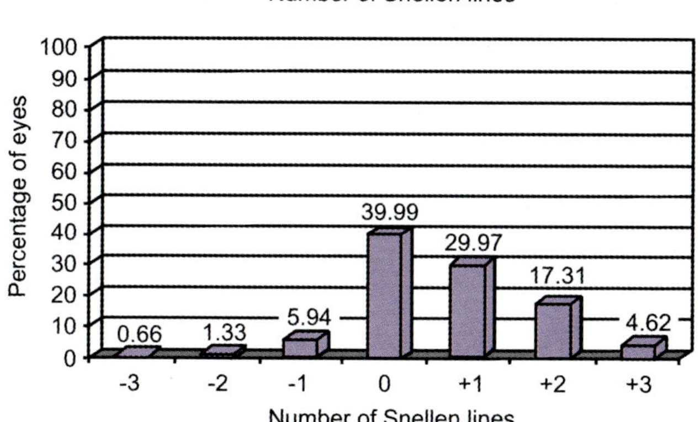

FIGURE 6.6: Shows changes in BSCVA 6 months post-operatively (Safety)

Efficacy

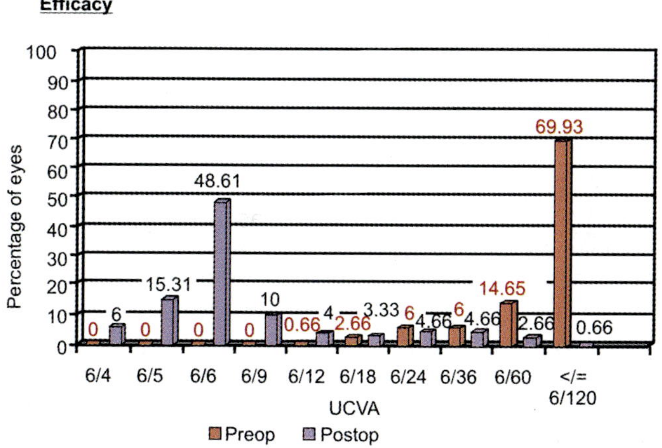

FIGURE 6.7: Compares preop and postop UCVA (Efficacy)

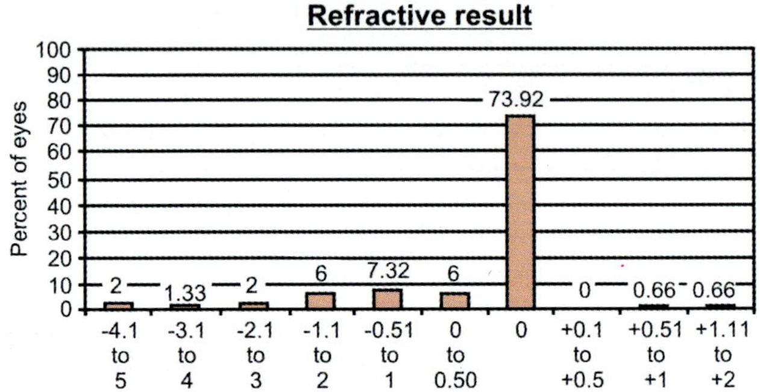

FIGURE 6.8: Shows the refractive results postoperatively after 6 months

or more and 126 eyes (83.91%) had UCVA of 6/12 or more.

Mean preoperative spherical equivalent was –5.25 D ± 1.68 D (Range -0.87 D to –15 D). Mean postoperative spherical equivalent (6 months) was –0.36 D ± 0.931 D (Range –4.25 D to +1.25). Difference between the two was statistically significant ($p<0.05$) (Figure 6.8). 132 eyes (87.91%) were within ±1.00 D of emmetropia while 120 eyes (79.92%) were within ± 0.05 D of emmetropia. 1 eye (0.66%) was overcorrected by > 0.5 D and 1 eye (0.66%) was overcorrected by >1D. The mean pupil diameter was 5.1 mm ± 0.62 mm. Preoperatively, 95 eyes (63.27%) had third order aberrations.42 eyes (28%) had second order aberration alone, while 13 eyes (8.65%) had fourth and fifth order aberrations. Postoperatively, 60 eyes (40%) had third order aberration.75 eyes (50%) had second order alone while 15 eyes (10%) had higher order aberrations.

DISCUSSION

Hartmann-Shack wavefront sensor was first used by Liang and colleagues to detect ocular aberrations.[11] They applied an adaptive optics deformable mirror to correct the lower and higher order aberrations of the eye. They reported a 6 times increase in contrast sensitivity to high spatial frequency when the pupil was large. This study demonstrated that correction of higher order aberrations could lead to supernormal vision in normal eyes.

In our series, using Zyoptix and Technolas 217 system, which is wavefront and corneal topography guided, we yielded results that are comparable to standard LASIK procedure.[12] In a series of 347 eyes, McDonald et al [12] reported a postoperative refraction of –0.29 ± 0.45 D (-0.36 ± 0.93 D in our series) with standard LASIK. 57 percent of the eyes in their series had postoperative UCVA of =6/6. In our study, 70 percent of the eyes had UCVA of =6/6, six months postoperatively.

Higher order aberrations were reduced post-operatively in our study. Third-order aberration (coma) was most common in our series, followed by second-order (defocus and astigmatism) and fourth-order (spherical aberration). Postoperatively, after 6 months, there was considerable decrease in third-order and fourth-order aberrations. While most of the eyes had only defocus and astigmatism (i.e. second -order aberration). A slight increase in fourth-order aberration (spherical) was noted. Spherical aberration is known to increase after LASIK.[13-15] Roberts has reported that cornea changes its shape in response to ablation and this change, along with wound healing effects have to be taken into account before customized correction can nullify higher-order aberrations.

Roberts and coworkers suggest that increase in spherical aberrations following LASIK may be caused by a biomechanically induced steepening and thickening that may occur in mid periphery of the cornea.[13] MacRae and coworkers have reported that simply creating a LASIK flap increases higher-order aberrations in unpredictable manner.[14] They suggest that improved results can be obtained using a surface ablation such as PRK or LASEK, or by doing a two-stage LASIK, with the second stage adjusting for the aberration created by the flap and initial ablation.

Scotopic visual complaints have been the bugbear of LASIK procedures, ranging from mild annoyance to server optical disability.[16, 17] Nighttime starbursts, reduced contrast sensitivity and haloes are the most common complaints.[16,17] Spherical aberration that is induced during LASIK may account for this scotopic complaints.[14] Pupil diameter is another factor that is important. When pupil diameter is large, as in young patients, dim light vision is improved after customized correction. [18, 19] In our series, 11 percent of the patients complained of haloes around light at night and difficult night driving. In dim light, the mean pupil diameter in these patients was 4.2mm while it was 5.9 mm in other patients. Smaller pupil diameter and induced higher-order aberration may account for these scotopic visual complaints.

Twenty-five percent of the patients in our series reported improvement in bright light vision, while 40 percent showed improvement in dim light vision. A similar improvement was noted by Cox and co-workers (presentation by Cox IG at Zyoptix Alliance meeting, 2002 reported in *Ocular Surgery News*, July 2002 volume 13, number 7). In our series, treatment optical zone ranged from 6 mm to 7 mm. Treatment with larger optical zones and transition zones as compared to conventional LASIK may be possible since entire corneal topography and not just the central cornea overlying pupil along with wavefront ablation in dilated pupil are considered during treatment. This may induce lesser spherical aberration post-LASIK and account for improved scotopic vision.

Though we did not measure contrast sensitivity and glare acuity postoperatively, our results suggest improved quality of vision and fewer glare problems with Zyoptix treatment. A more temporal appraisal of the procedure has to be carried out with comparison to standard LASIK. Short-term results suggest wavefront and topography guided LASIK may be a safe and effective procedure which improves the visual performance.

CONCLUSION

Wavefront and topography guided LASIK procedure leads to better visual performance by decreasing higher order aberration. Scotopic visual complaints may be reduced with this method.

REFERENCES

1. Helmholtz H. Handbuch der physiologischen optik. Leipzig: Leopold Voss.1867; 137-47.
2. Fyodorov S N, Durnev V V: Operation of dosaged dissection of corneal circular ligament
3. Binder PS, Waring GO III. Keratotomy for astigmatism. In Waring GO III (Ed.): Refractive Keratotomy for Myopia and Astigmatism. Mosby Year Book 1085–1198, 1992. in cases of myopia of mild degree. Ann Ophthalmol II: 1885 –90, 1979.

4. Kaufmann HE: Correction of aphakia Am J Ophthalmol 89: 1,1980
5. McGhee CNJ, Taylor HR, Garty DS et al: Excimer Lasers in Ophthalmology: Principles and Practice Martin Duntz: London, 1997.
6. MacRae S, Porter J, Cox IG, et al. Higher-order aberrations after conventional LASIK. ISRS: Dallas, Texas, 2000.
7. MacRae SM: Supernormal vision, hypervision, and customized corneal ablation. Guest Editorial J Cat Refract Surg Feb 26 (2) 2000.
8. Howland HC and Howland B, A subjective method for the measurement of monochromatic aberrations of the eye, J Opt Soc Am. 1977: 67:1508-1518
9. Liang J, Williams DR, Miller DT. Supernormal vision and high-resolution retinal imaging through adaptive optics. J Opt Soc Am 1997: 2884-2892
10. Fedor P, Kaufman S Corneal topography and imaging. eMedicine Journal, 2001;vol 2, no. 6.
11. Liang J, Williams D. Aberrations and retinal image quality of the normal human eye. J Opt Soc AM A 1997;14:2884-2892.
12. McDonald MB, Carr JD, Frantz JM, et al. Laser in situ keratomilieusis for myopia up to –11 diopters with up to –5 diopters of astigmatism with summit autonomous LADARVision excimer laser system. Ophthalmology2001; 108:309-316.
13. Roberts C. The cornea is not a piece of plastic. J Refract Surg 2000; 16:407-413.
14. MacRae SM, Roberts C, Porter J, et al. The biomechanics of a LASIK flap. ISRS Mid –Summer Meeting: Orlando, Florida, 2001.
15. Applegate RA, Howland HC, Klyce SD. Corneal aberration and refractive surgery. In: MacRae S (Editor). Customized Corneal Ablation. Thorofare NJ: Slack, Inc., 2001.
16. Holladay JT, Dudeja DR, Chang J. Functional vision and corneal changes after laser in situ keratomileusis determined by contrast sensitivity, glare testing, and corneal topography. J Cataract Refract Surg 1999; 25: 663-9.

17. Perez-Santonja JJ, Sakla HF, Alio JL. Contrast sensitivity after laser in situ keratomileusis. J Cataract Refract Surg 1998; 24: 183-9.
18. Applegate R, Howland H, Sharp R, et al. Corneal aberrations and visual performance after refractive keratectomy. J Refract Surg 1998; 14: 397-407.
19. Oshika T, Klyce S, Applegate R, et al. Comparison of corneal wavefront aberrations after photorefractive keratectomy and laser in situ keratomileusis. Am J Ophthal 1999; 127:1-7.

CHAPTER 7

"ORCA Wave"— Corneal Wavefront Guided LASIK

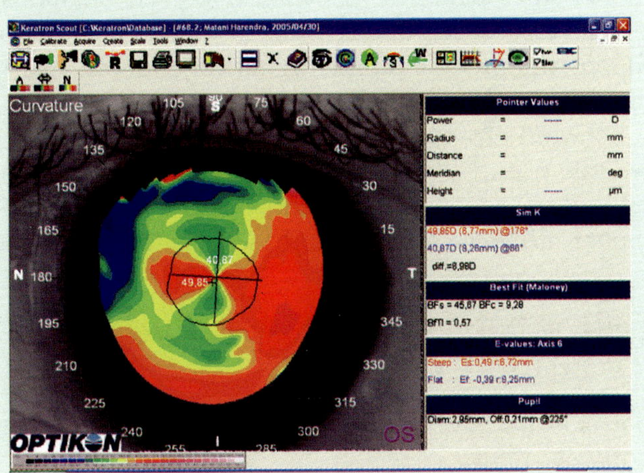

Cyres K Mehta
Keiki R Mehta
(India)

INTRODUCTION

LASIK has gained in popularity worldwide.New flying spot lasers with Gaussian beam profiles and high speed infrared trackers provide precise, predictable and consistent ablation leading to exceptional accuracy.

The promise of "supervision" is slowly becoming a reality with the availability of Hartmann Schack and Tscherning aberrometry systems,with linkages to excimer laser platforms.

The Wavelight company ,Germany,utilizes a Tscherning principle for its aberrometer. Bausch and Lomb provide the Orbscan Corneal analysis system, a projection based videokeratograph system which relies on slits of light,with the 217 laser platform. Schwind Eye Tech Solutions a Refractive Solutions and Excimer laser manufacturer out of Germany provide an interesting variation on Aberrometrically guided LASIK.

Schwind provides the COAS aberrometer as well as the ORK-W and ORK-CAM softwares which provide shot patterns based on the Optikon Keratron Scout Topographer, a Placido's principle based videokeratoscope.

A SHORT HISTORICAL ACCOUNT OF TOPOGRAPHY

1880: Placido invented a flat disk with alternating black and white rings.

1889: Javal placed the disks into his ophthalmometer, behind the arc that carried the ophthalmometric mires.

1896: Alvar Gullstrand from the Uppsala University invented the Photokeratoscope and made very accurate arc-step calculations , with an 'algorithm' to plot the corneal meridian profiles.This won him the Nobel prize in 1911.

1990s: Computerized corneal topography from EyeSys and a host of other companies basically all videokeratoscopes.

2001: Optikon 2000 an Italian company releases the Keratron Scout with a link to the Schwind ESIRIS flying spot laser.

TOPOGRAPHY AND WAVEFRONTS

A corneal topographer (CT) measures corneal shape while a Wavefront Analyser (WA) measures wavefront aberrations.

The Advent of the "corneal wavefront" ushers in a new era in refractive measurements.

The Concept of the Corneal Wavefront

The Corneal Wavefront is the part of the total aberrations of the eye, owed to the cornea.

So, Ocular Wavefront(OW)=Corneal Wavefront (CW) + Internal Wavefront (IW)

The Corneal Wavefront is easily calculated from the Corneal Topography by using an algorithm. An *'algorithm'* is the calculus procedure used to reconstruct corneal geometry from the calculation of the position of points on the corneal surface relative to axis or a reference sphere.

Ray tracing is used. Rays are traced from the fovea out of the eye.

Wavefront aberration is measured as the difference from a plane surface, at the entrance pupil,in object space.In *Ray tracing* we apply Snells law to the corneal surface to calculate (OPD) the Optical Path Difference. If a cornea is distorted (e.g. has a bulge in the surface) the rays of light spend a longer time in the cornea (where the bulge is) so the rays that enter air first, from the flatter regions of the cornea, accelerate and create a deformed wavefront.In the time a ray travels 3 micron in the cornea, it travels 4 micron in air. So if the cornea is distorted from its ideal shape,we can follow the ***"rule of 3"*****, i.e. every 3 microns of distortion from the ideal shape of the cornea will produce a +1 micron difference in the OPD map and a –1 micron difference in the wavefront error map.**

This Optical Path Difference, the basis of Corneal Wavefront theories,is the difference between the corneal wavefront and an Ideal wavefront. It is similar to the spherical offset which is the height difference between the cornea and a sphere.

Total aberration of the eye as measured by wavefront Analyzers depends on:

1. Size of the pupil: With the COAS analyzer,using a Hartmann Schack sensor,the aberrometric map depends as with any analyzer on pupil size.If the pupil opens only 5 mm, then the map generated is only 5 mm, an unacceptably small ablation diameter.
2. Effect of accommodation: Introduces another factor into the total wavefront, i.e the effect of the lens on the wavefront. As the lens changes shape to accommodate it itself induces aberrations.
3. Wavefront varies with age and from examination to examination and with epithelial factors.

In contrast, ***corneal aberrations*** are—

1. Relatively stable over time and serial measurements
2. Can be evaluated for different pupil diameters
3. Not affected by accommodation
4. More than 80 percent of the total wavefront aberrations are attributed to the Corneal Wavefront and this measurement is stable!

ORK CORWAVE also called **ORK-**W "Corneal Wavefront" Software-Link is successfully being used for:

- Treatment of virgin eyes
- Individual improvement of visual acuity (in case of corneal aberrations)
- Re-treatment of decentered ablations, by increasing the ablation diameter
- Re-treatment to enlarged optical zones to combat glare and haloes
- Re-treatment of irregular ablations and smoothing effect for irregular corneas.

Methods

The combination of the future oriented ESIRIS Excimer laser system for Refractive Surgery (200Hz pulse frequency, 330Hz active high speed eyetracking and 0.8 mm scanning spot with gaussian beam profile) together with the high resolution topography systems Optikon Keratron Scout shows us new possibilities of measuring and interpreting the cornea. With this an individual and true "customized ablation" may be performed with the Schwind Excimer Laser ESIRIS. An intelligent software (Schwind ORK software for Optimized Refractive Keratectomy), which realizes the transformation of the cornea into an individual, customized ablation profile, is the most important link between the diagnostic unit (topography system) and the Excimer laser for the treatment. A corneal wavefront generated by the software presents the cornea with its irregularities in form of a mathematic zernicke polynomial up to the 7th order. The projected "placido" rings and the information (data) resulting from it are the basis for the calculation. This is being described by the Optical Path Difference (OPD) with the help of ***Zernicke polynomials***. Corneal aberrations may now be calculated and compared with ocular aberrations.

ORK CORWAVE or "Corneal Wavefront Technology" delivers much more information about optical defects that may effect vision than just sphere and cylinder. It more or less describes the anterior corneal surface as a wavefront with its aberrations. Thus it is possible to qualify (describe) and quantify optical defects of the human eye. This information makes a real, individual ablation profile possible, which considerably increases and therefore improves postoperative visual quality of the patient.

Advantages of ORK CORWAVE(ORK-W)

- Pupil dilation of the patient,unlike aberrometry is not necessary for measurement
- Reliable measurement results, especially with irregular cornea, high astigmatism and "central islands."
- Selective simulation of corneal aberrations: Point Spread Function (PSF) - acuity chart or Modular Transfer Function (MTF - which relates to the contrast sensitivity)
- Individual treatment plan with decentrations and re-treatments

- Extended diagnostic possibilities by comparing the complete aberrometry of the eye with the corneal aberrations.
- ***Accommodation does not influence measuring results.***
- Treatment zone is ***not limited by the pupil.***

The Keratron Scout Manufactured by Optikon2000SPA (Rome, Italy).

It uses a small cone with 28 edges for the projection of Placido's rings.This allows us to measure at least 85 percent of the corneal surface which is indispensable for peripheral treatments like hyperopia and also for re-treatments by enlarging ablation diameter.

The software that connects the Laser to the Topographer is the Schwind ORK-W.

Steps in Performing a Corneal Wavefront Guided Ablation

1. Take a topographic picture from the Scout.Evaluate the picture for repeatability, artifacts, lashes, tear film abnormalities and adequate pupil recognition.
2. If the image meets the required criteria create a "Corneal Wavefront" map.

   The wavefront map can be broken down into and viewed as:

   a. Zernicke coefficients
   b. Point spread function
   c. Simulated vision chart
   d. Modulation transfer function (like contrast sensitivity).
   e. A street scene where the patient can see a street scene simulated preoperatively and postoperatively.

This is essential for patients undergoing treatment on higly aberrated corneas to realize the meaning of wavefront and how it adds "sharpness" to vision.

3. Export the measurements to the ORK-W software which creates a shot file (an ablation pattern).ORK-W creates a Prolate cornea.The Optical Zone can include the entire topographic map and not just pupil diameter (like a Wavefront analyzer)
4. Perform the ablation
5. A week and a month after treatment,put the patient back on the topographer and analyze the difference map.

OUR EXPERIENCE

Over a 4-month period with the Schwind ESIRIS laser and the Keratron Scout with ORK-W software for 110 cases which included 9 cases of highly aberrated eyes.

1. On many cases of virgin eyes, we were able to reduce postoperative aberrations by one-third to half, of the RMS value
2. Patients perceived the vision as sharp.No patient lost lines and a few experienced a one line gain in BCVA (14 patients)
3. Minimum treatment diameter was 6.5 mm with a 0.5 mm transition zone.Thus with Indian pupils we did not get any case of Haloes or Glare
4. Nine highly aberrated eyes, post-keratoplasty and post-trabeculectomy and post-ECCE were also treated with corneal wavefront.

Aberrations reduced by about a quarter in these complicated cases. Also in every case, the full cylinder was not eliminated. Postoperative BCVA, sometimes with spectacles (In cases where preoperative cylinder was as high as 10 D), improved about 1-2 lines in most cases (6 out of 9). No patient lost lines of BCVA!.So in our experience the system does work,in the sense that it provides better postoperative best corrected visual acuity.

What matters is the ability of the operator to choose the appropriate topographic map from the 4 maps the topographer presents every sequence for analysis. Every map which is exported for wavefront correction must be screened thoroughly, *not by a technician* but by the Laser surgeon, for tear film, lash and position defects and for adequate pupil recognition.

CASE STUDY

Patient HM aged 70 presented to us with a BCVA of 6/24 (no improvement on pinhole) in his one functioning left eye.

This eye had been operated previously elsewhere for ECCE and trabeculectomy 10 years ago. The pupil was a 3 mm non-dilating adherent pupil(to the PMMA IOL). Measured corneal thickness was 550 microns.

In Figure 7.1: notice that the Keratron scout topographer has measured the pupil at 2.95 mm and the cornea looks grossly distorted, with a measured astigmatism of 8.98 Diopters.

In Figures 7.2A and B: notice that the software using an arc step algorithm has generated a wavefront map. In the Zernicke coefficients map we can see that third order aberrations are significant and the astigmatism is 9.59. The total RMS value of the aberrations in the cornea is more than 11 microns (top left part of the picture).

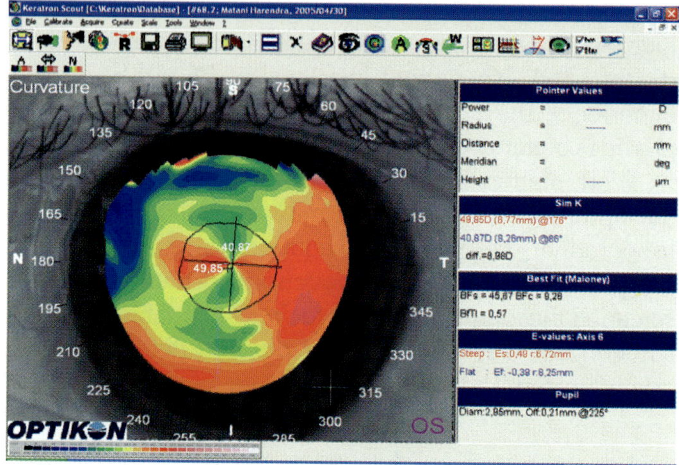

FIGURE 7.1: TOPO preoperative

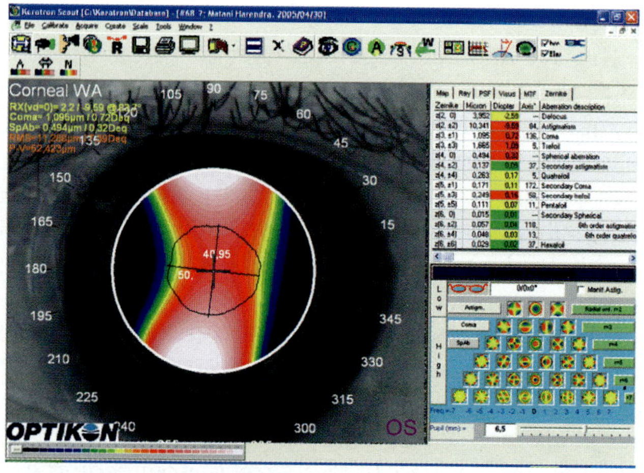

FIGURE 7.2A: Preoperative corneal wavefront map

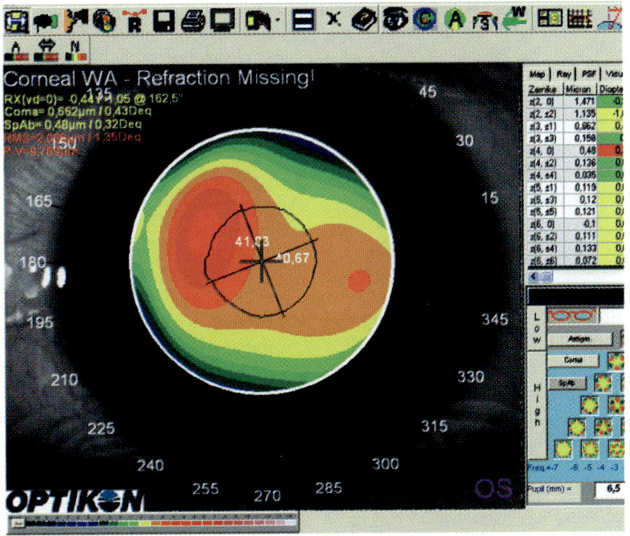

FIGURE 7.2B: Preoperative corneal wavefront map

In Figure 7.2C: notice that even though the patient accepts only +1-6D at 85 degrees, the topographer and software have decided the sphere to be 1.66 and cylinder to be –7.21. We have entered the ablation rate of 0.496 generated by the fluence test on the ESIRIS. The maximum height of ablation is determined to be 143.1 microns which is acceptable. The ZIP is slotted into the laser and the ablation performed on the eye under a 110 micron flap.

In Figure 7.3: Note the cylinder is greatly reduced to 4 D. *At week:* the cornea looks much 'smoother' with less rapid transitions.

In Figure 7.4: the RMS value is now reduced to 7 microns from 11, about a 30 percent drop. Astigmatism

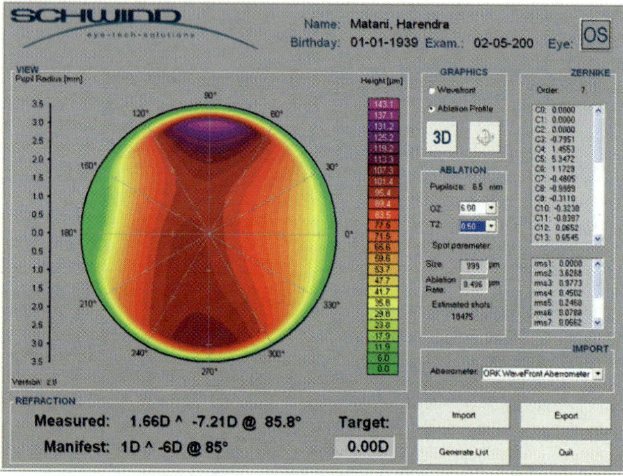

FIGURE 7.2C: Shot file generated with ORK-W software

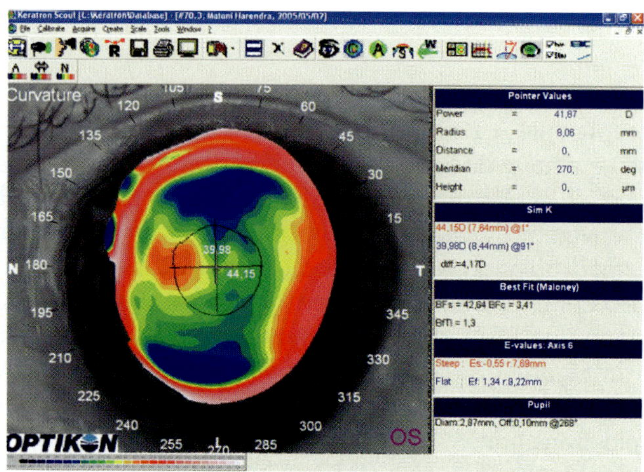

FIGURE 7.3: Postoperative TOPO

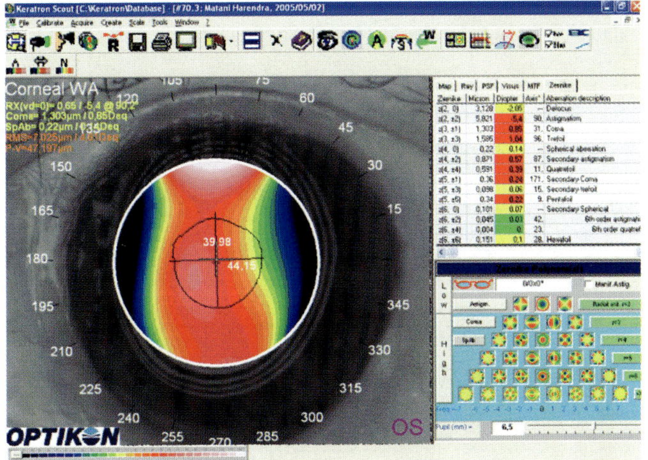

FIGURE 7.4: Postoperative wavefront

has dropped to 5 D from 9.4th order aberrations seem to have increased.We were baffled. Why? Reason.The flap had not yet perfectly settled.A month after the case the patient was 6/12 with only 2.5 cylinder!!

In Figure 7.5A: we can see that the simulated visual acuity is much better (the black and white picture) in the postoperative case. Both UCVA and BCVA have both improved by 50 percent a month postoperative.

Lets take a look at another case: This case underwent LASIK at another center that uses an ACS microkeratome that creates a nasal hinged flap.The flap was incomplete and part of the ablation fell on the hinge.Here even though the cylinder induced is barely 0.4 D (Figure 7.5B) the patient complained of glare and ghosting and distortion of images. She was referred for an evaluation.On topographic evaluation we can see the blue and red areas

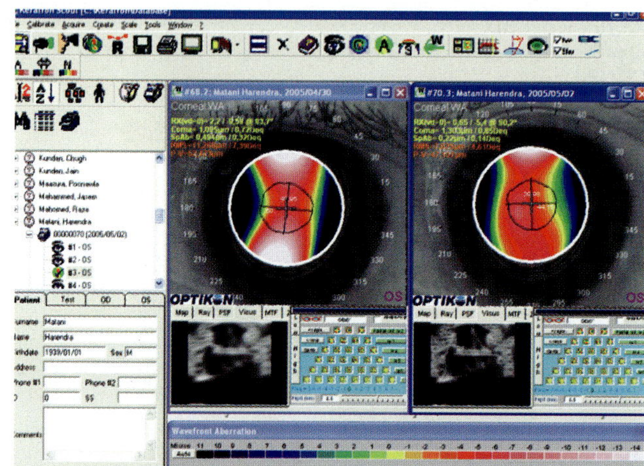

FIGURE 7.5A: Comparative visual acuity simulations

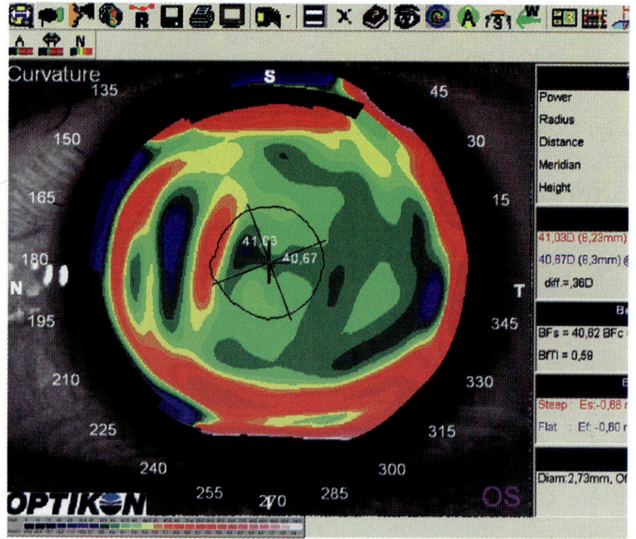

FIGURE 7.5B

where the flap was partial and laser energy fell on the upturned flap. Luckily for her pupil was only 3 mm in mesopic conditions.!

On corneal wavefront evaluation (Figure 7.5C) we realized that a large amount of COMA and spherical aberration had been induced with total value of aberrations crossing 2 microns where more than 1 micron is significant.This explains her loss of BCVA.She has lost one line of BCVA(6/9) due to the aberrations.She would benefit from the ORCA wave procedure.Thus corneal wavefront guided procedures have a definite role to play in retreatments.

I would like to share one more case series from Germany which demonstrates the strength of the system in *Retreatments.*

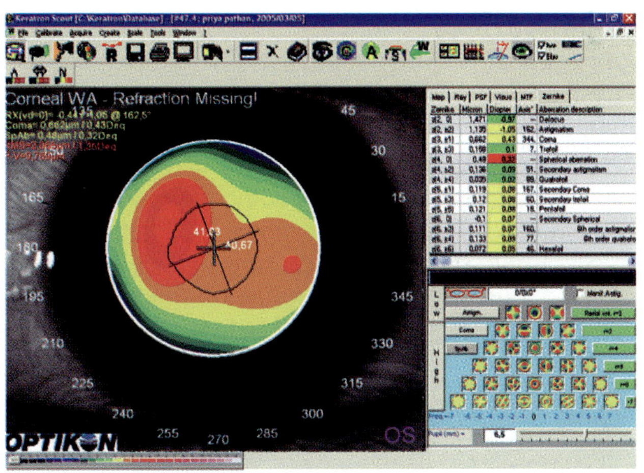

FIGURE 7.5C

Experience, Results, and Cases Treated:by Volker Rummelt, MD, Oberstenfeld, Germany, with the Schwind 200 Hz. Excimer laser, ORK-Software, and Optikon Keratron Scout Topography System. This experience is based on corneal wavefront data, which had been obtained from the Optikon Keratron Scout Topography System and the Schwind ORK software, on 12 eyes which had undergone LASIK treatment 11 months earlier, and who had been *retreated* from May–December 2002. There was a decentered ablation with a coma with 7/12 eyes preoperatively, a relatively small optical zone (6.0 mm) with 6/12 eyes with large pupil diameter at mesopic conditions with subjectively increased Halos at night and with 3/12 eyes there was an irregular astigmatism with a partially lasered flap (hinge) after LASIK.

The optical zone (OZ) of all retreated eyes was enlarged (6.5 mm), and, if possible, completed ***with a transition zone (1-1.5 mm).*** Post-ORK showed a **clear visual improvement** (vision median (UCVA) preoperative: 0.6; (UCVA) postoperative: >=1,0), a '**smoothing**' of the corneal ablation area and a decrease of selective corneal aberrations. From a subjective point of view, the visual acuity was considerably improved (increase of visual acuity and decreased perception of annoying Halos).

This shows us that—selective analysis of corneal wavefront permits an effective treatment of corneal ablation ***using the Schwind ORK-Software.***

CONCLUSION

LASIK has entered its golden era where retreatments are possible to correct past errors, aberrated eyes can be effectively treated and the entire process has become to

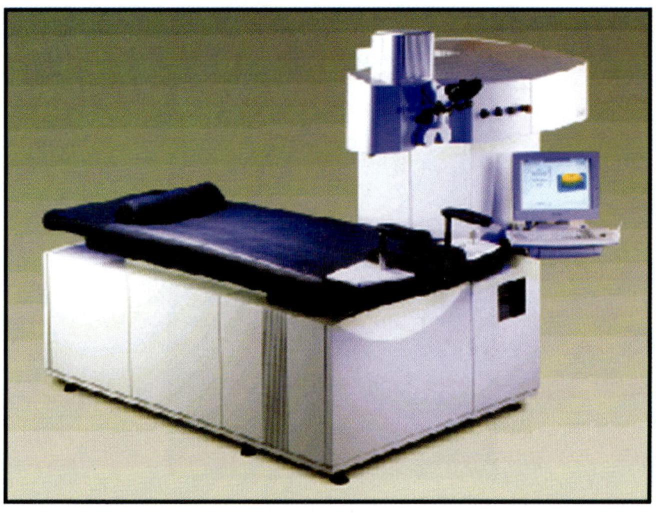

FIGURE 7.6: Schwind ESIRIS laser platform

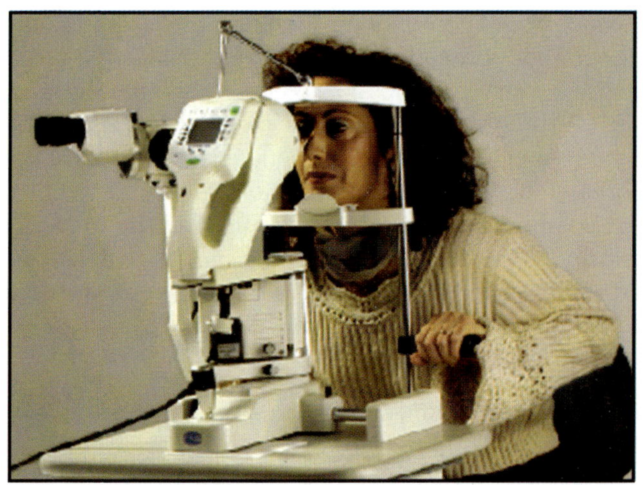

FIGURE 7.7: Keratron scout

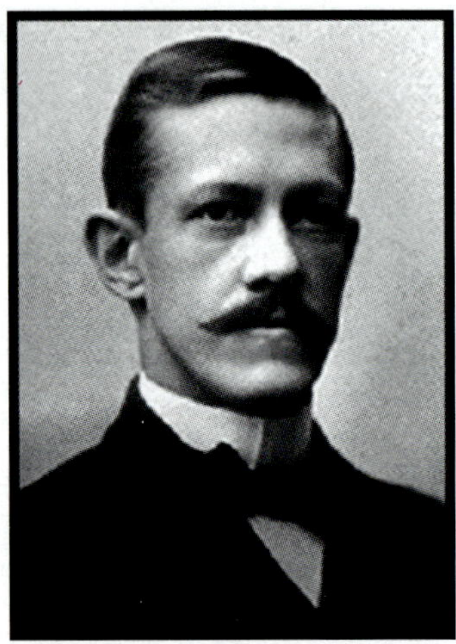

FIGURE 7.8: Prof Alvar Gullstrand—the father of corneal topography

a great extent "pain free for the Surgeon." With the new Topographic corneal wavefront ,the possibilities for further precise correction is possible. A newer software is under trial, ORK-CAM which will allow greater translation of the corneal wavefront into excimer energy allowing us to treat a greater percentage of aberration.

Evolution and revolution are the markers of human history. *"Its not the strongest of the species that survives, nor the most intelligent, but the one **most responsive to change**."* - Charles Darwin

BIBLIOGRAPHY

1. Artal P ,Berrio E,Guirao A,Piers P .Contribution of the cornea and internal surfaces to the change of ocular aberrations with age. J Opt Soc Am A 2002;19:137-43.

2. Guirao A,Artal P.Corneal wave aberration from videokeratography: accuracy and limitations of the procedure. J Opt Soc Am A 2000;17:955-65.
3. Gullstrand A.Photographic–Ophthalmometric and clinical Investigations of corneal refraction.Am J Optom Arch Am Acad Optom1966;43:143-214.
4. Koch DD,Foulks GN,Moran CT,Wakil JS.The corneal EyeSys system: accuracy analysis and reproducibility of first generation prototype.J Refract Corneal Surg1989;6:423-9.
5. Leven JR.The true inventors of the keratoscope and photokeratoscope. BJ History of Science 1965;2(8):324-42.
6. Mattioli R,Tripoli N.Corneal Geometry Reconstruction with the Keratron videographer.Optom Vis Sci 1997;74881-894.
7. Reinstein DZ,Srivannaboon S,Silverman RH,Sutton HFS,Coleman DJ.Limits of wavefront guided customized ablation:Biomechanical and epithelial factors. Invest Ophthalmol Vis Sci (Supple)2002;433-942.
8. Reynolds A. Introduction:History of corneal measurement. In Schanzlin D, Robin J (Eds): Corneal Topography Measuring and Modifying the Cornea. New York:Springer Verlag; 1991:vii-x.
9. Roberts C.The cornea is not a piece of plastic. Editorial J Refract Surg 2000;16:407-13.

Chapter 8

Wavefront Aberrometry for Irregular Astigmatism

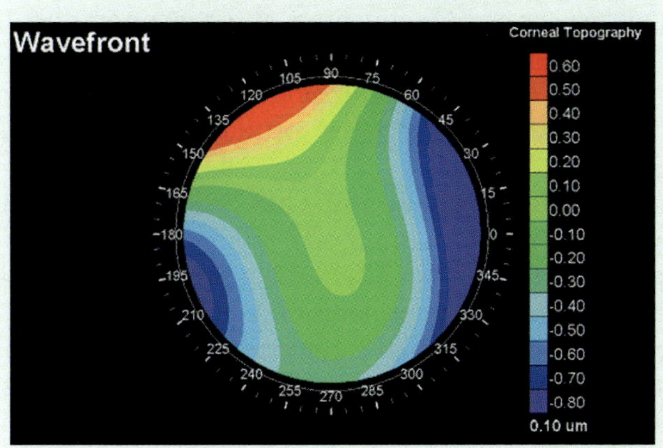

Jorge L Alió
Robert Montés-Micó
(Spain)

INTRODUCTION TO WAVEFRONT ABERRATION

Wavefront aberration is defined as the deviation between the reference wavefront that comes from a in ideal optic system and the wavefront that originates from a measured optical system. The unit used to measure it is microns of waves and it is shown as the root-mean-square (RMS). Wavefront analysis of the eye allows to determine the optical quality of the eye by evaluating the shape of its wavefront as wavefront aberrations.

There are several methods to evaluate the wavefront shape and are classified into the following three types:

1. Outgoing wavefront aberrometry (Hartmann-Shack sensor).[1]
2. Ingoing retinal imaging aberrometry (Cross cylinder aberroscope,[2] Tscherning aberroscope[3] and the sequential retinal ray tracing method).[4]
3. Ingoing feedback aberrometer (Spatially resolved refractometer[5] and the optical path difference method).[6]

When the wavefront shape has been obtained, using any of the previous methods, it can be analyzed by expanding it into sets of Zernicke polynomials to extract the characteristic components of the wavefront shape. In the Zernicke polynomial expansion, the different optical aberrations may be described by terms which are raised to different orders. First and second order terms describe tilt, astigmatism and spherical refractive error respectively; and third, fourth and higher-orders describe spherical aberration, coma and the rest of aberrations. Polynomials can be expanded up to any arbitrary order if sufficient numbers of measurements for calculations are made.

CORNEAL WAVEFRONT ABERRATIONS

Videokeratoscopes have enabled the measurement of the corneal shape and the determination of corneal first surface wavefront aberrations and their influence on visual performance.[7,8] To date, these methods have been used mainly to quantify the effects of refractive surgery on corneal aberrations and visual performance.

The corneal wavefront, which is one of the components of the total ocular wavefront, can be calculated from corneal topographic height data. The corneal wavefront can be fitted with a Zernicke polynomial decomposition in the same way that total ocular wavefront is measured by aberrometry and fitted with the same polynomial decomposition. Both decompositions allow inspection of the total ocular and corneal aberrations of the human eye, considering the contribution of the cornea to the total aberrations of the eye.

Using Zernicke polynomial decomposition we are able to examine the optical quality of the corneal surface generating the wavefront of the anterior surface of the cornea. Zernicke analysis is a sophisticated analytical method which is ideal for representing surfaces of any shape. It is based on a set of orthonormal polynomial developed by Zernicke. Using Zernicke's analysis, any surface can be described as the weighted sum of typical shapes represented by the polynomials. The series of polynomial is of increasing order and potentially infinite. The greater the number of polynomials used, the more detailed the surface representation. The components chosen by Zernicke are those specific for the wavefront aberrations. The orthonormal characteristics of this mathematical approach allow the analysis of the individual components of the different aberrations independently of each other, quantification of the prismatic component, the defocus component, the degree of regular astigmatism, the spherical aberration, coma and the rest of the higher order aberrations.

Figures 8.1A to E show the procedure for calculation of the optical characteristics of the corneal surface. From a topographic map (Figure 8.1A) it is possible to compute the corneal wavefront aberrations of the cornea, and to differentiate between second (defocus and astigmatism) and higher-order aberrations. Figures 8.1B and C represent the total wavefront aberrations and the higher-order aberrations, respectively, for a 3 mm pupil diameter. In the same way, Figures 8.1D and E show the same distribution but computed for a 6 mm pupil diameter. These plots show graphically the importance of the pupil diameter to calculate the optical quality of the cornea.

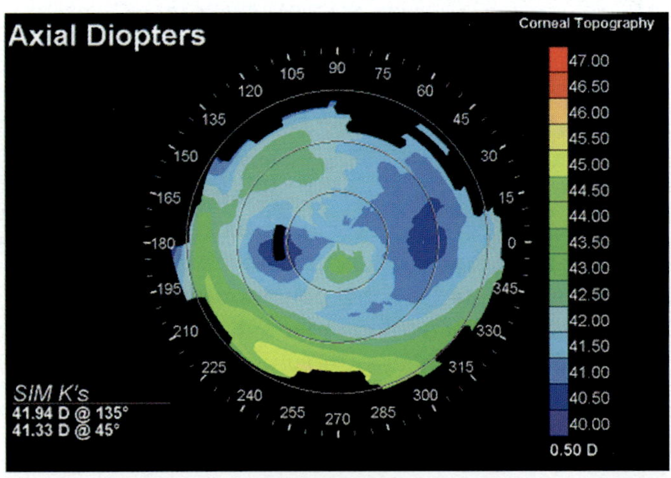

FIGURE 8.1A

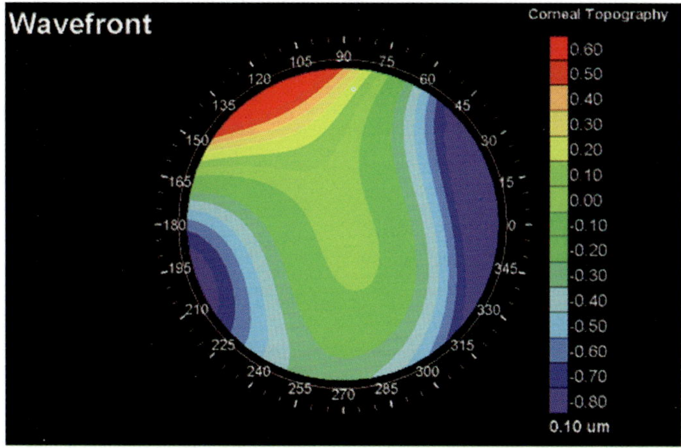

FIGURE 8.1B

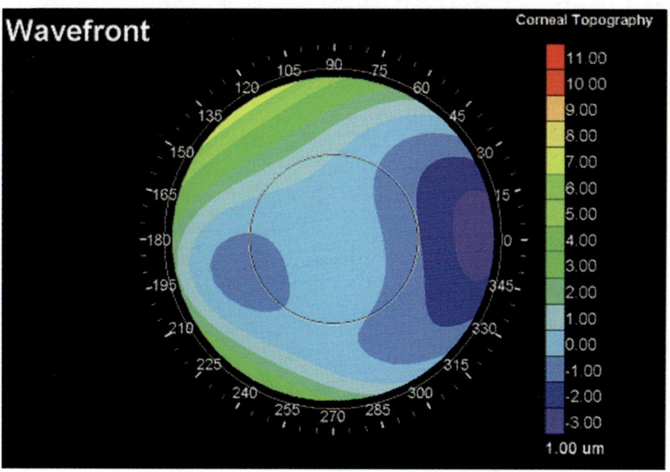

FIGURE 8.1C

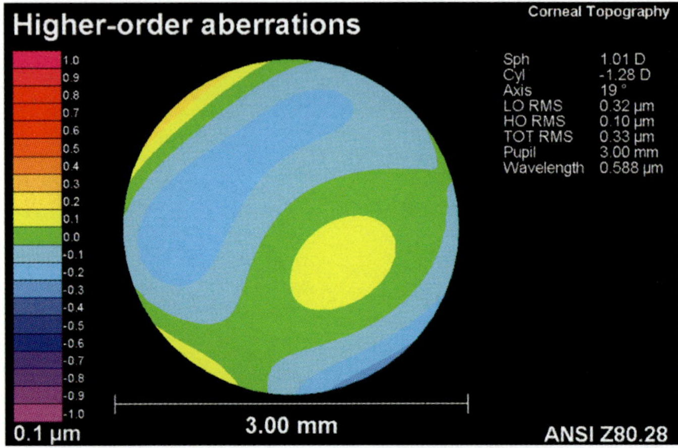

FIGURE 8.1D

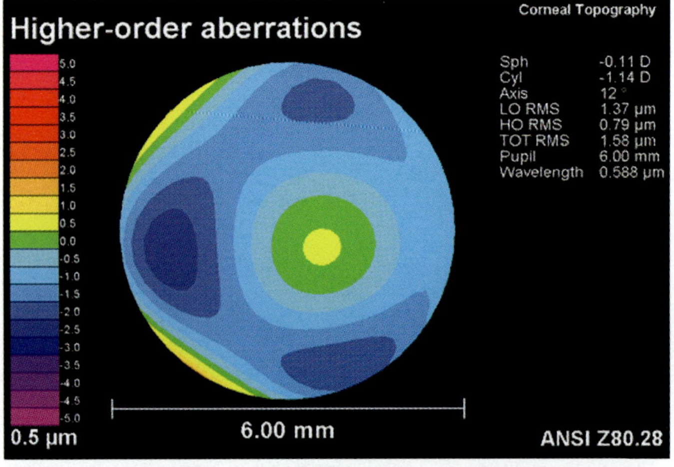

FIGURE 8.1E

FIGURES 8.1A to E: Corneal topographic map (A) and wavefront (B,D) and higher-order aberration maps (C,E) computed for a 3 and 6 mm pupil diameters (respectively)

In this specific case, the total root-mean-square (RMS) of higher-order aberrations varies from 0.10 to 0.79 microns, showing the variation in the optical quality of the cornea as a function of considering one pupil diameter.

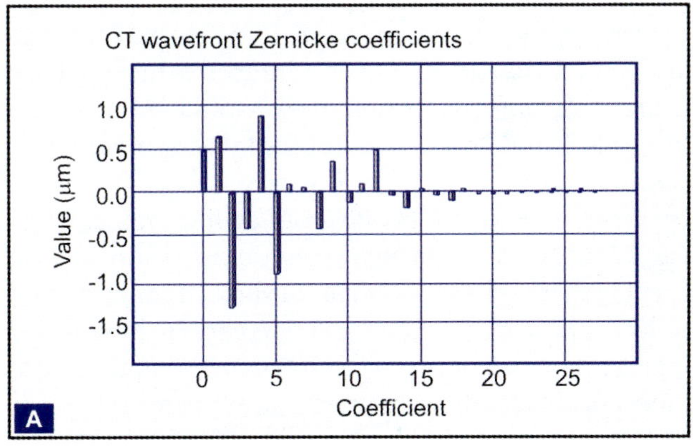

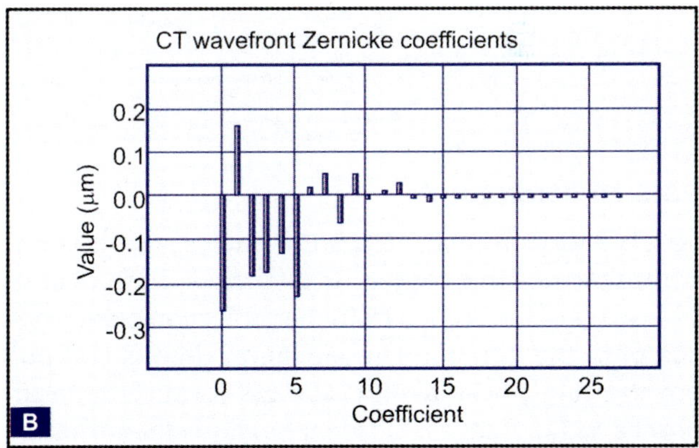

FIGURES 8.2A and B: Corneal topography Zernicke coefficient values computed for a 3 and 6 mm pupil diameter (A and B, respectively)

As we have commented previously, we can compute the different Zernicke polynomials and separately evaluate the contribution of the different coefficients to the final quality of the corneal surface. Figures 8.2A and B represent the corneal wavefront Zernicke coefficients of the topographic map of Figure 8.1 computed for a 3 and 6 mm pupil diameter. X-axis represents the coefficient number (tilt, defocus, astigmatism, spherical aberration, coma, etc.) and the Y-axis represents the value of the deviation from the reference wavefront in microns (advanced or delayed, positive or negative values). Large value of deviation indicates large deformation and poor optical quality of the corneal surface, then, from both graphs it is possible to observe an increase in the coefficient values and consequently a reduction in the optical quality of the cornea for a large pupil size (6 mm).

CORNEAL WAVEFRONT AS A GUIDE FOR THE CORRECTION OF IRREGULAR ASTIGMATISM

Basis of Treatment

The CSO topographer allows the analysis of the optical performance of the cornea. It measures a maximum of 6144 points of the cornea from the projection of 24 placido rings onto the cornea. The elevation data is computed from the ring positions and surface location measured from the video images. Corneal height is then translated into corneal wavefront and fitted into Zernicke polynomials. These corneal aberrations do not depend on accommodation and pupil size.

Corneal aberrations contribute to approximately 80 percent of the total ocular aberrations in normal eyes and to an even greater value in corneas with irregular astigmatism. Corneal aberrometry is a revolutionary tool for the evaluation of quality of vision, and can be advantageously used to treat irregular astigmatism causes by a previous corneal refractive surgery.

For this prospective, non-randomized pilot study, we evaluated 18 patients (18 eyes): 10 males and 8 females. Mean age of the patient was 38.5 ± 7.3 years (range 25 to 63 years). All these patients had a previous uneventful corneal refractive surgery and they were diagnosed of macroirregular or mixed (macro and micro) irregular astigmatism caused by the previous corneal refractive surgery. We evaluated the results obtained after a follow-up of 3 months. All surgical procedures were performed by the same surgeon (JLA) at the Instituto Oftalmológico de Alicante (Alicante, Spain).

The criteria for the selection of the patients were: corneal irregular astigmatism induced by previous corneal refractive surgery, decreased best spectacle-corrected visual acuity (BCVA), glare, ghost images and distorted vision, intolerance or absence of motivation to use contact lenses. We waited for a period of 6 months to confirm both the complete stabilization of the subjective refraction, the corneal topography and the tear film.

Clinical Examination

For each visit a comprehensive preoperative ocular examination was performed on each patient. This included previous ocular medical report, slit-lamp biomicroscopy, applanation tonometry, ultrasonic pachymetry. Subjective evaluation of quality of vision was assessed by asking the patients whether halos, glare, and monocular diplopia were reduced after surgery with best spectacle correction. Uncorrected visual acuity (UCVA) and BCVA were tested preoperatively, 1 and 3 months follow-up. Refraction was measured preoperatively and postoperatively under cycloplegia and using the high plus technique.

Corneal topography and corneal aberration is a very important diagnostic and treatment tool and was obtained under proper tear film conditions before treatment, 1 month and 3 months after treatment.

Surgical Technique

Preliminary step of the procedure included obtaining the corneal topography by means of the CSO (CSO Ophthalmics, Milano, Italy). For this process, both the alignment and the stability of the pre-corneal tear film are extremely important. As mentioned above, the CSO topographer is able to convert the elevation data in terms of Zernicke polynomials to quantify the corneal wavefront aberrometry. The root-mean-square (RMS) was used as a measure of the optical quality before and after customized corneal wavefront analysis.

After capturing and analyzing corneal aberrations up to the 7th Zernicke order, this data is processed by the ORK-W software (Schwind), which transforms this corneal aberration data into an adequate ablation profile. The software enables the surgeon to take an active part in the decision-making process, selecting the best solution for each patient. The software also allows the exclusion of specific aberrations according to specific surgical criteria and the choice of wide optical and transition zone.

Finally, customized ablation is performed with the Schwind ESIRIS Excimer-Laser. It is a scanning spot laser technology with a spot of 0.8 μm and a repetition rate of 200 Hz guided by its 330 Hz video based eye-tracking system.

Results

Efficacy

UCVA improved in 81 percent of the patients, from 0.3±0.15 (range from 0.7 to 0.1) logarithm of minimum angle of resolution (logMAR) preoperatively to 0.2±0.27 (range from 0.8 to 0.00) logMAR at 3 months follow-up (Figure 8.3) with an efficacy index of 1.08 (Figure 8.4). The mean gain of lines of postoperative UCVA was 1.81±1.5 lines.

Safety

At 3 months follow-up 55 percent gained one line of BCVA, 27 percent gained two lines, 11 percent gained

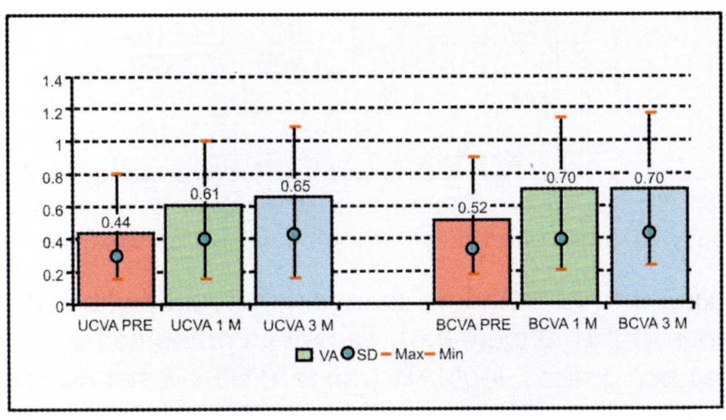

FIGURE 8.3: UCVA and BCVA before an after corneal aberration oriented ablation

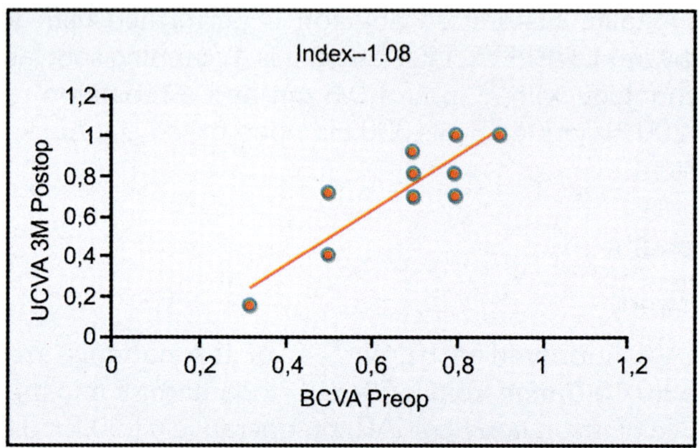

FIGURE 8.4: Efficacy index

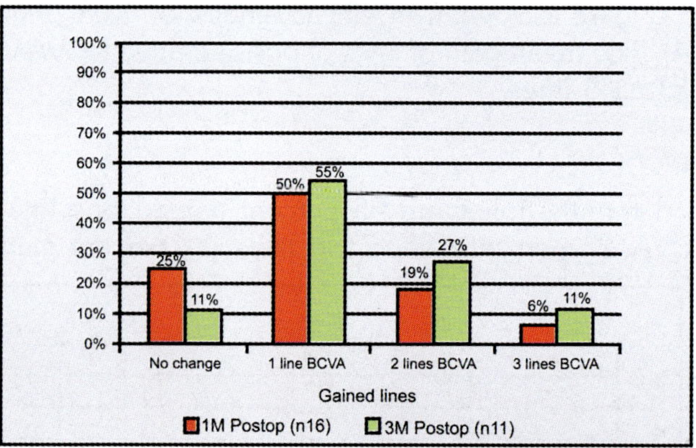

FIGURE 8.5: Safety. Change in best spectacle-corrected visual acuity (1 month and 3 months after ORK-W treatment)

3 lines and 11% had no change (Figure 8.5) with a safety index of 1.16 (Figure 8.6). The mean preoperative BCVA was 0.2 ± 0.17 logMAR (range 0.5 to 0.1) and mean postoperative BCVA was 0.10 ± 0.23 logMAR (range 0.5 to 0.0). Then mean gain of lines of postoperative BCVA was 1.09± 0.7 lines.

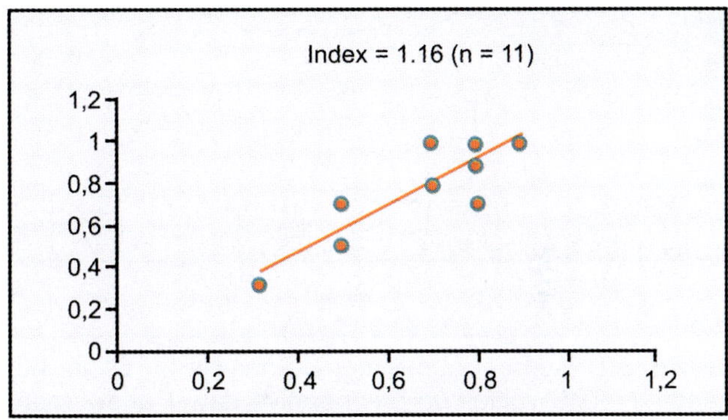

FIGURE 8.6: Safety index

Predictability

Mean preoperative SE was –0.29 D (range 1.75 D to –2.00 D; SD 1.04); at last postoperative examination, mean SE was –0.20 D (range –0.50 D to –2.25; SD, 0.62).

Higher Order Aberrations

The preoperative and postoperative changes in the root-mean square (RMS) values of the corneal higher-order wavefront aberration (total, spherical and coma-like aberrations) are shown graphically in Figure 8.7. All the data was analyzed for a 6 mm pupil. After ORK-W, there was a statically significant decreased in total higher order aberration.

Total Higher Order Corneal Wavefront

After ORK-W, there was statistically significant change in total higher order corneal wavefront aberration. Total

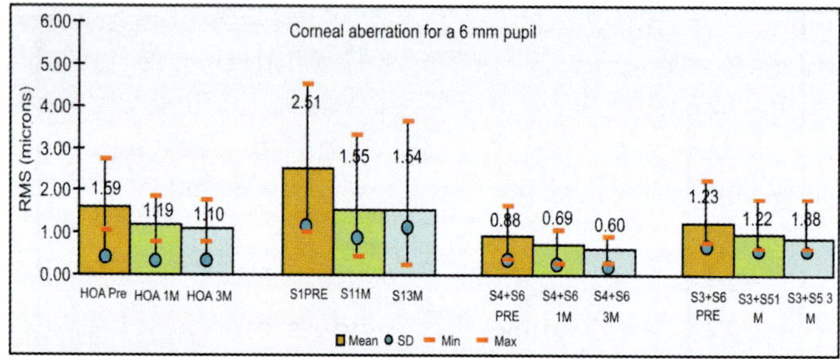

FIGURE 8.7: Corneal aberrometric analysis for 6 mm pupil. Change in RMS values on preoperative day, 1 and 3 months after ORK-W treatment

higher order aberration reduced by a factor of 1.34 and 1.45 at 1 month and 3 months of surgery respectively. (Paired t-test; $p<0.005$ for 1 and 3 months follow-up).

First Order Aberrations

Although ORK-W treatment does not affect directly in first order aberration, all the patients have shown statically significant changes in first order aberration. First order corneal aberration reduced by a factor of 1.62 and 1.54 at 1 and 3 months after surgery respectively (Paired t-test; $p<0.005$ for 1 and 3 months follow-up).We may suggest that this improvement in first order aberration could be as a consequence of recentration in the ablation profile.

Coma-like Aberrations

Third order and fifth order Zernicke coefficients are indicators of coma-like aberrations. For a 6 mm pupil, the root-mean-square (RMS) of the wavefront aberration decreased significantly at 1 and 3 months by a factor 1.34 and 1.38 respectively. In all cases the reduction in coma-like corneal wavefront aberration was statistically significant (Paired t-test; P<.005 for 1 and 3 months).

Spherical-like Aberration

Fourth order Zernicke coefficients are indicators of spherical-like aberrations. The RMS values decreased significantly 1 and 3 months after surgery by a factor of 1.27 and 1.47 respectively.

CASE REPORT

A 33-year-old white male was referred to our clinic with an ocular history of refractive surgery in both eyes. He complained of poor quality of vision, ghost images and halos especially at night in his right eye. He had a history of moderate myopia (–3.75 –1.00×115°, 20/20 visual acuity) before LASIK treatment. After we examined the patient, his uncorrected visual acuity (UCVA) was 20/40 with a manifest refraction of –1.75 –0.75×170°, 20/30 visual acuity. Corneal thickness measured by ultrasonic pachymetry was 482 µm. Preoperative corneal higher order aberration revealed a RMS of 1.19 µm (largest component was coma-like aberration with a RMS of 1.12 µm). Analysis of the RMS values shows that the major improvement was for tilt and coma-like aberration (Figure 8.8). After pre-evaluation the patient underwent corneal wavefront-guided custom ablation (ORK-W). Figure 8.9 shows the ablation pattern used by the laser according to corneal wavefront data. The differential

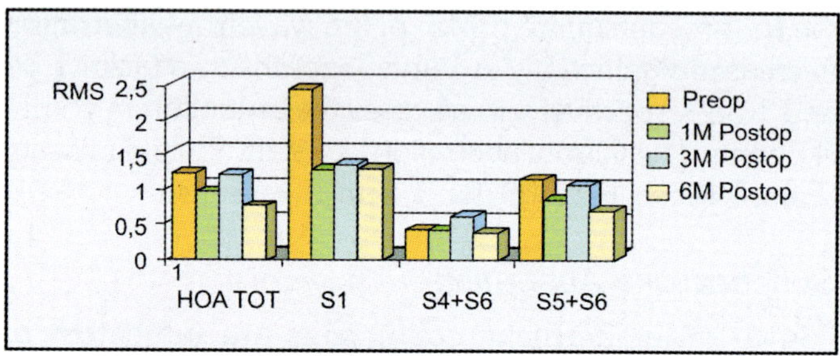

FIGURE 8.8: The bar graph above shows the magnitude (RMS) of each higher order corneal aberration (total, tilt, spherical- and coma-like aberrations) for 6 mm pupil, before and after ORK-W treatment (1,3 and 6 months postop) for these patient

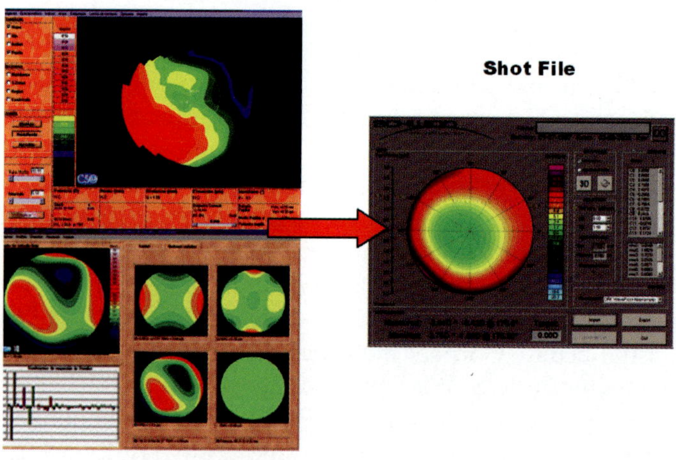

FIGURE 8.9: Clinical case. Treatment ablation profile

instantaneous map is shown in Figure 8.10 and demonstrates the efficacy of the treatment. At 6 months after ORK-W treatment UCVA was 20/20 with a manifest refraction of OD: –0.50×180° (20/20). The RMS was 0.72 μm for Total HOA and 0.63 μm for coma-like aberrations.

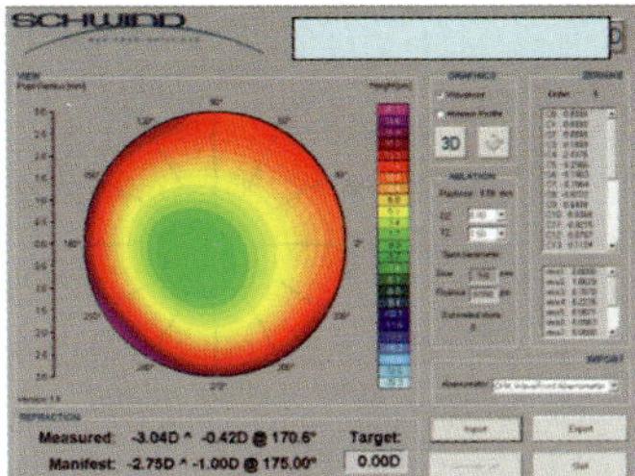

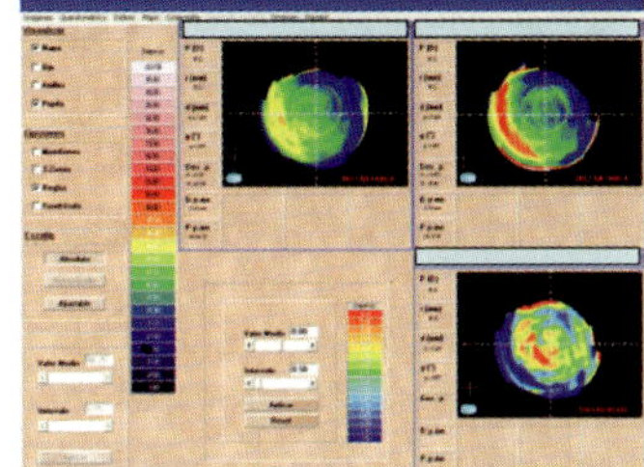

FIGURE 8.10: Clinical case. Differential Instantaneous map at preop an 6 months postop

CONCLUSIONS

The extensive use of corneal refractive surgery has increased the number of patients with corneal irregularities.[7,8] Correction of irregular astigmatism remains a challenge to refractive surgeons. Irregular astigmatism can be one of the most difficult and frustrating problems in refractive surgery. Treatment of irregular astigmatism oriented by corneal wavefront aberration has proved to be a successful technique. We have observed a significant improvement of uncorrected visual acuity, best corrected visual acuity and RMS values of HOA. These objective results also correlate with an improvement of patient visual symptoms after ORK-W treatment.

Corneal wavefront guided laser may be an excellent tool for correction of irregular astigmatism induce by previous corneal refractive surgery. In our hands preliminary results have shown that both visual and corneal irregularity improvements are better with corneal wavefront oriented treatment ORK-W compared to topography oriented treatment (TOPOLINK).[8]

REFERENCES

1. Liang J, Grimm B, Goelz S, Bille JF. Objective measurement of wave aberrations of the human eye with the use of a Hartmann-Shack wave-front sensor. J Opt Soc Am A 1994;11:1949-57.
2. Howland B, Howland HC. Subjective measurement of high-order aberrations of the eye. Science 1976;193:580-2.
3. Mrochen M, Kaemmerer M, Mierdel P, Krinke HE, Seiler T. Principles of Tscherning aberrometry. J Refract Surg 2000;16:S570-1.
4. Molebny VV, Panagopoulou SI, Molebny SV, Wakil YS, Pallikaris IG. Principles of ray tracing aberrometry. J Refract Surg 2000;16:S572-5.
5. Burns SA. The spatially resolved refractometer. J Refract Surg 2000;16:S566-9.
6. MacRae S, Fujieda M. Slit skiascopic-guided ablation using the Nidek laser. J Refract Surg 2000;16:S576-80.
7. Alió JL, Artola A, Rodriguez-Mier FA. Selective zonal ablations with excimer laser for correction of irregular astigmatism induced by refractive surgery. Ophthalmology 2000;107:662-73.
8. Alió JL, Belda JI, Osman AA, Shalaby AM. Topography-guided laser *in situ* keratomileusis (TOPOLINK) to correct irregular astigmatism after previous refractive surgery. J Refract Surg 2003;19:516-27.

CHAPTER 9

Presbyopic LASIK

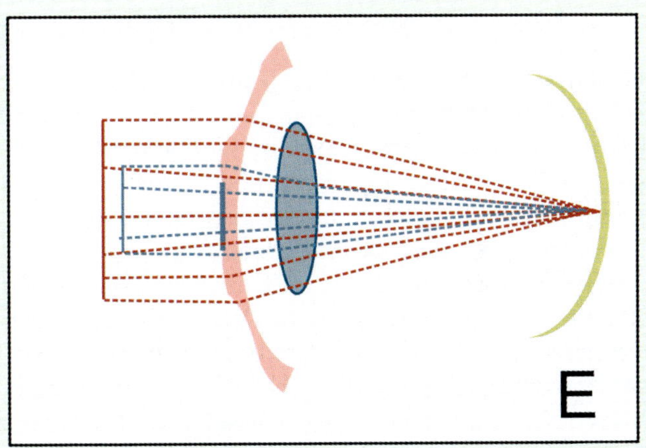

Amar Agarwal (India)
Athiya Agarwal (India)
Sunita Agarwal (India)
Guillermo Avalos-Urzua (Mexico)
Ashok Garg (India)

INTRODUCTION

Presbyopia, is the final frontier for an ophthalmologist. In the 21st century the latest developments, which are taking place, are in the field of presbyopia. In presbyopia, the nearest point that can be focused gradually recedes, leading to the need for optical prosthesis for close work such as reading and eventually even for focus in the middle distance.

PREVIOUS EXCIMER LASER TECHNIQUES

Presbyopic photorefractive keratectomy (PRK) has been tried. In this using the excimer laser, a mask consisting of a mobile diaphragm formed by two blunt blades was used to ablate a 10 to 17 micron deep semilunar-shaped zone immediately below the papillary center, steepening the corneal curvature in that area.

Monofocal vision with LASIK has also been tried to solve the problem of presbyopia. The goal in such cases is to make the patient anisometropic. In this one eye is used for distance vision and the other for near vision. This is obviously not indicated in all subjects. The residual consequences are partial loss of stereopsis, asthenopia, headache, aneisokonia and decreased binocularity.

HISTORY

Guillermo Avalos[1,2] started the idea of presbyopic LASIK. This is called the PARM technique. He held a live surgical conference in Mexico where he had invited the Agarwals to perform phakonit and the no-anesthesia cataract surgery technique. There he discussed with them the idea of presbyopic LASIK and when they came back they started the technique.

PRINCIPLE

The objective is to allow the patient to focus on near objects while retaining his ability to focus on far objects, taking into account the refractive error of the eye when the treatment is performed. With this LASIK technique the corneal curvature is modified, creating a bilateral multifocal cornea in the treated optical zone. A combination of hyperopic and myopic LASIK is done aiming to make a multifocal cornea. We determine if the eye is presbyopic plano, presbyopic with spherical hyperopia or presbyopia with spherical myopia. These may also have astigmatism in which case the astigmatism is treated at the same time.

PROLATE AND OBLATE CORNEA

It is important for us to understand a prolate and oblate cornea before we progress further on the technique of presbyopic LASIK. The shape of spheroid (a conoidal surface of revolution) is qualitatively prolate or oblate, depending on whether it is stretched or flattened in its axial dimension. In a prolate cornea the meridional curvature decreases from pole to equator and in an oblate cornea the meridional curvature continually increases. The optical surfaces of the normal human eye both cornea and lens is prolate. This shape has an optical advantage in that spherical aberration can be avoided. Following LASIK the prolateness of the anterior cornea reduces but is insufficient to eliminate its spherical aberration. Thus one should remember the normal cornea is prolate. When myopic LASIK is done the cornea becomes oblate. When hyperopic LASIK is done the cornea becomes prolate.

Every patient treated with an excimer laser is left with an oblate or prolate shaped cornea depending upon the myopia or hyperopia of the patient. The approach to improve visual quality after LASIK is to apply geometric optics and use the patient's refraction, precise preoperative corneal height data and optimal postoperative anterior corneal shape in order to have a customized prolate shape treatment.

TECHNIQUE

First of all a superficial corneal flap is created with the microkeratome. The corneal flap performed with the microkeratome must be between 8.5 and 9.5 mm in order to have an available corneal surface for treatment of at least 8 mm. In this way, the laser beam does not touch the hinge of the flap. In India the Bausch and Lomb LASIK machine is used and in Mexico the Apollo machine is used. Once the flap has been created a hyperopic ablation in an optical zone of 5 mm is done (Figure 9.1). The treated cornea now has a steepness section. The cornea is thus myopic, prolate. This allows the eye to focus in a range that includes near vision but excludes far vision.

With this myopic-shaped cornea, one now selects a smaller area of the central cornea that is concentric with the previous worked area. The size of the area is a 4 mm optical zone. A myopic LASIK is now done with the 4 mm optical zone (Figure 9.2). The resulting cornea now has a central area (oblate) that is configured for the eye

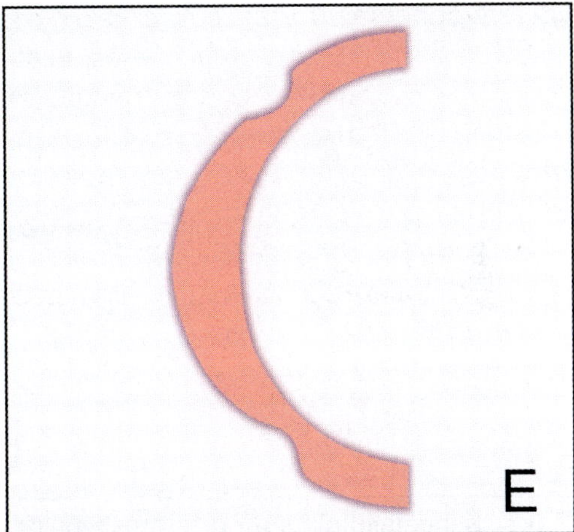

FIGURE 9.1: Hyperopic LASIK done on the cornea. Myopic prolate cornea produced

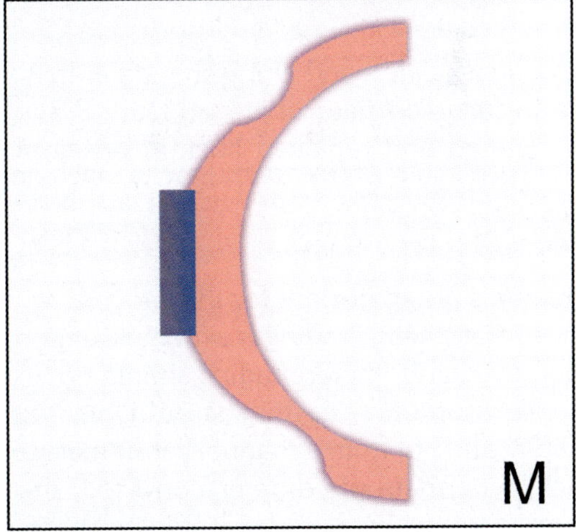

FIGURE 9.2: Myopic LASIK done. Myopic ablation of 4 mm optical zone performed to create a central oblate cornea

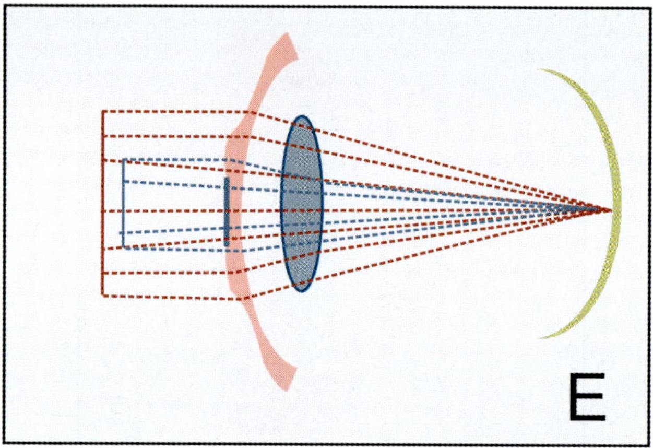

FIGURE 9.3: Schematic diagram of a presbyopic cornea in which hyperopic and myopic LASIK has been done. The patient can thus focus for near and distance

to focus on far objects and a ring shaped area that allows the eye to focus on near objects (Figure 9.3). The flap is now cleaned and replaced back in position.

KERATOMETRY AND PACHYMETRY

Pachymetry is not important for this procedure. The preoperative keratometry reading is extremely important. The postoperative keratometer reading should not exceed 48 D. The keratometer reading should be taken from topography and not from a manual keratometer machine. For each hypermetropic diopter corrected, the corneal curvature increases in 0.89 keratometric diopters as an average. It is recommended to treat patients with keratometry in the range between 41 and 43 D to obtain postoperative curves under 48 D. If the cornea is more than 48 D, it produces undesired optical alterations like glare, halos, decreased visual acuity and decreased contrast sensitivity. The preoperative and postoperative keratometer readings should be nearly the same for the patient to be comfortable.

ASTIGMATISM

If astigmatism is present, it is recommended to use as a limit 2.5 D. One should also remember there is an induced astigmatism of 0.5 to 0.75 D created by the corneal shape after the surgery and this can decrease one or two lines of uncorrected visual acuity.

Plano Example

Now let us look at treating presbyopic patients who are basically plano for distance.

Example 1

Let us take a patient who is plano for distance and is 20/20. For near on addition of + 2 D the patient is J1. The preoperative keratometer let us say is 41 D.

There are three steps in the presbyopic LASIK treatment.

1 STEP—For distance—No treatment is required as the patient is plano 20/20.

2 STEP—For near—Hyperopic LASIK is done of + 2 D. A 5 mm optical zone is taken. We have already mentioned that each diopter of hyperopia corrected changes the corneal curvature by 0.89 D, which is approximately 1 D.

So the keratometer changes from 41 to 43 D (approximately).

3 STEP—Myopic LASIK of minus 1 D with a 4 mm optical zone. So keratometer now becomes 42 D.

Regression occurs for hyperopia treatment to about 1 D, so we have done myopic ablation of minus 1 and not minus 2 D. The preoperative keratometer reading was 41 D and postoperative keratometer reading is 42 D, which is nearly the same.

Hyperopic Example

Now let us look at presbyopic LASIK being performed in a hyperopic eye.

Example 2

Let us take a patient who is hyperopic for distance and is 20/20 with + 1 D. For near on addition of + 3 D the patient is J1. The preoperative keratometer let us say is 42 D.

There are three steps in the presbyopic LASIK treatment.

1 STEP—For distance—Hyperopic LASIK is done of + 1 D with a 5 mm optical zone. So keratometer changes from 42 D to 43 D.

2 STEP—For near—Hyperopic LASIK is done of + 3 D. A 5 mm optical zone is taken. We have already mentioned that each diopter of hyperopia corrected changes the corneal curvature by 0.89 D, which is approximately 1 D. So the keratometer changes from 43 to 46 D (approximately).

3 STEP—Myopic LASIK of minus 2 D with a 4 mm optical zone. So keratometer now becomes 44 D.

Regression occurs for hyperopia treatment to about 1 D, so we have done myopic ablation of minus 2 and not minus 3 D. The preop keratometer reading was 42 D but after making the patient plano it is 43 D. The postoperative keratometer reading is 44 D, which is nearly the same.

Though we have to correct totally 4 D for hypermetropia we take it in two steps. One should not do it in one step as that much hyperopia corrected in one step makes the central cornea too steep to perform the myopic ablation.

Example 3

Let us take a patient who is hyperopic for distance and is 20/20 with + 3 D. For near on addition of + 3 D the patient is J1. The preoperative keratometer let us say is 44 D.

The preoperative keratometer reading is 44 D and we have to correct 3 D for distance and 3 D for near. So if we do presbyopic LASIK we will make the keratometer reading 50 D. So, one should not treat such patients with presbyopia LASIK.

Myopic Example

Now let us look at myopic patients.

Example 4

Let us take a patient who is myopic for distance and is 20/20 with minus 2 D. For near on addition of + 2 D the patient is J1. This means the patient is plano for near. The preoperative keratometer let us say is 43 D.

There are three steps in the presbyopic LASIK treatment.

1 STEP—For distance—Patient is myopic so no treatment is required.

2 STEP—For near—Hyperopic LASIK is done of + 2 D. A 5 mm optical zone is taken. We have already mentioned that each dioptere of hyperopia corrected changes the corneal curvature by 0.89 D, which is approximately 1 D. So the keratometer changes from 43 to 45 D (approximately).

3 STEP—Myopic LASIK of minus 3 D with a 4 mm optical zone. So keratometer now becomes 42 D.

Regression occurs for hyperopia treatment to about 1 D, so we have done myopic ablation of minus 3 and not minus 4 D. The preoperative keratometer reading was 43 D but patient was myopic by 2 D, so actually the keratometer reading should be 41 D. The postoperative keratometer reading is 42 D, which is nearly the same.

We did myopic ablation of 3 D, as patient is myopic of 2 D and presbyopic of 2 D. Regression factor taken is 1 D.

SUMMARY

This idea of presbyopic LASIK is not the end of it all. This technique needs further improvizations to become the technique of choice for one and all.

REFERENCES

1. Guillermo Avalos: Presbyopic LASIK- the PARM technique in Amar Agarwal's Presbyopia: A Surgical Textbook. Slack Inc, USA, 2002.
2. Agarwal T, et al. Presbyopic LASIK- the Agarwal technique in Amar Agarwal's Presbyopia: A Surgical Textbook. Slack Inc, USA, 2002.

CHAPTER 10

Intacs

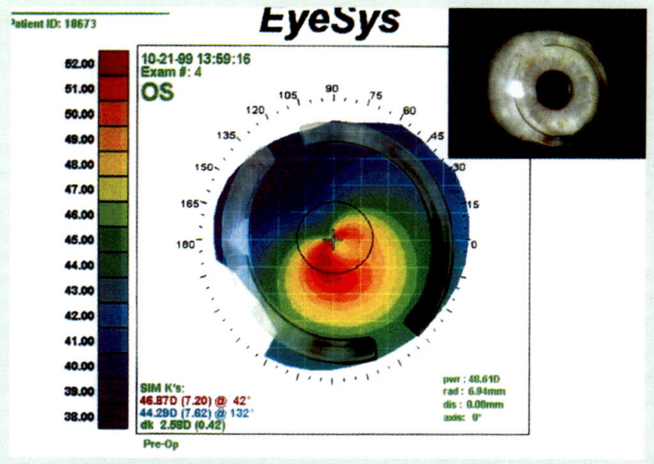

George D Kymionis
Charalambos Siganos
Ioannis G Pallikaris

(**Greece**)

INTRODUCTION

Barraquer made the first attempts for biocompatible material implantation intrastromally to the cornea in 1949.[1] Since then, a remarkable improvement has been made. In April 1999, the U.S. Food and Drug Administration (FDA) approved Intacs (Intacs; Addition Technology Inc., Fremont, California, USA) for sale in the United States for the correction of low myopia[2,3] (Table 10.1). The potential advantage of Intacs implantation over the current existed refractive techniques such as reversibility (reverse treatment effects), maintaining the natural prolate corneal shape and the preservation of cornea stroma are the main reasons for the expand of Intacs' treatments indications.

TABLE 10.1: Ring segment description

- Made of PMMA
- Outer diameter: 8.1 mm
- Inner diameter: 6.77 mm
- Arc length: 150°
- Positioning holes diameter: 0.28 mm
- Ring cross section: Hexagonal
- Each package contains two segments: Right and left

THE TECHNIQUE

The procedure is performed under topical anesthesia (anesthetic drops). The surgeon marks the geometric center of the cornea (11 mm zone marker-Sinskey hook) and measures corneal thickness at the site of the planned incision. An incision, 1.2 mm in length is made with a diamond blade at the 12 O'clock position, approximately 2.0 mm from the limbus. Using a diamond knife set at

70 percent of the corneal thickness at the incision site (calibrated diamond knife with 15° angled-pivot knife) and 2 intrastromal corneal pockets are created using a pocketing hook, stromal spreader, and clockwise and anticlockwise dissection glides, under suction created by a vacuum centering guide (step 1:400 mBar-step 2: 600 mBar). The 2 polymethylmethacrylate segments (150° crescent-shaped inserts) are implanted in the clockwise and counterclockwise tunnels, maintaining a space of 2.0 mm between their ends and 1.5 mm between the opposite edge of each segment and the edge of the incision. After the stromal pocket is carefully washed with balanced salt solution, the incision is being closed with a single interrupted 10-0 nylon suture. Postoperatively, all eyes receive antibiotic/steroid combination eye drops 4 times per day for 1 week. In addition, all patients are instructed to use preservative-free artificial tears frequently. The sutures are removed 2 weeks after surgery.

The thickness of the Intacs is based on the attempted correction according to the nomogram (five different thickness inserts, 0.25, 0.30, 0.35, 0.40 and 0.45 mm, are currently available). The nomogram for Intacs inserts selection is described in Table 10.2.

TABLE 10.2: Intacs nomogram for myopia

Thickness	*Average correction*
0.25	-1.3 D (1-1.6)
0.30	-2.0 D (1.7-2.3)
0.35	-2.7 D (2.4-3.0)
0.40	-3.4 D (3.1-3.7)
0.45	-4.1 D (3.8-4.4)

INTACS FOR LOW MYOPIA

Indications for Intacs implantation are: patients older than 21-year-old and stability of refraction for at least 12 months prior to the preoperative examination. Intacs inserts are contraindicated in patients with collagen vacular, autoimmune or immunodeficiency diseases, in pregnant or nursing women, presence of ocular conditions, such as keratoconus, recurrent corneal erosion syndrome or corneal dystrophy, that may predispose the patient to future complications, in patients who are taking at least one of the following medications: isotretinoin, amiodarone, sumatriptan.

The results from phase II and phase III[4] clinical protocols showed that at 1 year, 97 percent of patients who completed follow-up had 20/40 or better uncorrected visual acuity (UCVA). Seventy-four percent of patients had 20/20 or better UCVA. Ninety-two percent of eyes were within ±1 D of intended refractive correction, and 69 percent were within 0.5 D of intended refractive correction. At 3 months, 90 percent of patients had less than 1.0 D of change from the previous examination performed at 1 month. The ocular complication rate was 11 percent at 12 months. Nearly 9 percent of patients requested to have their inserts removed and a total of 3.8 percent of patients required a secondary surgical intervention (Table 10.3).

Recently, a bioptics procedure[5] (combined LASIK and ICRS implantation) reported engouraging results for patients with low pachymetric values or high myopia. Post-Intacs implantation complications are: under- or over-correction, migration of segments toward the wound, neovascularization, extrusion and visual side effects (glare or haloes).

TABLE 10.3: Potential complications during Intacs implantation

Complications	*Cause-precautions*
Abnormal lamellar dissection	Improper stromal channel
Rings on significant different levels	Improper stromal channel
Decentered channel	Slipping of vacuum
Decentered ring placement	Incision placement maker
Corneal perforation (anterior surface)	Slipping of vacuum
Corneal perforation (posterior surface)	Too deep incision (pachymetry)
Perilimbal hemorrage	Vacuum centering guide
Breakage of the ring	Handle with care
Incision gape	Suture incision
Ring ends overlap	Push with sinskey hook
Incomplete ring advancement	Push with sinskey hook
Conjunctival chemosis	Vacuum centering guide

INTACS FOR KERATOCONUS-PELLUCID MARGINAL DEGENERATION

Intacs were designed to achieve a refractive adjustment by flattening the central corneal curvature while maintaining clarity in the central optical zone. Patients must have clear central corneas. Exclusion criteria are: previous intraocular or corneal surgery; history of herpes keratitis; diagnosed autoimmune disease; and systemic connective tissue disease.

Several studies have demonstrated the efficacy of Intacs in correcting low myopia, while several studies reported encouraging results in keratoconic eyes and post-LASIK corneal ectasia. In the year 2000, Colin and associates[6] first published an article about their preliminary results regarding the management of keratoconus with Intacs. One year later, the same authors published a series of 10 keratoconic patients 1-year after Intacs implantation where they support that Intacs reduced the corneal steepening and astigmatism, while visual acuity was improved in almost all eyes[7]. Recently, Siganos et al[8] reported similar results in keratoconic patients. The surgical procedure is almost the same as myopia correction except the thickness of segments (0.45 mm) and the position of Intacs implantation. Two Intacs segments of thickness are inserted according to the topographic image, aiming at embracing the keratoconus area to try to achieve maximal flattening. With mean follow-up of 11.3 months, intracorneal ring segments implantation improved UCVA and BCVA in the majority of the keratoconus patients. In conclusion, Intacs seem to offer a minimally invasive alternative treatment before PKP for keratoconic patients with clear corneas and contact lens intolerance, especially in early stages of the disease with less topographic irregularities.

Pellucid marginal degeneration (PMD) is a bilateral, noninflammatory disorder characterized by a peripheral band of thinning of the inferior cornea. The disease is usually asymptomatic except for the progressive deterioration in uncorrected visual acuity and best spectacle-corrected visual acuity caused by the irregular astigmatism induced by the corneal ectasia. Recently, Kymionis et al[9] reported a 42-year-old man that had Intacs implantation for early pellucid marginal degeneration (PMD). Two Intacs segments (0.45 mm thickness) were inserted uneventfully in the fashion typically used for low myopia correction (nasal temporal). Eleven months after the procedure, the uncorrected visual acuity was 20/200, compared with counting fingers preoperatively, while the

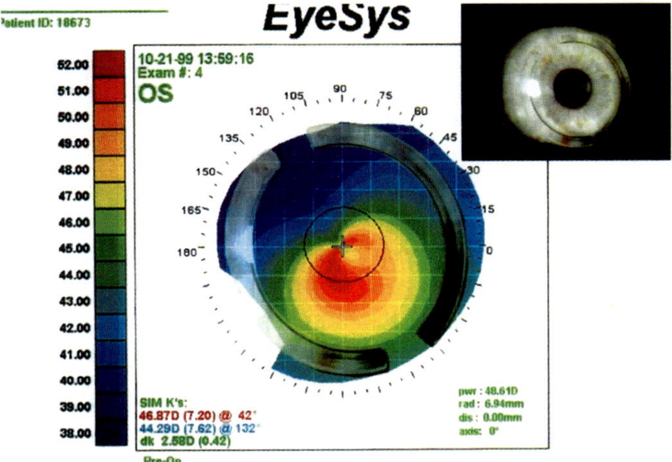

FIGURE 10.1: Preoperative topography and Intacs position of insertion (top right) of a keratoconic patient

best spectacle-corrected visual acuity improved to 20/25 from 20/50. Corneal topographic pattern was also improved. Although the results are encouraging, concern still exists regarding the long-term effect of this approach for the management of patients with PMD.

INTACS FOR POST-LASIK CORNEAL ECTASIA

The main advantage of Intacs is that, unlike excimer laser refractive techniques, they preserve corneal tissue while maintaining clarity in the central optical zone. In this way, Intacs may represent an interesting surgical alternative for patients with corneal ectasia after LASIK. The procedure is similar to low myopia or keratoconus. The thickness of the Intacs is based on the attempted correction. Using a diamond knife set at 70 percent of the corneal thickness at the incision site, a 0.9 mm radial incision is created, and 2 intrastromal corneal pockets are created using a pocketing lever, stromal spreader, and clockwise and anticlockwise dissection glides. Two tunnels (right and left) are created using clockwise and anticlockwise dissectors under suction created by a vacuum centering guide. The 2 polymethylmethacrylate segments are implanted in the clockwise and counterclockwise tunnels, maintaining a space of 2.0 mm between their ends and 1.5 mm between the opposite edge of each segment and the edge of the incision. Because of the standard 7 mm optic zone diameter of the ring segments, Intacs segments are inevitably ended up more central and deeper to the LASIK flap edge.

In a recent article, Kymionis et al[10] reported that Intacs implantation in post-LASIK cornea ectasia results in statistically significant reduction in spherical equivalent error (pre-Intacs, mean +/– SD: –4.81 +/– 3.24 Diopters (D) (range, –13.75 to –2.50 D) to –0.96 +/– 2.93 D (range, –8.75 to 2.50 D) (P<.001). Pre-Intacs uncorrected visual acuity was 20/100 or worse in all eyes (range, counting fingers to 20/100) while at the last follow-up examination, 9 (90%) of 10 eyes had uncorrected visual acuity of 20/40 or better (range, counting fingers to 20/20). Three eyes maintained the pre-Intacs best spectacle-corrected visual acuity while the rest of the eyes (7) experienced a gain of 1 to 2 lines. The mean difference between pre-Intacs and last follow-up best spectacle-corrected visual acuity was a gain of 1.00 +/– 0.82 lines. In conclusion, Intacs implantation improved uncorrected visual acuity and best spectacle-corrected visual acuity in patients with post-LASIK ectasia. Even though the results are encouraging, concern still exists regarding the long-term effect of such an approach for the management of post-LASIK ectasia.

REFERENCES

1. Burris TE. Intrastromal corneal ring technology: Results and indications. Curr Opin Ophthalmol 1998;9: 9-14.
2. Schanzlin DJ, Asbell PA, Burris TE, Durrie DS. The intrastromal corneal ring segments. Phase II results for the correction of myopia. Ophthalmology 1997;104:1067-78.
3. Nose W, Neves RA, Burris TE, et al. Intrastromal corneal ring: 12-month sighted myopic eyes. J Refract Surg 1996;12: 20-8.
4. Rapuano CJ, Sugar A, Koch DD, et al. Intrastromal corneal ring segments for low myopia: a report by the American Academy of Ophthalmology. Ophthalmology 2001;108(10): 1922-8.
5. Primack JD, Azar DT. Laser in situ keratomileusis and intrastromal corneal ring segments for high myopia. Three-step procedure. J Cataract Refract Surg 2003; 29(5): 869-74.
6. Colin J, Cochener B, Savary G, Malet F. Correcting keratoconus with intracorneal rings. J Cataract Refract Surg 2000;26:1117-22.
7. Colin J, Cochener B, Savary G, Malet F, Holmes-Higgin D. Intacs inserts for treating keratoconus: one-year results. Ophthalmology. 2001;108:1409-14.
8. Siganos CS, Kymionis GD, Kartakis N, et al. Management of keratoconus with Intacs. Am J Ophthalmol 2003;135(1): 64-70.
9. Kymionis GD, Aslanides IM, Siganos CS, Pallikaris IG. Intacs for early pellucid marginal degeneration. J Cataract Refract Surg. 2004;30(1):230-3.
10. Kymionis GD, Siganos CS, Kounis G, et al. Management of post-LASIK corneal ectasia with Intacs inserts: One-year results. Arch Ophthalmol 2003;121(3):322-6.

CHAPTER 11

Contact Lens Fitting in Refractive Surgery

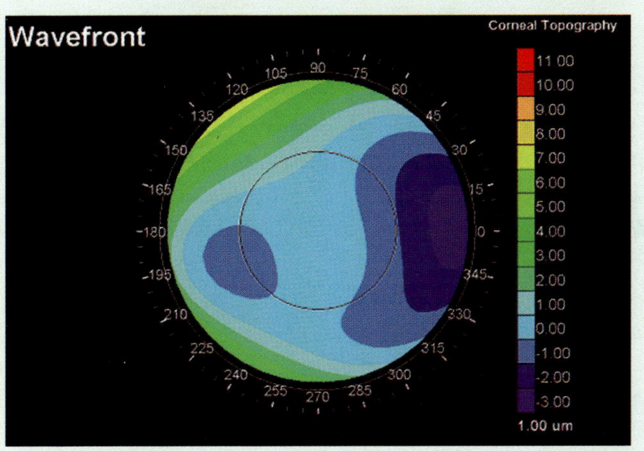

Ashok Garg (India)

INTRODUCTION

Contact lenses have significant role to play in the modern refractive surgery, whether it is radial keratotomy, photo refractive keratectomy (PRK) and latest LASIK surgery, no system is yet so perfect to achieve 100 percent uncorrected emmetropia. In such situations patients are weary of putting spectacles again for over corrected/under corrected visual acuity and astigmatism. Contact lenses are the only viable effective way to achieve 20/20 visual acuity.

Let me discuss here the significance and usefulness of contact lens fitting in various refractive procedures being practiced by ophthalmologists worldwide.

CONTACT LENS FITTING AFTER RADIAL KERATOTOMY

Till the last decade radial keratotomy was the treatment of choice for curing myopia and to certain degree of hypermetropia. Although this technique is now out of favor in developed countries but still in developing countries RK surgery is treatment of choice for more than 50 percent of patients. This may be due to high cost factor in modern LASIK surgery.

Despite advancements in diamond knife and techniques of radial keratotomy about 15 to 20 percent of patients remain under corrected or over corrected (1 D or greater). Such patients are ideally suited for contact lens fitting to achieve 20/20 vision.

Indications for Contact Lens Fitting in RK Surgery

- Overcorrection
- Undercorrection
- Irregular astigmatism
- Regular astigmatism
- Anisometropia
- Fluctuating vision

Contact lens fitting following RK surgery poses difficulty to both patient and ophthalmologist because of post RK corneal topography. Patient is emotionally down due to unfulfilled expectations of free of spectacles and contact lenses.

Computerized corneal topography shows the central corneal flattening which reduces the myopia power of eye alongwith relative steepening of peripheral cornea. Epithelium may show dystrophic changes, hypoesthesia and punctate lesions.

In intersecting incisions there may be marked surface irregularity which may lead to decentration, central pool, intermediate touch and marked ocular irritation due to lifting of edges. Tear pool stagnation may result in hypoxic damage.

In such corneas contact lenses tend to slip themselves over the steeper part of the cornea which leads to decentration and improper vision.

Fitting Procedure

It is generally recommended to wait atleast for 3 to 6 months after. Radial keratotomy before contact lens fitting. Generally large rigid gas permeable lenses (RGP lenses) are lenses of choice in post RK condition because these lenses provide excellant oxygen transmission, move perfectly on the cornea and provides good tear exchange and good visual acuity. These lenses are fitted by hit and trial method on the basis of following primary requisites:

- Good tear exchange
- Lens should not move excessively
- Lens weight should be uniform over a large part of cornea
- Proper centration to achieve optimal vision.

Choice of RGP Trial Lenses

If post RK corneal flattening is not excessive (about 38 D or greater) than regular RGP lens (Spherical or aspheric) and of high oxygen transmissibility can be fitted usually a large lens of 9.5 mm diameter is selected on the basis of choosing a trial lens 2.5 D steeper than the postoperative keratometry. Final fitting is done on the basis of fluorescein pattern. Preferably select a large diameter RGP lens and achieve optimal fitting by changing the base curve. Trapped air bubbles may be dealt with fenestration.

For extreme central corneal flattening a number of special lenses are commercially available. Menicon's Plateau lens is an ideal one in which the lens periphery is steeper than the base curve. This configure suits the post RK cornea's profile.

The following steps may be used when fitting RGP lenses following RK surgery.

- Large lens diameter (9.5-11 mm) is generally recommended.

- Optic zone should be small relatively in relation to over all lens diameter (7 mm optic zone is recommended for a 9.5 mm overall lens diameter).
- Thin lenses should be used for optimum oxygen transmission. If a problem of lens flexure arises, switch to thicker lens design.
- Base curve of RGP lens after RK = 6.5 + 0.9 post-operative K / where K is average postoperative keratometry). Usually the contact lens should align with superior midperipheral cornea. Some times post-operative K readings may result in excessive lens movement and centration problems.
- RGP lenses generally have flatter peripheral curves than the base curve.
- Generally lens power is calculated equal to preoperative spherical equivalent or over refraction is done. Minus power must be added in final contact lens fitting as in post RK there is gap between the flat central cornea and the contact lens which is filled with tears thus creating a plus power.
- Decentration is a common problem in post RK contact lens fitting. If the lens slips too high than prism may be added or lens diameter can be increased. If the lens rides low a lenticular lens can be used or lens diameter can be decreased.
- Toric lenses may be given to correct the residual astigmatism.
- Therapeutic lens can be fittted in high myopia cases showing postoperative under correction. These lenses may be used to mould the cornea (orthokeratology).
- If air bubble become trapped. Under the lens in the gap of central flattened cornea and contact lens and

tears may pool due to poor tear exchange than corneal edema may develop leading to poor visual acuity. In such situation lens diamter may be decreased, base curve is flattened or the lens is fenestrated.

- Reverse curve lens is available commercially for reshaping the flattened apical cornea with steeper peripheral curves. These lenses may be used in post RK fitting.

Fitting Technique

- First fit the flattened central area. Choose the trial lens 1 D steeper than the flattest curve. Assess the fit using fluorescein staining for centration and alignment. Generally 7.5-8 mm of optic zone is standardized but can be altered depending on lateral lag.

If lag is less than smaller optical zone is preferred.

- The reverse curve should be 3 D steeper than the base curve with a variation between 2 and 4 D.
- Fit the peripheral curve zone so that there is touch in the transition zones and a minimal edge stand off of 0.1mm.
- Soft contact lenses should be reserved for sensitive cases and should be prescribed with a great caution because of potential risk of infection and vasculari-sation. If soft lenses are to be fitted than select lenses with high oxygen transmission. Lens care compliance should be monitored and lenses should be replaced frequently.

Postfitting Complications and Failures

- Besides the general problems associated with contact lens fitting, sometime corneal vascularization may develop which ascends into the incisions from the limbus. The reported incidence of neovascularization is as high as 32 to 58 percent.

- There is reporting of contact lens failure which may be due to irritation, fluctuating vision, neovascularization and changes in refractive error.

CONTACT LENS FITTING AFTER PHOTOREFRACTIVE KERATECTOMY (PRK)

In last decade photo therapeutic keratectomy was procedure of choice for refractive surgery. Since the inception of sophisticated LASIK surgery and PRK procedure shortcomings, it has also gone out of favor among ophthalmologists.

In PRK surgery contact lens fitting has a significant role specially postoperatively.

In excimer laser PRK it involves an average 50 to 100 um deep ablation over a 5 to 6 mm wide area of central cornea which results in central flattening and reduced myopia. However mid peripheral corneal topography remains unchanged.

Indications for Post PRK Contact Lens Fitting

- Bandage contact lens to reduce pain in immediate post-surgical period. Following PRK patient experiences marked ocular pain for 48 to 72 hours which can be sharply reduced by giving bandage contact lens.
- To restore binocular vision by fitting the lens in the fellow eye in conditions when one eye is only operated or patient himself is reluctant for second eye PRK surgery in the same sitting.

- To correct over or under correction to achieve 20/20 vision.

As compared to RK surgery, lesser PRK surgery patients need post-surgical refractive correction due to regression, irregular astigmation or under correction. Generaly PRK patients have predictable post-surgical corneal topography.

Usually post PRK refractions are stable at 6 months interval. RGP contact lenses should be fitted ideally 18-24 weeks after surgery. RGP lenses are generally fitted in post PRK stage because of their high oxygen transmissibility. The lens parameters in preoperative phase are the best predictors of the lens parameters in post PRK stage. If the patients has not worn any lens prior to PRK procedure the non-operated eye or preoperative keratometric (K) reading can be safely used for the initial lens selection. Rigid gas permeable lenses can be fitted with either lid attachment or interpalpebral fit. Lens movement shall vary with the fitting approach—a lid attachment fit may move < 1 mm with each blink while an interpalpebral central fit may move more.

Fitting technique of contact lens in post PRK phase is mentioned as below:

- Evaluate pre-surgical cornea by 'K' reading or corneoscopic mapping.
- Trial RGP lens fit should be assessed by an alignment Fluorescein pattern analysis with marked pooling over the 6 mm laser area.
- Do over refraction to determine optimal visual acuity. By computerized corneal topography select flattest reading of topography at the 5 mm zone for initial base curve.

As the midperipheral corneal topography remains unchanged after PRK procedure so it is relatively easier to fit contact lenses after PRK as compare to post RK surgery. Care should be taken to ensure proper tear exchange under the lens (Avoid tear pooling) to allow for venting of debris.

Apart from RGP lenses, hydrogel contact lenses with High oxygen transmission can also be fitted following PRK procedure as the post PRK cornea is least susceptible to neovascularization.

CONTACT LENS FITTING IN LASIK SURGERY

Contact lenses have significant role to play specially post operatively in modern refractive surgery like LASIK surgery.

Despite a lot of technological advancements being made in the field of LASIK Surgery and other refractive surgeries like New Wave Front Technology, custom ablation technology, laser Microkeratomes, Aberrometers, LASEK and conductive keratoplasty (CK). No system is yet not completly perfect to achieve 100 percent uncorrected 20/20 visual acuity. Contact lenses provides an excellant alternative to achieve post LASIK emmetropia. Here I shall describe the role of contact lenses preoperatively and postoperatively in LASIK surgery.

Contact Lens Fitting Before LASIK Surgery

There are certain indications preoperatively where we can fit contact lenses to the patients.

Fellow Eye

Usually LASIK surgery is performed bilaterally. Sometime patient is anxious and wishes to have only one eye performed in single sitting followed by second eye few weeks later. In such cases contact lenses are fitted in the fellow (unoperated) eye to achieve binocular vision and emmetropia. This is temporary arrangement of lens fitting in non-lasered eye till the patient is operated upon for the second eye. This arrangement restores binocular vision and confidence and safety in patient while driving and in out door movements.

Corneal Warpage

In day-to-day practice we have seen patients wearing rigid or semi rigid gas permeable lenses (RGP) showing symptoms of corneal warpage leading to induced irregular astigmatism. In such cases RGP lenses are replaced by soft contact lenses. Patients have to wait for 18 to 24 weeks before any LASIK surgery is performed in such eyes to provide time to the cornea to recover from the warpage effects and returns to its normal anatomical shape. As the cornea reshaping takes place. It is preferable to change the soft contact lenses every two months. After achieving healthy cornea switch the patient to spectacles till the three consistent and stable topography and refraction readings are obtained before performing LASIK surgery.

Contact Lens Fitting in Post-LASIK Phase

Immediate Post-LASIK Surgery Period

Following LASIK surgery patient experiences considerable amount of pain which may persist for 48 to 72 hours. Bandage contact lenses are advised in immediate post

LASIK period in conjunction with topical non-steroidal medication (Diclofenac sodium, Ketorolac tromathamine or suprofen) to reduce pain discomfort appreciately. Bandage contact lenses are currently being prescribed routinely in immediate post-LASIK period for 48 to 72 hours with excellant results.

Early Post-LASIK Surgery Period

In early post-LASIK period contact lenses are given for:

i. Over correction under correction and astigmation (regular and irregular) to achieve optimal vision.
ii. For epithelial defects to provide healing of the cornea.
iii. For high myopia if residual number remains.

Usually soft contact lenses are prescribed which acts as a conformer. Inspite of modern LASIK surgery a number of patients are still confronted with over correction, under correction or astigmatism.

For post LASIK contact lens fitting integrity of the flap after 12 weeks of surgery is considered sufficient to withstand the minor trauma and movement of an RGP lens. By 12 weeks refraction and corneal thickness changes get stabilized.

Epithelial defect develop as a result of epithelial basement dystrophy or excessive instillation of topical anesthetic drops prior to the use of microkeratome. This may result in epithelial sloughing. The microkeratome blade slides across the epithelium and denudes a portion of the epithelium. In epithelial defect cases contact lens is prescribed to hold the flap firmly in place when there is myopia of more than 6 diopters. This prevents wrinkles and leads to good conformity of corneal flap to the underlying corneal stroma.

iv. *For proper molding:* Soft contact lenses are fitted as conforming shall have a smoothing effect specially in irregular cornea and reduces the risk of wrinkles and folds to the minimum.

v. *Unilateral LASIK procedure:* When one eye is treated by LASIK for more than one specific reasons including patient unwillingness, contact lens in the fellow eye is fitted to obtain binocular vision and emmetropia.

vi. *Pre-enhancement fitting:* In certain situations one eye remains under corrected and needs enhancement after a duration of 8 to 24 weeks. In such cases contact lens is fitted to achieve emmetropia so that patients may lead normal life specially in relation to driving, reading and TV viewing, etc. Contact lenses are specially useful when these are central islands that requires sometime to disappear.

vii. *Induced keratoconus:* Keratectasia or induced keratoconus develops as a result of too little stroma left after LASIK surgery. This condition is although rare and develops specially in high myopia, contact lenses specially tailored for keratoconus are often fitted in such cases.

viii In LASIK surgery contraindicated cases when patients are unfit for LASIK surgery due to physiological and pathological conditions, their refractive error can be corrected by contact lenses which is an excellant option to achieve optimal vision without spectacles.

Usually low pachymetry readings, Slit-lamp abnormalities and abnormal corneal topography observations are main cause of LASIK surgery contraindications. Developing cataract, corneal pathology and associated retinal pathologies are other factors for contraindication of LASIK surgery.

In following clinical conditions contact lenses are treatment of choice and are preferred to refractive surgery.

- Healed keloids which may be adversely affected by LASIK surgery.
- Patients with thin and irregular corneas leading to keratoconus.
- Patients having systemic collagen diseases.
- Highly anxious and nuisance patients who expect only 20/20 vision after LASIK surgery.
- High myopes (15-20 diopters) when LASIK surgery is contraindicated and patient is not willing to undergo alternate surgical procedures.
- When corneas are extremely thinned for second laser enhancement.

For achieving emmetropia prospects of contact lenses in refractive surgery are quite bright. Custom designed contact lenses, bifocal contact lenses of disposable type, Extended wear and non-disposable type shall help the patient to maintain optimal vision.

BIBLIOGRAPHY

1. Agarwal A, et al. 4 Volume Textbook of Ophthalmology: New Delhi: Jaypee Brothers Medical Publishers, 2002.
2. Agarwal A, et al. Refractive Surgery: New Delhi: Jaypee Brothers Medical Publishers, 2000.
3. Agarwal A, et al. LASIK and Beyond LASIK. Highlights of Ophthamology, Panama, 2001.
4. Stein H. Contact lenses in refractive surgery. Highlights of Ophthalmology, 2002; 1:10-3.
5. Stein H, et al. Contact Lenses. New Delhi: Jaypee Brothers Medical Publishers, 1997.
6. Dada VK, et al, Textbook of Contact Lenses. New Delhi: Jaypee Brothers Medical Publishers, 1996.

CHAPTER 12

Ocular Pharmacokinetics in LASIK and LASEK Surgery

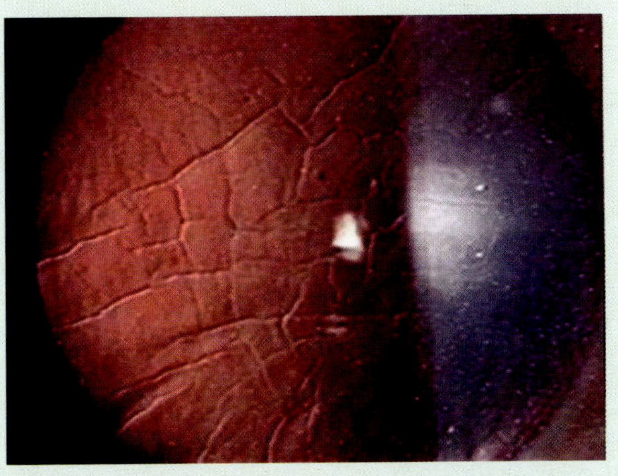

Ashok Garg (India)

INTRODUCTION

Every since Theo Seiler in 1987 and Marguerite McDonald in 1988 did the first corneal ablation in normal sighted eye, Excimer Laser Refractive Surgery has produced revolutionary changes in the field of ophthalmology. Refractive surgery is certainly a high tech advancement in the field of ophthalmic surgery of the last decade of this millenium which has come as a great boon to spectacle weary patients all around the world.

LASIK (Laser-assisted in Situ Keratomileusis) and LASEK (Laser-assisted Subepithelial Keratectomy) offer a unique opportunity to provide ametropia to patients with refractive error ranging from –20.00 D of myopia to +8.00 D of hyperopia. The rapid visual recovery and decreased incidence of complications associated with LASIK and LASEK make them far superior to both excimer photoablation (PRK) and automated Lamellar Keratoplasty (ALK).

LASIK and LASEK provides an extra-ordinary accurate method of tissue removal (0.20-0.25 μm tissue per pulse). The extreme pain, haze, regression and slow visual rehablitation of PRK are absent thus the minimum use of post precedure medications specially topical steroids and its potential adverse effects.

Although pre-procedure medications are same in Lasik and Lasek as those in PRK surgery while post-procedure medications are drasticaly reduced in Lasik and Lasek surgery leading to quick visual rehabilitation of patient post-operatively.

Development of automated micro Keratome Hansatome and Laser Microkeratome has make LASIK and LASEK surgery more safe even in the hand of novice refractive surgeon. Indeed the LASIK and LASEK surgery have come of age.

Here, now I shall discuss the ocular therapeutics used in LASIK and LASEK surgery before and after the procedure.

PREPROCEDURE THERAPEUTIC MEDICATIONS

Preoperatively patient is given broad range topical antibiotic eyedrops (Preferably Gatifloxacin (0.3%) or Moxifloxacin (0.5%) at 4 hourly interval starting 24 hours prior to surgery.

A mild oral sedation (diazepam 3-10 mg) is given in all cases. Bilateral simultaneous surgery is done in all cases.

Topical Anesthesia

For Lasik/Lasek Surgery, refractive Surgeon prefer to give topical anesthesia because of rapid onset of action and lesser irritation to the patient.

2-5 minutes prior to the surgery any of the following topical anesthetic agent can be safely used.

- Proparacaine HCl – 0.5%
- Benoxinate HCl – 0.4%
- Tetracaine HCl – 0.5%

Proparacaine is most commonly used anesthetic agent followed by Benoxinate and tetracaine. Other topical agent like Xylocaine (4%) is less commonly used due to problems of irritation, allergy, etc.

Proparacaine, benoxinate and tetracaine have rapid onset of action and cause little tingling sensation and irritation to the patient.

Onset of anesthetic action starts with in 15 to 20 seconds with these agents and effects last for 15 to 20 minutes sufficient for the completion of LASIK/LASEK Surgery. Proparacaine or Benoxinate are given topically in the dosage of 2 drops in each eye 2 to 3 times repeated at the interval of one minute.

After topical anesthesia some refractive surgeon prefer to instill Pilocarpine 1 percent in the eye to aid in marking the optical axis.

Pachymetry is performed and patients is carefully centred and eyelids are cleaned with betadine solution (Iodine solution) and operative eye is given a sterile plastic ophthalmic drape to cover the eyelid margins and the cilia.

POSTPROCEDURE THERAPEUTIC MEDICATIONS

The biggest advantage of LASIK and LASEK over PRK is the minimum use of ocular therapeutic in postoperative phase. The visual recovery in LASIK and LASEK is virtually immediate owing to the preservation of the epithelium of the cornea. Typically recovery is painless and post-procedure refractions and vision are remarkably stable during the postoperative period. Postprocedure medications are quite significant for early visual rehabilitation and recovery of the patient. During the initial active post-operative phase. Refractive Surgeons prefer to give –

a. Oral antibiotic (Gatifloxacin 400 mg OD or Levofloxacin 500 mg OD for 5 days).
b. Topical Fluorometholone (FML, 0.1%) eyedrops four times a day for two weeks.

c. Topical lubricant like polyvinyl alcohol liquifilm tear drops 4 times a day for two weeks.
d. Topical antibiotic (Moxifloxacin 0.5%). QID for a week. Immediately after LASIK/LASEK procedure some surgeon prefer to give patch for 2 to 3 hours. While other view is to ask the patient to wear a clear eye shield nightly for a week.
e. Oral analgesic (Tab. Diclofenac 75 mg SR BD for three days if needed but not in routine).

Patient operated for LASIK/Lasek surgery is called for follow up on –

- 2nd day post procedure
- Ist week
- 2nd week
- 3rd week

One each follow up following examination are done

- Vision check up
- IOP with noncontact tonometer
- Slit Lamp Examination for Haze
- Topography to see corneal profile.

Corneal wound healing and its modulations after LASIK/LASEK surgery have multiple components. LASIK/LASEK is a refractive surgical procedure that is performed in several steps and each step involved a different structure of cornea.

PHASES OF HEALING

Following LASIK/LASEK injury healing occurs in several phases. The earliest phase involves the healing of epithelial injury and is characterised by the migration of epithelium which occurs 12 to 24 hr after prcedure 2.3 days after the insult, epithelial cell proliferation is evident. Six months after the surgical insult the development of fibrous metaplasia is complete. Throughout these phases of healing the types of cytokine communication are operating to create an integrated repair of injured corneal areas.

Although LASIK/LASEK is safe and reliable procedure yet it is susceptible to all the complications noted in PRK procedure which includes overcorrection, undercorrection, decentration, infection, loss and displacement of flap, central islands and epithelial in growth.

Cornea healing following LASIK/LASEK should be considered as a combination of events involving the response to injury of the epithelium and stroma.

Understanding these events and the molecules that regulate the wound healing response should enable the refractive surgeon to induce fewer complications and aid in developing therapeutic modalities to alter would healing precisely.

Close follow up and attention to postoperative medications and surface lubrication will enable the surgeon to achieve better results.

FURTHER READING

1. Agarwal Amar, Textbook of Ophthalmology, ed.1, New Delhi: Jaypee Medical Publishers, 2002.
2. Bartlett JD. Clinical Ocular Pharmacology, ed.4, Boston: Butterworth-Heinemann,2001
3. Bartlett JD. Ophthalmic Drug Facts. Lippincott – William and Wilkins, 2001.
4. Crick RP, Trimble RB, Textbook of Clinical Ophthalmology. Hodder and Stoughton, 1986.
5. Duane TD. Clinical Ophthalmology, ed. 4. Butterworth – Heinemann, 1999.

6. Duvall, Ophthalmic Medications and Pharmacology: Slack Inc, 1998.
7. Ellis. PP, Ocular Therapeutics and Pharmacology, ed. 7: C.V. Mosby, 1985.
8. Fechner, Ocular Therapeutics: Slack Inc., 1998.
9. Fraunfelder, Current Ocular Therapy, ed. 5: W.B. Saunders, 2000.
10. Garg A, Current Trends in ophthalmology, ed. 1, New Delhi: Jaypee Medical Publishers, 1997.
11. Garg A, Manual of Ocular Therapeutics, ed. 1, New Delhi: Jaypee Medical Publishers, 1996.
12. Garg A. Ready Reckoner of Ocular Therapeutics, ed.1, New Delhi: 2002.
13. Goodman. LS, Gilman. A, Pharmacological Basis of Therapeutics, ed.7, New York: Macmillan, 1985.
14. Havener's, Ocular Pharmacology, ed. 6: C.V. Mosby, 1994.
15. Kanski, Clinical ophthalmology, ed. 4: Butterworth – Heineman, 1999.
16. Kershner. Ophthalmic Medications and Pharmacology. Slack. Inc., 1994.
17. Olin BR, et al. Drugs Facts and Comparisons: Facts and Comparisons, St. Louis, 1997.
18. Onofrey, The Ocular Therapeutics. Lippincott-William and Wilkins, 1997.
19. Rhee, The Wills Eye drug Guide. Lippincott – William and Wilkins, 1998.
20. Steven Podos, Textbook of Ophthalmology. New Delhi: Jaypee Medical Publishers, 2001.
21. Zimmerman, Textbook of Ocular Pharmacology. Lippincott and William and Wilkins, 1997.

CHAPTER 13

Presby-LASIK for Myopia and Hyperopia A New Optical Theory: The Hypermultifocality of Cornea

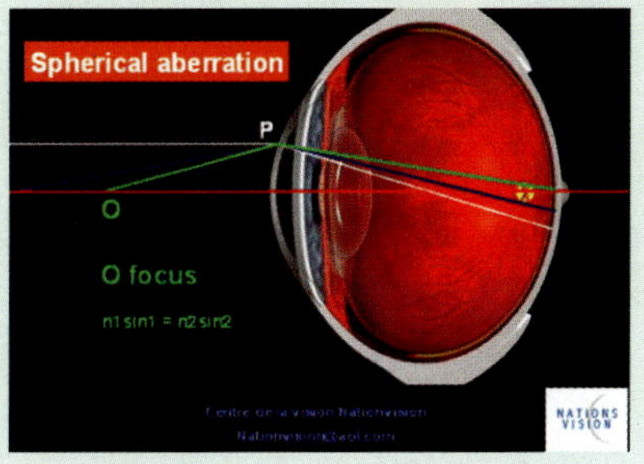

Frederic Hehn (France)

INTRODUCTION

Many techniques like: conductive keratoplastie, scleral incisions,[6] scleral expension band,[5] laser presbyopia reversal,[4] multifocal phakic IOL,[2] try to compensate presbyopia. Excimer laser is one of them.[3]

Cornea takes a great part of the accommodation process,[8] and then it doesn't astonish that some variations of the cornea shape can be used to compensate presbyopia.

Since many years, good results have been obtained in hyperopic eyes with excimer laser[1] for the both near and distant vision; in using central cornea for near vision and medium cornea for distant vision. But often this technique induce a little myopia and some discorfort for driving car due to the myosis in photopic conditions. This concept of distant vision in medium cornea and near vision in the center is not available in myopic eye.Then we tried to compensate presbyopia with the contrary concept: distant vision in central cornea and near vision in medium cornea like some authors do.[3]

THEORETICAL BASEMENT

We propose a new optical theory: the hypermultifocality of cornea to explain our excellent results in presby-LASIK.

George O Waring[7] has described 4 anatomic zones of the cornea: central optical 0 to 4 mm OZ (optical zone), paracentral "medium" 4 to 8 mm OZ, peripheral 9 to 11 mm OZ and limbal 12 mm OZ. We have to describe 3 refractive optical zones.

In central cornea there is no spherical aberration. Infinity focus on macula without using lens accommodation. In central cornea, with the lens accommodation, the near vision is very precise because there is a lot of luminosity then also a good contrast sensitivity.

But is there another way to see a middle or near object without using lens accommodation? Yes there is, it's the "hyper-multifocality" of cornea due to the spherical aberration. It's well known that spherical aberrations are bad for distant vision because they give a big blur circle.

On the contrary, spherical aberration can be useful for middle vision. If you choice a P point of the medium cornea more than 4 mm OZ, of course there are spherical aberration, and the infinity do not focus on macula, but focus in front of the macula.

Due to the Fresnel-Descartes law n1sin1 = n2sin2 we can find a "O" object which can focus on macula without lens accommodation. Many others object can focus on macula also without using lens accommodation.

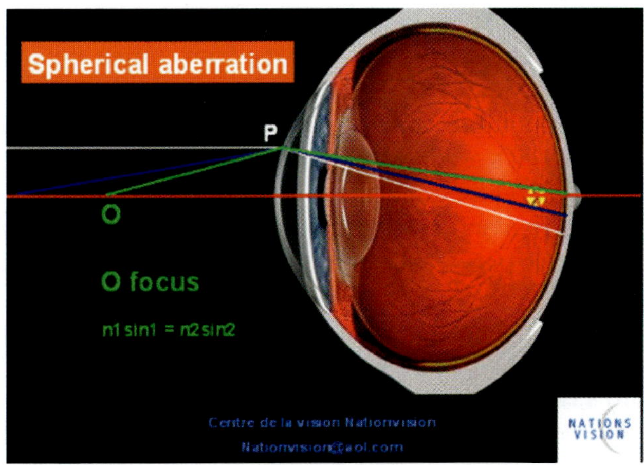

FIGURE 13.1

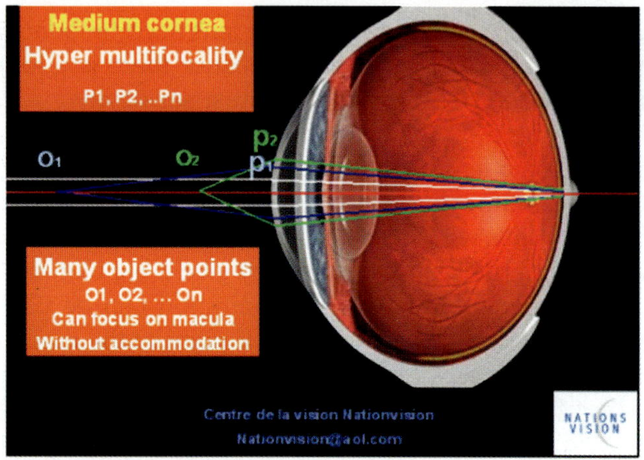

FIGURE 13.2

That's I call "hypermultifocality" of the medium cornea. Then at any time many object's planes focus together on macula without accommodation. The choice of the sharp image on the retina is a brain selection.

The hypermultifocality of the medium cornea expands the depth of focus. Evidently the nearest of the eye the object is, the more peripheral on the cornea is the focus point. Then it's a limited process, if the object is too near of the eye, the theoric focus point will be too peripheral on the cornea and give no retinal image due to the pupil filter and the very low level of luminosity entrance inside the eye.

A proof ? I can give you more than one. If you use a pin hole you lost depth of focus; it's very simple and every body can perform it.

A second proof is in concern with the pseudophakic emmetropic patient. Evidently it occurs in this case a very

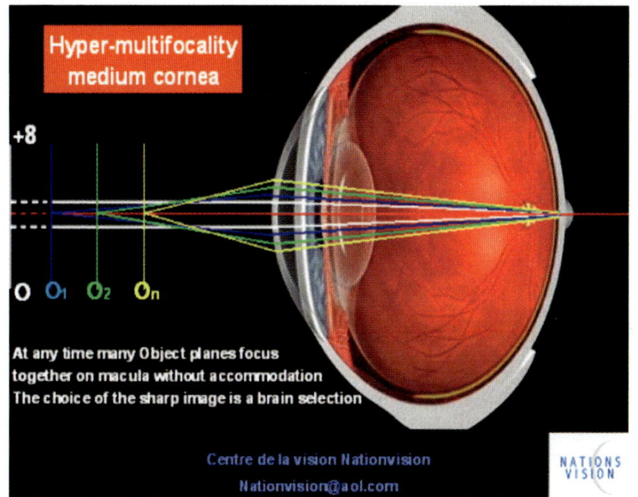

FIGURE 13.3

good distant vision, but also a good middle vision with a useful depth of focus, the only lake is the near vision. This good middle vision and depth of focus cannot be due to the central cornea and then consequently are due to the natural hypermultifocality of the medium cornea. Then I affirm: "In using spherical aberration it's possible to see a midle distant or a near object by medium cornea without using lens accommodation".

With this new concept, I had to find a constant keratometric zone, that's to say, a spherical cornea zone to use spherical aberration. We have analyzed 50 non astigmatic cornea, and found a constant keratometry on a 6.0 mm OZ [min 5.00, max 7.00]

We find 3 optical zones for 3 refractive effects.

1. **Central [0 to 4]** for distant vision

2. **Medium [4 to 6]** spherical aberrations give hyper-multifocality for midle and near vision
3. **Peripheral [6 to 12]** there are spherical aberrations but the negative asphericity and Pupil filter give no refractive effect. It's only useful for visual field, luminosity and contrast sensitivity

PRESBY-LASIK TECHNIQUE

Our Presby-LASIK technique enhance natural property of hyper-multicality of the medium cornea to focus on near objects without lens accommodation.

We are using now the high speed and precision wavelight allegretto Eye Q. The ablation profile is aspheric due to the wavefront optimized ablation profile. In central cornea a circular beam is being projected on the cornea but in medium and peripheral cornea the ellipse surface of the excimer laser treatment covers a larger area, resulting in a lower energy density. The lower ablation rate causes a spherical aberration resulting in poor night vision. The allegretto wave algorithm compensates for this.

The presby-LASIK first step is to steepen medium and central cornea for near and middle vision by a hyperopic 6.5 mm OZ treatment and 9.00 mm total treatment zone. The second step is to flatten central cornea for distant vision by a myopic 5.0 mm OZ treatment and 5.60 mm total treatment zone.

With this presby-lasik technique, you can treat plus 3 diopters even at forty five years old to treat the present and the future presbyopia. Because the more you steepen the medium cornea, the more you can flatten the central cornea.

Presby-LASIK is only possible if the mesopic pupil size is less than 5 mm width. That's often the case in patients more than 50 years old.

We treat patients from 45 years old until 70 years old with the same technique.

RESULTS

We show only 2 clinical results. Case one, an hyperopic eye +1.00 of a 55 year old female. After laser there is a very good point spread function.

The corneal topography before and after laser show a perfect centration.

Good results: 18/20 J2 monocular UCVA.

Case two, a 60 years old female, myopic –5.50 diopter. There is no increase in high order aberration after laser, but a gentle increase of second defocus (C12) C twelve = Z°4 "spherical aberration".

It remains also a C4 defocus – 3.25. It's only an aberrometric measurement but not a real value because the clinical refraction is plano. This measure is due to the steep curve of the medium cornea induced by the presby-LASIK treatment.

The corneal topography is perfectly centred and progressive with smooth transitions. The result is perfect, a very little point spread function. Patient has no glare and no halos. 20/20 J1 monocular UCVA.

DISCUSSION

In one hand, this kind of middle or near vision, in using the hypermultifocality of the medium cornea, is tiredless

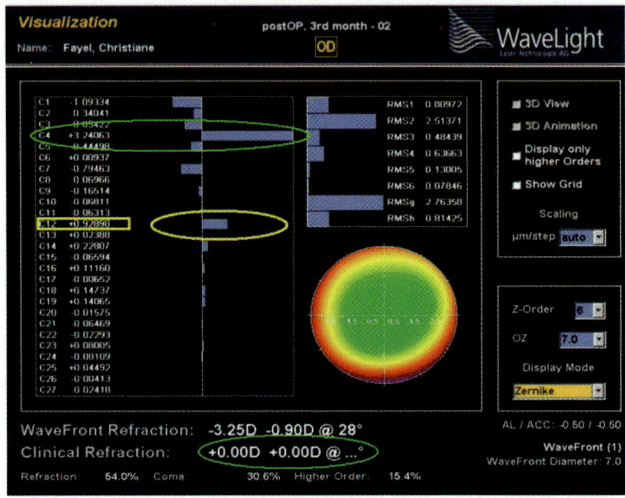

FIGURE 13.4

because there is a passive view. But this view mode needs a lot of luminosity for a good contrast and depends on pupil size. In another hand the near vision in central cornea which use lens accommodation is tiredness because it's due to a muscular effort; but this kind of near vision is more precise because more luminosity can go inside the eye by central cornea than it can by medium cornea.

The results were good in the both myopic and hyperopic eye, because distant vision in central cornea and near vision in medium cornea seems to be more efficient than the contrary concept, because it's use the natural property of hypermultifocality of medium cornea to focus on middle and near vision, without using lens accommodation.

As the transitions zones are very, very progressives and smooth, patients get no glare and no halos. The pupil size has been controlled before laser treatment, and must be less than 5.00 mm width in mesopic condition. This technique give a good vision for distant vision whatever are the luminosity conditions.

The only restriction is the necessary of getting enough luminosity for a good contrast to near vision.

CONCLUSION

Our presby-lasik technique build not a bifocal cornea but a continuous multifocal aspherical cornea that expand depth of focus to correct presbyopia. The next step is to treat pseudophakic eye with this presby-lasik technique. Further studies must be done to confirm the hyper-multifocality theory and clinical results.

REFERENCES

1. Alio JL, Cimberle M, Presby-LASIK is an option for hyperopic presbyopic patients, surgeon says. Ocular surgery news, 30, November 2004.
2. Baikoff G, Matach G, Fontaine A, Ferraz C, Spera C. Correction of presbyopia with refractive multifocal phakic intraocular lenses. J Cataract Refract Surg 2004; 30: 1454-1460.
3. Bruce Jackson W, Agarwal A, Avalos G, Multifocal LASIK offers multitude of options for treating presbyopia. Eurotimes, 31, October 2003.
4. Kadambi V, Lin JT. Clinical results of laser presbyopia reversal using the Optivision infrared laser in: Agarwal A, ed, Presbyopia; a Surgical Textbook. Thorofare, NJ, Slack, 2002; 133-135.
5. Mathiews S. Scleral expension surgery does not restore accommodation in human presbyopia. Ophthalmology 1999, 106; number 5, 873-877.

6. Schachar RA. Cause and treatment of presbyopia with a method for increasing amplitude of accommodation. Ann Ophthalmol 1992; 26:445-447, 452.
7. Waring III GO. Refractive keratotomy for myopia and astigmatism. Mosby – year book 1992, Chapter 3 page 49.
8. Yasuda A, Yamaguchi T, Ohkoshi K. Changes in corneal curvature in accommodation. J Cataract Refract Surg 2003, 29: 1297-1301.

CHAPTER 14

RELASIK (LASIK Enhancement)

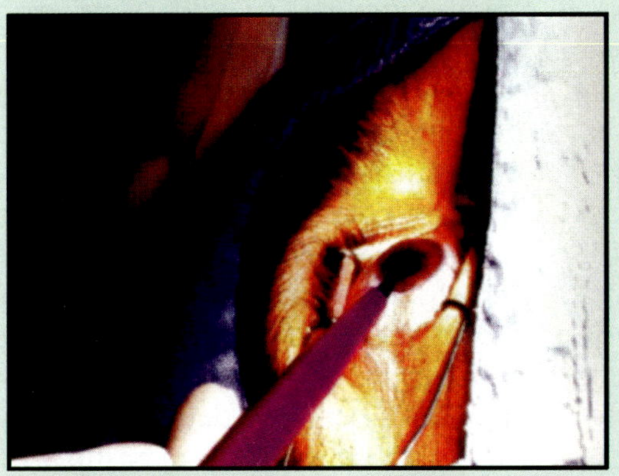

Guillermo Avalos-Urzua
Ariadna Silva-Lepe
(Mexico)

INTRODUCTION

LASIK (laser in situ keratomileusis) is, nowaday, probably the safest and most predictable refractive surgery available.

Patients believe that the procedure will permanently and completely eliminate their refractive defect.

It is the refractive surgeon's responsibility to inform the patient that the procedure is intended to eliminate their dependency on glasses or contact lenses, and that the degree of correction obtained will depend on several variables as the diopters the patient has, as well as the combination of different types of refractive errors (myopia with astigmatism, hyperopia with astigmatism, etc). The sum of all factors will have an impact on the final corrective results.

Inevitable sometimes we'll have to "redo" some eyes. Depending on the postoperative characteristics of the cornea, it may be necessary and useful to do an enhancement in order to improve the results obtained during the first surgery. Enhancement rates in USA range from 6 to 15 percent; with millions of people undergoing LASIK, this translates into hundreds of thousands of enhancements being performed annually.[1]

LASIK surgery is performed intrastromally, allowing the surgeon to perform a second ablation to correct any under or overcorrection. Furthermore it allows us to do retreatment (enhancement of the first procedure, of any defect which may have occurred during the first surgery, such as the inducement of astigmatism or the production of irregular astigmatism, or the presence of regression, which is common in the majority of refractive procedures.

Regression has been reported by many authors. Guell and Muller[2] report higher rate of regression after LASIK for high myopias in comparison to moderate myopias. Chayet et al[3] observed early postoperative regression that stabilized between 3 and 6 months after treatment in myopias with MSE –14.02 D. One regression mechanism is the proliferation of keratocytes in the corneal stoma, while another possible mechanism is epithelial hyperplasia.

The majority of refractive surgeons are in agreement that the limit of myopic correction with LASIK is –12.00 D since the corneal flatness in high myopias is excessive and generates poor optic quality corneas.

As the degree of myopia increases, the amount of regression and the subsequent need for enhancement procedures increase as well. The typical maximal regression occurs between two and four weeks postoperative, after which relative stability is achieved. A smaller amount of regression is generally noted one two three months postoperatively.

Qi et al[4] evaluated the results of excimer retreatment for undercorrection or regression after LASIK. They studied 2 149 eyes that were divided into 2 groups according to their degrees of pre-First LASIK myopia spherical equivalents. Group I was </= 10.00 diopters (D) (41 eyes); group II was > 10.00 D (47 eyes). The retreatment ratio was 4.1 percent among the 2 149 eyes. In group II, the ratio was 2.3 times that of the group I. In the comparison with other eyes, the eyes received retreatment no difference in sex, laterality and age. Over 50.0 percent had pre-First LASIK diopters >/= 10.00 D, and 73.9 percent had astigmatism correction in first LASIK. After retreatment, no undercorrection or regression occurred in group I, but there was undercorrection in group II. The ratio within +/- 1.00 D of emmetropia after 1 year was 68.3 percent in group I and 51.1 percent in group II. The UCVA above 0.5 was over 90.0 percent in all eyes. Eight eyes (9.0%) lost two or more lines of BCVA. The serious complication after retreatment was keratoconus of 3 eyes in group II. They concluded that the risk factors which lead to retreatment after first LASIK are high myopia with astigmatism before first LASIK and the reaction to the operation.

In this study, retreatment was safe, effective, predictable and accurate for </= –10.00 D correction in first LASIK. But, to prevent the occurrence of serious complication such as keratoconus, it is better not to perform retreatment for > –10.00 D in first LASIK.

Other factors that increase chances of LASIK retreatment are higher initial corrections, astigmatism and older age of patients, as shown by Hersh et al[5] in their study that included 2,485 eyes (1,306 patients) who underwent LASIK surgery for myopia, hyperopia or astigmatism. Of the 2,485 patients, 288 eyes of 233 patients underwent one retreatment, and 3 eyes of 3 patients required two retreatment procedures.

They stated that the overall 1-year incidence of retreatment was 10.5 percent. They concluded that higher initial corrections and residual astigmatism were associated with a significantly higher rate of retreatment. Patients older than 40 years were at greater risk for retreatment. No gender difference was evident.

All of the previously discussed was also emphasized by Perlman and Reinert.[6] In their paper these authors tried to confirm that enhancements after primary LASIK are effective in dealing with residual refractive errors, and to determine if any variables prior to or during the primary LASIK procedure predisposed eyes to require subsequent enhancement. They concluded that enhancements were an effective way of dealing with residual refractive errors after primary LASIK. Age greater than 45 years or a history of recent rigid contact lens use was significantly associated with the need for enhancement in patients with myopia or myopic astigmatism.

Factors associated to LASIK enhancements:

PATIENT DISSATISFACTION

While some patients may be happy with 20/25 or 20/35 corrected vision, others won't be as content. Durrie[7] strives for "20/happy" for his patients, maintaining that it's all right to enhance a patient at 20/25 or even 20/20 if the patient has stable refraction and topography that can be corrected with current technology. Regarding patient perceptions, "The rule of thumb is that there is no rule of thumb" enhancements depend on the patient's needs.

Speaker[1] gives the patient a contact lens to simulate the intended result. He postulates that particularly in pre-presbyopic or presbyopic patients, sometimes the effect can't be anticipated unless the patient tries out the contact first.

PATIENT AGE

When evaluating the patient's request for an enhancement, take his or her age into consideration. It is said that a younger patient who is undercorrected will generally be more inclined to be persistent about the enhancement, while undercorrected patients who are prepresbyopic and presbyopic may find it advantageous to have a broad range of vision preserved so that the only time they would need glasses would be to drive at night.

On the other hand, people in their 20s and 30s can still see well if they are slightly overcorrected, but in presbyopic patients who are overcorrected, they don't see well either distance or close, and they are persistent in wanting the correction.

EFFECT OF ENVIRONMENTAL FACTORS

Walter KA, Stevenson AW[8], determined whether environmental factors affect LASIK enhancement rates. They found that the 2-week-preoperative mean outdoor relative humidity, procedure room relative humidity, outdoor temperature, and procedure room temperature may have to be considered during LASIK planning. The effect of these environmental variables on LASIK outcomes warrants further evaluation.

OTHER

Some authors have designed formulas to predict the probability of LASIK enhancement as Hu et al[9]. They developed a formula to predict a patient's need for LASIK enhancement. Multivariate logistic regression analysis was used to determine a formula for the probability of enhancement surgery. Age ($P < .0001$), preoperative cycloplegic sphere ($P < .0001$), and surgeon ($P < .0001$) were the statistically significant factors for predicting retreatment. The predictive formula derived from these factors had a sensitivity of 79 percent, a specificity of

61 percent, and positive and negative predictive values of 31 percent and 93 percent, respectively. Older age, higher preoperative cycloplegic sphere, and surgeon significantly influenced a patient's likelihood for LASIK retreatment. A formula based on these predisposing factors helps to more accurately predict the need for retreatment.

INDICATIONS

Clinical indications[1] for re-treatment include residual or induced astigmatism and under- and overcorrection. It is very important that surgeons and ophthalmologists evaluate patients with induced astigmatism and who may have lost a line of best-corrected visual acuity to make sure the induced astigmatism isn't caused by striae, or wrinkles in the flap. If astigmatism is caused by striae, and the ophthalmologist plans to do an enhancement by lifting the flap, the result is unpredictable. One should be careful not to lead patients to believe that a small amount of laser correction will restore a quality of vision as it may not.

The amount of residual defect recommendable for treatment for a second ablation is greater than 0.75D.

EVALUATION

All patients who undergo enhancement should first have their cycloplegic refraction evaluated as well as an ultrasonic pachymetry and a corneal topography.

PACHYMETRY

The primary factor that determines whether or not to do an enhancement is the result of the pachymetry, which can differ if you are doing an enhancement in a patient with a preoperative correction greater or lower than –6.00 D. As a safety measure, the surgeon should always leave 250 microns of stroma plus an average of 160 microns of thickness of the corneal flap, leaving us with a total of 410 microns. As a basic principle, reablations should not be performed if the cornea shows a total pachymetry of less than 410 microns. If the preoperative correction in the original surgery is less than –6.00 D, the undercorrection is usually between –0.5 and –1.50 D. Since first ablations are usually less than 80 microns, surely a second ablation of 20 microns can be performed without any inconvenience. If we have a cornea of 530 microns and remove 160 microns the flap plus an additional 80 microns of the ablation, we are left with a stroma under the flap of 290 microns, leaving us with 40 microns for the second ablation.

In myopias greater than –6.00 D, for example with –11.0 D, also with a cornea of 530 microns, we do a first ablation of approximately 130 microns which leaves us with a residual stroma of 240 microns and a total pachymetry of only 400 microns.

In this case an enhancement is not an option since the surgeon needs to recognize the potential risk of creating corneal ectasia.

In their paper Muallem et al[10] evaluated whether flap thickness changes after the primary LASIK procedure and assessed the accuracy of intraoperative pachymetry and ablation depth measurements in predicting stromal bed thickness before enhancement in eyes that have had primary myopic LASIK. They concluded that the flap thickness tended to be thicker at enhancement than at primary LASIK. Intraoperative pachymetry and ablation depth measurements proved to be precise tools to predict stromal bed thickness before enhancement in eyes that had had primary myopic LASIK. They suggested that this information may help in planning LASIK enhancements.

Two methods were compared for estimating residual stromal bed thickness before repeat LASIK, by Randleman et al.[11]

They compared two methods of calculating residual stromal bed (RSB) thickness after repeat LASIK, to determine which method generates more conservative RSB thickness estimates, and to determine any factors related to the discrepancy between these 2 calculation methods. This group compared calculated RSB thickness after second and third LASIK using either original corneal thickness (CT) minus flap thickness and all ablations (original CT method) or pre-enhancement CT minus flap thickness and enhancement ablation (repeat CT method). They conclude that using original preoperative CT measurements provides a more conservative and thus safer approach than using CT measurements obtained before repeat LASIK to calculate RSB thickness after repeat LASIK.

TOPOGRAPHY

Another important factor is the topography. Kanellopoulos[1] referred in his publication that topography-guided LASIK enhancement using the *Allegretto Wave system* appears to be safe and effective for improving poor quality of vision associated with small, eccentric ablations and irregular astigmatism after previous refractive surgery.

Based on data collected of 17 consecutive eyes during a mean follow-up period of 6.5 months, he concluded the topography-guided enhancement resulted in improved topography accompanied by a reduction in the mean asphericity value toward a more desirable level. There was good cylinder correction and reasonable spherical adjustment, accompanied by marked improvement in night vision quality. Patients eligible for the procedure had to present with a small optical zone, decentered ablation, irregular astigmatism, or night vision problems and have a residual SE ± 1.50 D. In addition, they were required to have estimated postenhancement thicknesses of 280 μm in the stromal bed and 400 μm for the total cornea. As an additional criterion, patients needed to have highly reproducible topography maps. Only topographies with =75 percent of the corneal surface mapped were included. Re-treatment was performed with flap lifting, not cutting, and ultrasonic pachymetry measurements were obtained preoperatively and after flap lifting to verify that patients fulfilled the criteria for residual stromal and corneal thickness.

TIMMING

Stability is imperative before an enhancement can be considered. Stability of postoperative refraction in LASIK, when you have treated myopias lower than –6.00 D, is two months. For this reason, with this group of patients it is appropriate to do the enhancement after two months. When treating myopias greater than –6.0 D the stability of the postoperative refraction can prolong itself up two 6 months, and any intent of reablation should be done after this time. If you are going to do a retreatment due to an overcorrection of a myopic LASIK, you should wait at least 6 months, since in the first few weeks post-LASIK there may exist overcorrections that progressively diminish in the first two months. Before this time, if overcorrections exist we should manage them with medication (pilocarpine 0.5% or 1%) for several months in order to induce myopia or whith the application of soft contact lenses since this stimulates the epithelial hyperplasia and in some cases we can obtain regression of the overcorrection. After six months, if the overcorrection persists we should think of doing hyperopic LASIK. Hersh et al[5] found that the average length of time between initial treatment and enhancement was 7.3 +/– 6.4 months; 85 percent of retreatments took place within 1 year.

CONTRAINDICATIONS

Contraindications for enhancement include the thickness of the cornea. Simon[1] cited 250 microns as the minimal bed thickness in order to perform either the primary surgery or an enhancement. Durrie[17] considers the total corneal thickness, which includes 160 microns for the flap and 250 microns for the bed.

As for other contraindications, it has been cited[10] uncontrolled blepharitis, dry eye and epithelial basement membrane dystrophy.

REOPERATION TECHNIQUE

The best option for correcting residual defects induced during the first LASIK surgery is a second LASIK procedure. One of the primary advantages of LASIK is its adjustability, which allows for the possibility of a future reablation (enhancement).

The original surgeon should have the characteristics of the cut registered such as de diameter, thickness, hinge, size or free cap and if the cut was regular or irregular as well as the reason for the complication of the cut.

Diameter: It is important to know the diameter of the cut in order to avoid making an error in lifting a flap that was partial or insufficient in diameter; especially if the reablation is going to be hyperopic to treat an over-correction.

Thickness: Thin flaps (130 microns or less) shrink easily when being lifted, producing striae or folds, which result in visual postoperative defects.

Hinge: When doing a hyperopic retreatment with a large hinge you will obtain an appropriate ablation since the hinge will be blocking the treatment zone.

Free cap: The greatest of care is required when lifting the flap in order to avoid a second free cap and the future risk of displacement.

Regular or Irregular surfaces: It is preferable to treat whatever irregularity of the cut on the same level in order to obtain a better result in your retreatment. If the original procedure was done by another surgeon, it is necessary to do a careful study of the corneal disk with the slit lamp. The best way of doing this is to install a drop of anesthesia and with a round instrument 4 to 5 mm in diameter (the author uses the Caro/Avalos Flap Smoother) apply pressure to the center of the cornea which makes the cut in the cornea evident. In this way you can evaluate the diameter of the cut while having a good idea of the size of the hinge. It is very difficult to visually appreciate the thickness of the cut with the slit- lamp, if it is 130 or 160 microns; this is a personal judgment call. With the slit-lamp (biomicroscopic examination) it is very difficult to know if the cut was partial or not, we can only visualize the border of the cut and attempt to appreciate its limits. Regularity or irregularity of the cut is preferably observed with the topography since the flap makes it impossible to see irregular areas in the stroma. The LASIK surgeon generally achieves good exactitude in the correction of the refractive problem. When there is an undercorrection it could be due to an insufficient ablation or to regression. In low myopias (less than -6 D) if a significant under-correction is present and we did not do the original surgery, we should assume that probably problems existed in the cut. Irregular astigmatism in the topography or haze in the interface can confirm that it was not a good quality cut and in this case a retreatment should be performed by means of a second cut.

There are two options for performing the reablation: a) a second cut, b) relifting the flap

SECOND CUT

It has been mentioned that 6 months after the original procedure the process of healing between the flap and the stroma is complete, making it difficult to lift the flap. Lifting the flap increases the risk of producing epithelial ingrowths in the interface. A new cut can be made at the same depth of the anterior cut or it can be deeper (180 or 200 microns).

A second cut could produce a free lamellar tissue that could cause disastrous refractive conditions that are not easily resolved. As well, a second cut causes a double interface, which can produce diminution of the BCVA and ghosts in vision. If the first cut had irregularities in the corneal stroma doing a second cut on another depth will not correct this stromal abnormalities, since they need to be treated on the same level in which they occurred.

In my opinion, one of the fundamental aspects of doing a retreatment is to know if I performed the original LASIK procedure or if it was performed by another surgeon.

RELIFTING THE FLAP

It is generally believed that it is easer to lift the flap six months after the original procedure, it has also been mentioned that you can lift the flap even after three years.[12] In our clinic it has be done after three years without difficult, by using an appropriated technique. Other motives for recommending the management of the original flap is that the intrinsic risk of the microkeratome (thin flap, free cap, holes, etc) are not present.

Domniz et al[13] compared enhancement techniques following LASIK. Recutting was performed on 263 eyes and the flap was lifted in 55 eyes that had LASIK for simple myopia or myopic astigmatism. The time interval between LASIK and retreatment was 340+/–46 days in the recutting group and 215+/–36 days in the flap lifting group. In the recutting group, mean spherical equivalent refraction improved from –1.48+/–1.25 D to –0.49+/–0.88 D at 6 months. In the flap lifting group, mean spherical equivalent refraction improved from

–1.05+/–1.49 D to –0.45+/–0.39 D at 6 months. Refractive cylinder did not change significantly in either group.

There was a significant increase in uncorrected visual acuity UCVA of 6/6 in each group. In the recutting group, UCVA of 6/6 increased from 3.8 to 65.2 percent at 6 months, and in the lifting group from 3.6 to 71.1 percent at 6 months. In the recutting group, seven free flaps and three macerated flaps that required removal occurred. One eye in the recutting group and two in the lifting group developed significant epithelial ingrowth. No patient lost more than one line of BSCVA. Their conclusion was that procedures were safe, effective, and highly predictable for enhancements, but flap complications may be more likely with recutting.

In Hersh et al[5] study nearly all (285) of the 288 retreatments performed, were accomplished using a manual flap lift approach; 3 eyes required a repeat microkeratome cut.

Netto et al[14] at The Cole Eye Institute analyzed the results achieved with LASIK retreatment after lifting the original flap in a large series of patients. LASIK retreatment was performed in 334 eyes, and the mean time between initial procedure and retreatment was 8.2+/–6.2 months. The mean spherical equivalent (SE) improved from –1.2+/–0.6 diopters (D) (range, –4.2 to +1.2 D) before retreatment to +0.2+/–0.4 D (range, –3.1 to +1.1 D) after the retreatment. The uncorrected visual acuity (UCVA) after retreatment was 20/20 or better in 58 percent and 20/40 or better in 92 percent of eyes. The mean SE was within +/–1.0 D in 96 percent of the patients and within +/–0.5 D in 80.5 percent after retreatment. Eighteen eyes (5%) lost 1 line of best-corrected visual acuity, and 4 eyes (1%) lost 2 lines. In this study, LASIK retreatment surgery performed by relifting the flap was a useful procedure for correcting residual refractive errors after the primary LASIK procedure. It provided good uncorrected visual acuity, predictable results, good refractive stability, and few complications.

SURGICAL TECHNIQUE

Enhancements should be treated the same way as the first LASIK procedure; the same rules of the asepsis are applied to the second treatment. During surgical cleaning, the patient face is washed with betadine solution and they are given their first dose of anesthetic (proparacaine). This is followed by drops of ciprofloxacin. They are then placed on a stretcher where a drape is placed over their face in order to isolate the eyelids and eyelashes from the ocular globe. Once on the stretcher, a second dose of anesthetic is applied and the speculum is placed. A mark is made in the corneal epithelium whith the side of a 25 G needle followed by the application of a gentian violet color mark, this mark is radial and is extended from the border of the pupil to the limbus. Once this has been done, excess color should then be cleaned away with a wet sponge.

With a round instrument, pressure is apply to the center of the cornea, in order to observe the border of the corneal disk cut or flap through the microscope, for this purpose I use a glass rod or I recommend using the Caro/Avalos compressor instrument. Occasionally in light colored iris this can be difficult to observe. In both eyes, the easiest zone of the flap to observe is the temporal inferior sector of the cornea. Once this has been located, use a thin slightly curve spatula and attempt to insert it under the edge of the corneal disk in a parallel movement, without withdrawing the round instrument that is applying pressure to the eye. This will help to overcome epithelial resistance. Once the point of the spatula is under the corneal flap, steer it towards the center of the pupil. Then, in a rotating movement while maintaining the instrument in a fixed position in the center of the pupil, rotate above and below trying to loosen it at least 180 degrees. During this movement the spatula should not be withdrawn or reinserted, in order to avoid inserting epithelial cells in the interface. Once it has been loosened 180 degrees, withdraw the spatula and with a non toothed forceps lift the corneal flap in a semicircular movement (upwards and downwards) in order to finish loosening the corneal flap until you arrive at the hinge, then fold the disk back over the conjunctiva. One should be careful when lifting the flap to be sure to withdraw the tag of the epithelium in order to avoid inserting it under the flap toward the interface. With a dry sponge clean the entire length of the stromal border of the cornea while making sure that the sponge does not pass toward the stroma. I recommend dampening the stromal face of the flap to avoid dryness caused by exposure to the environment, which will form striae and folds. I do not recommend the use of saline solution to separate the disk from the stroma since it modifies the hydration of the stroma and consequently the ablation as well as the adhesion between the flap and the posterior stroma.

Perez-Santonja et al[15] in their paper describe a refinement technique for LASIK re-treatment called circular flap rhexis, based on a careful flap edge identification, linear epithelial tear for minimizing epithelial irregularities and defects, and a delicate flap replacement to promote a strong adhesion between the flap edge and the stromal bed. Their LASIK re-treatment with this flap rhexis technique was performed in 43 eyes at 3 or 6 months after the primary LASIK. After a 12 month follow-up, the epithelial ingrowth and flap melting rates were recorded. Epithelial growth was found in 9.3 percent of the cases (4 out of 43 eyes) and flap melting in 2.3 percent of the cases (1 out of 43) at 12 months after LASIK re-treatment by circular flap rhexis. These disorders were always peripheral and did not affect visual acuity or corneal astigmatism.

They concluded that LASIK re-treatment using circular flap rhexis is an effective technique to decrease the epithelium related complications after LASIK re-treatment.

Once the stroma is exposed, align the eye with the lasers aiming beam in order to proceed with your re-treatment in regards to the quantity of the ablation, it should be performed the total amount correction for patients between 20 and 35 years old. From 35 to 45 years decrease 10 percent of the correction and from 45 years onwards decrease by 20 percent of the total amount to be corrected.

When finalizing the ablation you should irrigate the stroma to eliminate all the debris from both the previous and current ablation. Clean the flap especially around the edge in order to avoid leaving epithelial remains. Once the flap has been collocated in its correct position and is properly aligned, dry the border with a wet sponge and use the Caro compressor in the central portion of the flap, applying pressure for 15 seconds, which would produce good adhesion between the flap and the stroma and avoids its posterior displacement if, when lifting the flap, you produce a significant epithelial defect you should apply a soft contact lens for 3 to 5 days which allows complete healing. If there are not epithelial defects, the postoperative indications should be the same as in the original procedure, apply drops containing dexamethasone and antibiotics (fluoroquinolones), add nonsteroidal drops if you choose in order to decrease postoperative sensation. It is the surgeon's decision whether or not to use a patch for several hours.

The postoperative regimen is normal, including the use of steroids and antibiotics for 8 days and artificial tears for a month.

After an enhancement, the patient needs to be treated with steroids and antibiotics to prevent against infection or diffuse lamellar keratitis, which occurs in the interface between the flap and the stromal. Suresh and Rootman[16] reported a case of bilateral infectious keratitis occurring as a complication of bilateral simultaneous LASIK enhancement procedures. Corneal scraping from the interface of both eyes grew Staphylococcus aureus. The infection cleared after treatment with fluoroquinolones. The patient was left with bilateral paracentral corneal scars.

They concluded that when bilateral surgery is performed, bilateral infection may occur as a rare complication.

Therefore, the patient should be seen by their surgeon frequently, with special attention been paid to epithelial healing at the edge of the flap as well as periodic follow-up each month to observe the possibility of the appearance of epithelial ingrowth. If epithelial ingrowth appears at some postoperative stage, you can apply laser YAG

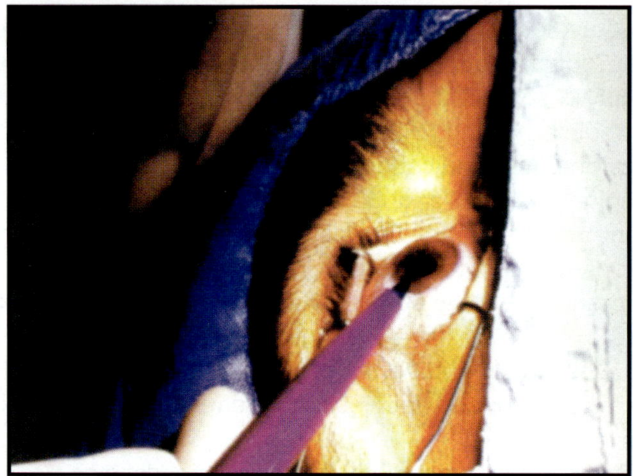

FIGURE 14.1: Reference mark

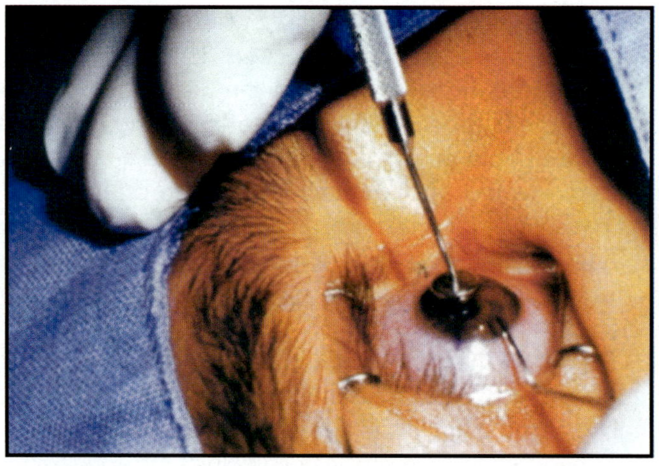

FIGURE 14.2: Use a thin slightly curve spatula, attempt to insert

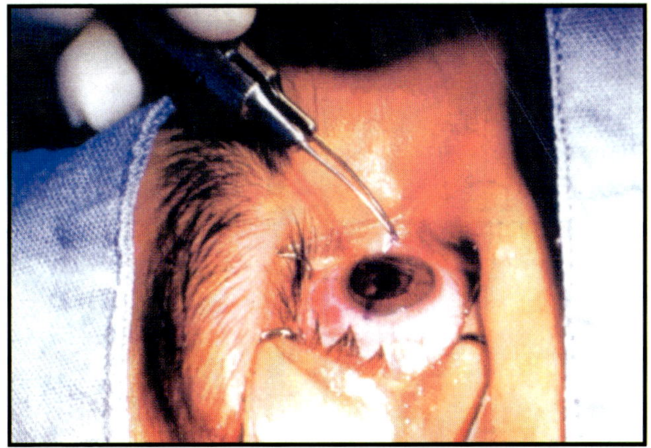

FIGURE 14.3: Lift the flap with fine forceps

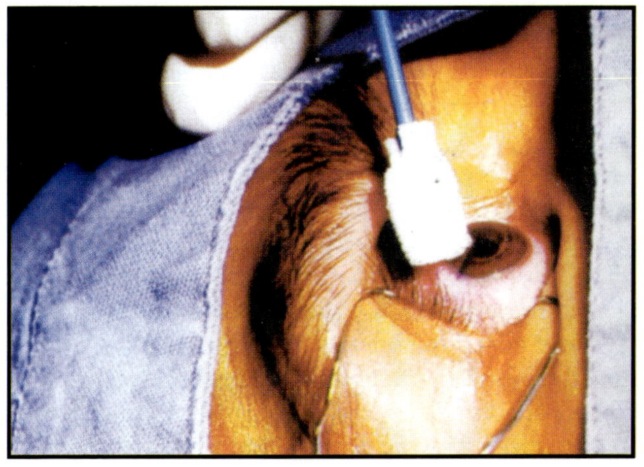

FIGURE 14.4: Recollocate the flap and dry the border with a wet sponge

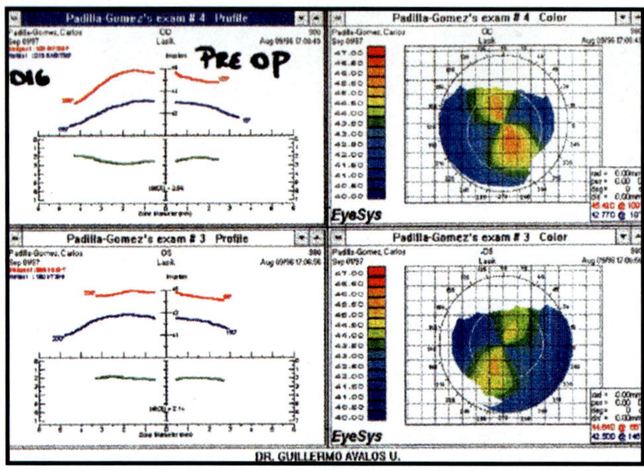

FIGURE 14.5: Patient 1 preoperative

(yttrium-aluminum-garned) on the area in order to destroy epithelial cells and to avoid relifting the flap.

I have been doing this procedure for the past 10 years with very successful results (Figures 14.1 to 14.5).

Rubinfeld et al[17] reported serious complications caused by recutting LASIK flaps for enhancement and reconsider the current preferred method of LASIK enhancement. In this retrospective noncomparative nonconsecutive case series comprised LASIK patients in the private practices of 9 experienced refractive surgeons and those reported in a survey of refractive surgeons. Case histories, refractions, corneal topographies, slit-lamp photographs, and measurements of uncorrected and best corrected (BCVA) visual acuity after recutting LASIK flaps were collected. Surveys of refractive surgeons and an analysis of changing practice trends among the authors and these surgeons were assessed. In 12 cases, significant loss of BCVA and subjective visual difficulties resulted from recutting LASIK flaps. Most surveyed surgeons had changed their practice from recutting to lifting flaps even 9 to 10 years postoperatively with good results. They concluded that recutting flaps for enhancement should be avoided unless other alternatives are unavailable.

We can establish various principles or rules before doing our re-treatment:

- Do a cornea topography and ultrasonic pachymetry
- If the characteristics of the original cut are known and it was a normal cut, always lift the flap.
- The time since the original surgery is not important. In this respect, you should be cautious if a cut of a large diameter appears near the limbus. In this zone scarring is very pronounced due to the perilimbic vessels which make it difficult to find the edge of the flap and to lift it.
- In this particular case I do recommend a second cut. If the characteristics of the first cut are unknown, and the cornea studies do not give enough information about the initial cut, you can opt to do a second cut.
- Do a second cut if you find irregular astigmatism in the topography, haze or multiple metallic particles in the interface, since this tells us that there were problems with the cut
- Do not do a retreatment in high myopias if the total pachymetry is less 460 microns.
- Wait six months to do a second cut.
- Be careful whith flat corneas (less than 39 D) because of the risk of a thin cut, small diameter cut and free cap when doing a second cut

- Do not irrigate below the flap when lifting it, this hydrates the stroma and the ablation is not properly performed.
- Carefully study the cornea doing topography and pachymetry revision on several occasions since some cases of progressive regression can mean ectasia

COMPLICATIONS

- Flap dehydration and shrinkage
- Laminated cut with a loose lamellar stromal tissue
- Epithelial ingrowth
- Striae
- Haze in the interface
- Dislodged flap
- Ectasia

Two of the complications previously mentioned produce very significant visual defects, the loss of stromal tissue during a second cut and ectasia postLASIK.

Fortunately I have no experienced the loss of stromal tissue during a second cut after LASIK. However, I have had a case when doing LASIK on a patient who previously had had lamellar keratectomy.

I would like to exemplify a complication (ectasia) with the following pictures (Figures 14.6 to 14.12).

Outcomes after Laser in situ Keratomileusis Retreatment

Alka et al[18] evaluated the refractive and visual performance after (LASIK) retreatment. They studied 33 eyes of 23 patients who underwent LASIK retreatment for residual myopia with or without astigmatism. The mean spherical

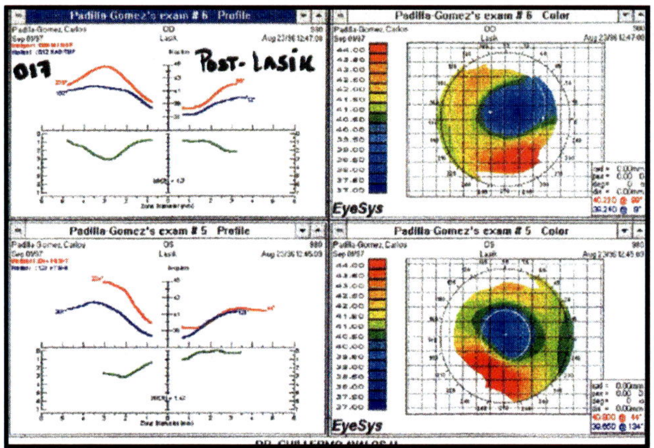

FIGURE 14.6: Patient 1 postLASIK

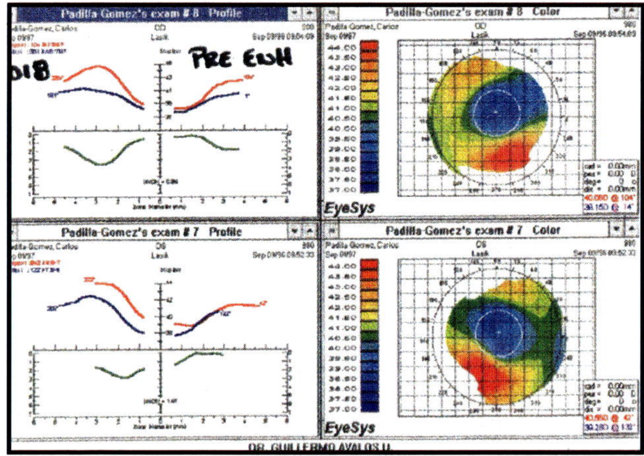

FIGURE 14.7: Patient 1 pre-enhancement (undercorrection)

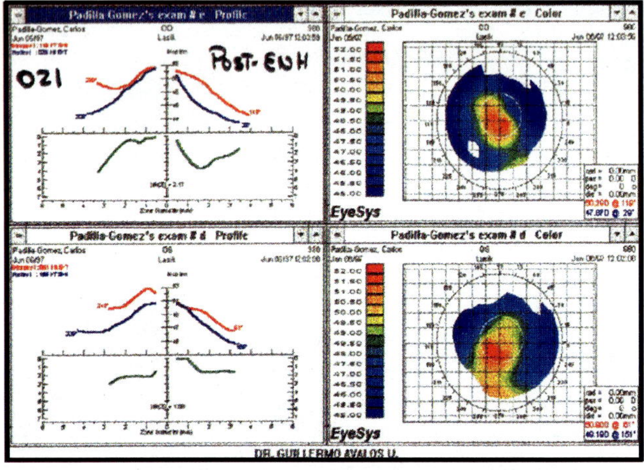

FIGURE 14.8: Patient 1 Post-enhancement (9 months later)

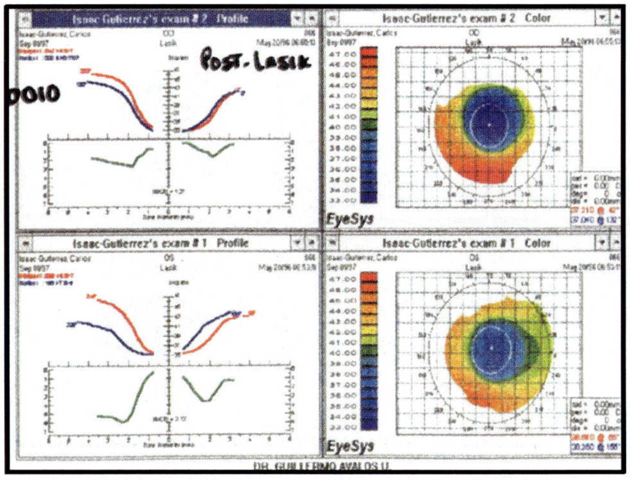

FIGURE 14.9: Patient 2 PostLASIK

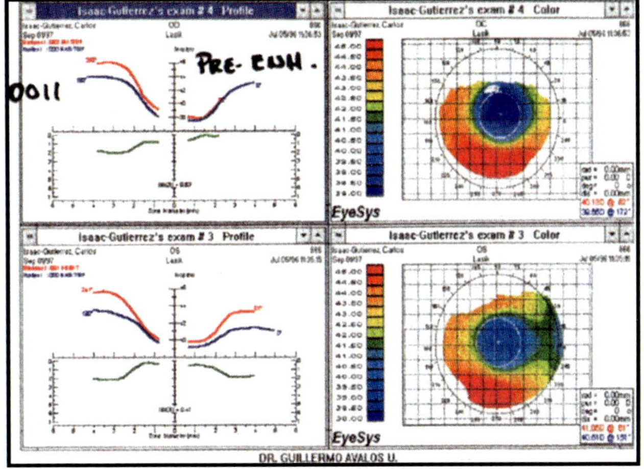

FIGURE 14.10: Patient 2 Pre-enhancement (undercorrection)

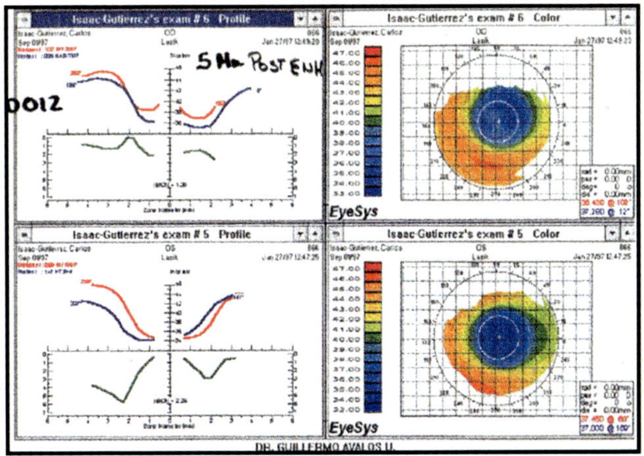

FIGURE 14.11: Patient 2 Post-enhancement (5 months later)

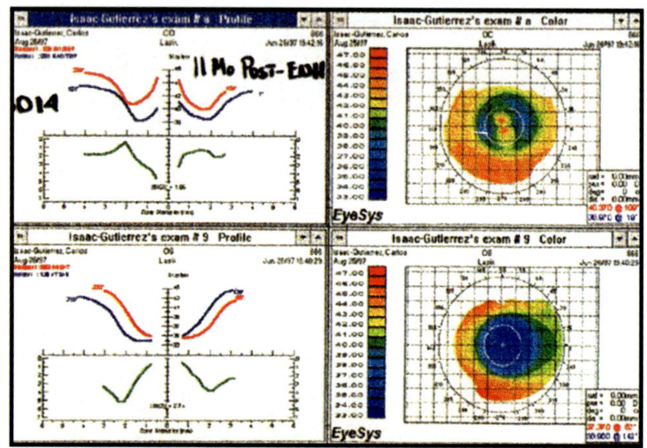

FIGURE 14.12: Patient 2 Post-enhancement (11 months later)

equivalent refraction was –2.85 ± 2.17 D. They found that ablation zones following retreatment should be ≥ 5.00 mm and remain unchanged to improve visual performance.

Like much of medicine, there are no hard-and-fast rules to LASIK enhancement. Each surgeon has his or her own guidelines on why, when and how to re-treat. Many times, the need for enhancement is based purely on patient perception; but in some circumstances, there may be a clinical indication. In any case, LASIK enhancement is an integral part of the refractive surgeon's practice.[19]

SUMMARY

LASIK improves refractive predictability, since the residual defects can be improved or corrected, simply by lifting the flap and applying a new ablation. If this procedure is done following the correct parameters of time and technique, we can be assured of obtaining excellent optical and surgical results.

REFERENCES

1. Guttman, C. Topography-guided LASIK enhancement advantageous. Quality of vision enhanced in eyes with small eccentric ablations, irregular astigmatism. Ophthalmology Times Apr 1, 2005 . Available at http://ot.adv100.com/ophthalmologytimes/article/articleDetail.jsp?id=153461. Accessed April 22, 2005.
2. Guell JL, Muller A: Lasik in situ keratomileusis (LASIK) for myopia from -7.00 to -28.00 diopters. J Refractive Surgery 1996;12:228-38.
3. Chayet A, Assil K, Montes et al: Regression and its mechanism after laser in situ keratomileusis in moderate and high myopia. Ophthalmology 1998;105:1194-9.
4. Qi H, et al. Excimer retreatment for undercorrection or regression after laser in situ keratomileusis. Zhonghua Yan Ke Za Zhi 2002;38(2):72-5.
5. Hersh PS, Fry KL, Bishop DS. Incidence and associations of retreatment after LASIK. Ophthalmol 2003;110(4):748-54.
6. Perlman EM, Reinert SE. Factors influencing the need for enhancement after laser in situ keratomileusis. J Refract Surg. 2004 Nov-Dec;20(6):783-9.
7. Durrie DS, Vande Garde TL. LASIK enhancements. Int Ophthalmol Clin. 2000 Summer;40(3):103-10
8. Walter KA, Stevenson AW. Effect of environmental factors on myopic LASIK enhancement rates. J Cataract Refract Surg. 2004 Apr;30(4):798-803.
9. Hu DJ, et al. Predictive formula for calculating the probability of LASIK enhancement. J Cataract Refract Surg. 2004 Feb;30(2):363-8.

10. Muallem MS, et al. Flap and stromal bed thickness in laser in situ keratomileusis enhancement. J Cataract Refract Surg. 2004;30(11):2295-302.
11. Randleman JB, et al. A comparison of 2 methods for estimating residual stromal bed thickness before repeat LASIK. Ophthalmology. 2005 Jan;112(1):98-103.
12. Suarez E: KMSG Hotline 1999.
13. Domniz Y, et al. Recutting the cornea versus lifting the flap: comparison of two enhancement techniques following laser in situ keratomileusis. J Refract Surg 2001; 17(5):505-10.
14. Netto MV, Wilson SE: Flap lift for LASIK retreatment in eyes with myopia. Ophthalmology 2004 Jul;111(7):1362-7.
15. Perez-Santonja JJ, et al. Circular flap rhexis: a refinement technique for LASIK re-treatment Arch Soc Esp Oftalmol 2001;76(5):303-8.
16. Suresh PS, Rootman DS. Bilateral infectious keratitis after a laser in situ keratomileusis enhancement procedure. Cataract Refract Surg. 2002 Apr;28(4):720-1.
17. Rubinfeld RS et al. To lift or recut: changing trends in LASIK enhancement. J Cataract Refract Surg. 2003 Dec;29(12): 2306-17.
18. Alka R, Ramamurthy B, Namrata S, et al: Outcomes After Laser in situ Keratomileusis Retreatment in High Myopes. J Refract Surg 2003; 19:159-64.
19. Schena L. LASIK Enhancement: Why, When and How. EyeNet Magazine. Available at http://www.aao.org/aao/news/eyenet/archive/06_01/refract.html. Accessed April 22,2005.

Chapter 15

LASIK: Complications and Management

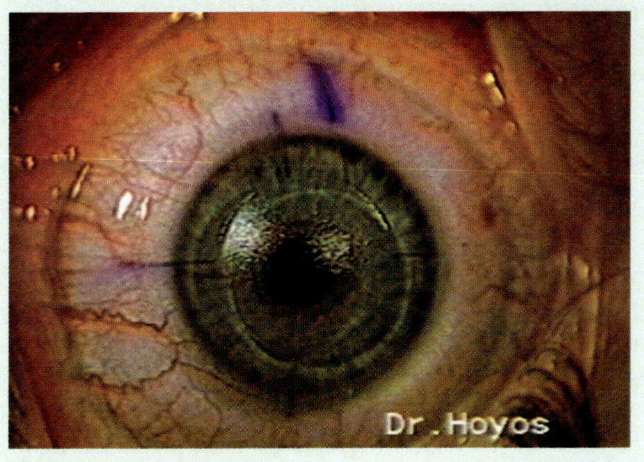

Melania Cigales
Jairo E Hoyos
Jairo Hoyos-Chacon
(Spain)

INTRODUCTION

In the last few years, owing to the speed of surgery and visual recovery along with a good visual outcome, LASIK has become the most popular refractive technique. However, like all surgical procedures, LASIK is not without its possible complications. These complications can be intraoperative, arising while creating the flap with the microkeratome or during ablation with the excimer laser. The incidence of these complications diminishes throughout the surgeon's learning curve and with each technological development. However, even when surgery is successfully undertaken, complications may also appear in the postoperative period. Herein, we discuss the most common complications of LASIK and their management.

MICROKERATOME COMPLICATIONS

One of the most important steps when performing LASIK surgery is creating the corneal flap using the microkeratome. A good corneal flap needs to be smooth and even, of an appropriate thickness including the epithelium, Bowman's membrane and anterior stroma, and of a diameter that allows the exposure of sufficient stromal bed to perform the ablation. At times, the characteristics of flap obtained are not those desired, and we should be very aware of the possible complications that can arise while creating the flap using the microkeratome. In this way, we will be able to prevent them or suitably resolve any complications that do occur.

Free Cap

To create the flap, we must stop the motion of the microkeratome before it completes its full stroke, or alternatively use a stopper. When the corneal disk finishes up unattached to the cornea by a hinge, then we have what is called a free cap (Figure 15.1). Perhaps the most frequent cause of a free cap is, however, a very flat cornea. Patients with flat corneas and a mean keratometry of less than 41 diopters present a higher risk of a free cap occurring.[1] A flat cornea will protrude relatively less into the suction ring compared to a steep cornea, and this will give rise to a smaller diameter disk and a free cap. This problem only affects primary flat corneas since a flat cornea secondary to refractive surgery will behave exactly as the original cornea curvature. Some microkeratomes include calibration lenses that help calibrate the stopper

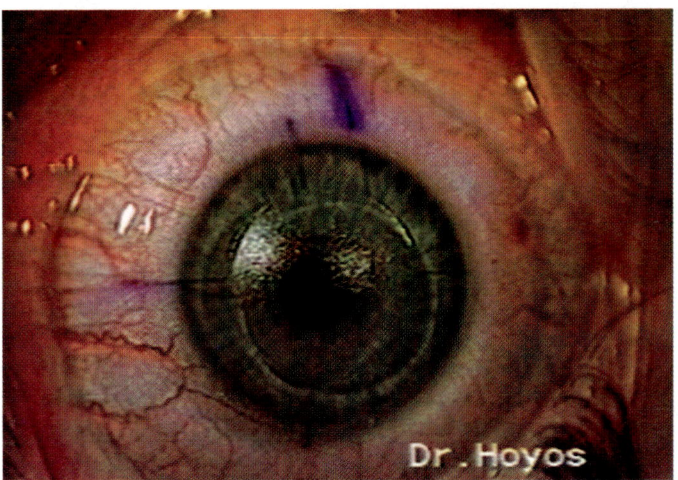

FIGURE 15.1: Free cap

depending on the diameter predicted for the flap. Other instruments have several suction rings and stoppers which are selected according to the keratometric readings.

When a free cap is obtained, we are confronted with two potential complications during the surgical procedure. The most serious of these is that it is often impossible to differentiate between the epithelial and stromal sides of the disk.[2] If the disk is replaced with the epithelial side face-down, there is a risk of epithelialization of the interface and loss of the disk. A further complication arises from the difficulty of repositioning the disk in its exact position. If the disk is rotated on the stromal bed, this commonly gives rise to astigmatism. Every LASIK surgeon must be aware of the possibility of a free cap and must be prepared for this complication by always using the epithelial reference markings.

When a free cap occurs, we can continue with the surgical procedure and place the disk in an anti-desiccation chamber with the epithelial surface facing downwards[3] during the ablation step. Once the ablation is complete, the disk can then be repositioned and the markings aligned until the disk has attached to its bed.

Incomplete Flap

During a keratectomy, the microkeratome can stop before completing its stroke and give rise to an incomplete flap and a corneal bed of insufficient size to perform an ablation (Figure 15.2). Some microkeratomes have a protection mechanism whereby they automatically stop if there is a loss of suction pressure while conducting the keratectomy, designed to impede continuous cutting and greater complications.[4] However, at times the driving

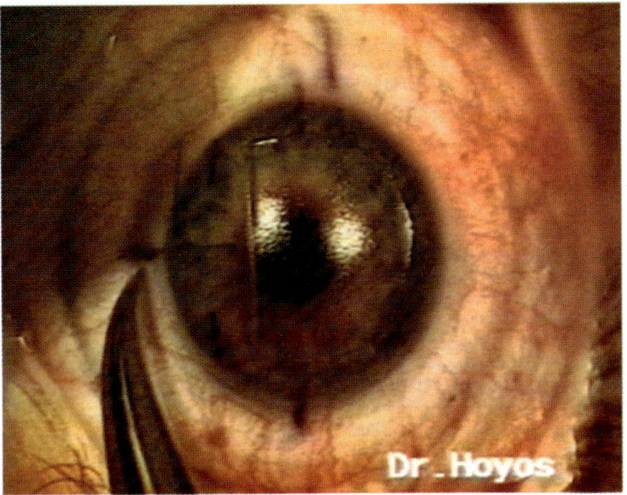

FIGURE 15.2: Incomplete flap

motor of the instrument may fail.[4] One of the most common reasons for an automatic microkeratome with an electric motor to breakdown is entry of the water used to help the instrument slide. It is, therefore, recommended that we have the microkeratome checked by the manufacture on a routine basis. In other cases, the microkeratome becomes blocked by the blepharostat, the eyelashes or eyelids.[1] It is thus essential that we prepare the surgical field well, covering eyelids and eyelashes with adhesive strips so that they do not interrupt the microkeratome stroke. Also, only use blepharostats that open the eye widely.

The size of the exposed corneal bed can be measured with callipers to check whether is will be large enough for the ablation. We could even perform the ablation by slightly decreasing the optical zone and protect the hinge to avoid its ablation. However, when the exposed bed is insufficient for ablation, surgery should be suspended; we should not attempt to prolong the keratectomy by manual dissection because this induces irregular astigmatism which is not easily resolved.[5] A few months later, a slightly deeper keratectomy can be attempted. If we make it shallower and part of the first flap remains on the bed, during ablation, tissue might be moved and lost provoking irregular astigmatism and intense hyperopization.[6]

Thin Flaps, Buttonholes and Irregular Cuts

It is widely accepted by LASIK surgeons that the ideal flap thickness is 130-160 microns. This measure is determined by the plate in the microkeratome head. However, most microkeratomes generally produce thinner cuts than expected and several pachymetric studies have indicated a high degree of variability in the thicknesses achieved.[7] Thin flaps are commonly associated with the complication of a central hole known as a buttonhole (Figure 15.3). The most common causes of thin flaps, buttonholes and irregular cuts are: inadequate suction, poor blade quality, steep corneas and microkeratome malfunction.[8]

The suction ring induces an ocular hypertension above the 70-100 mmHg required to perform the keratectomy. A lack of pressure may be due to inadequate fitting of the suction ring on the eyeball. This commonly occurs in the case of small sunken orbits or astigmatic eyes, over which it is difficult to place the ring.[8] If suction is completely lost and the microkeratome continues to function, we will obtain a free, irregular and small cut possibly affecting

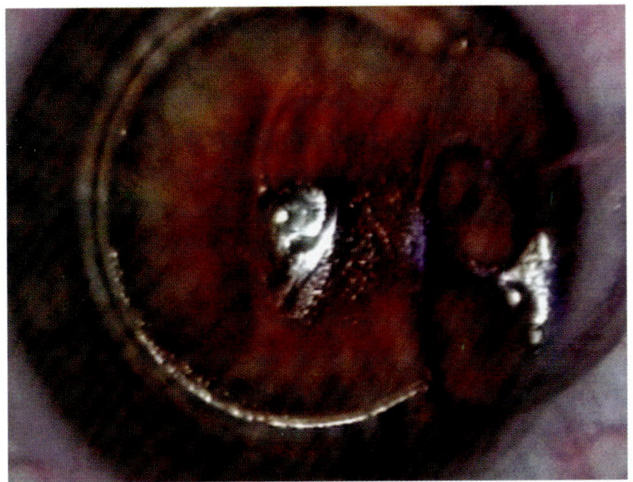

FIGURE 15.3: Buttonhole

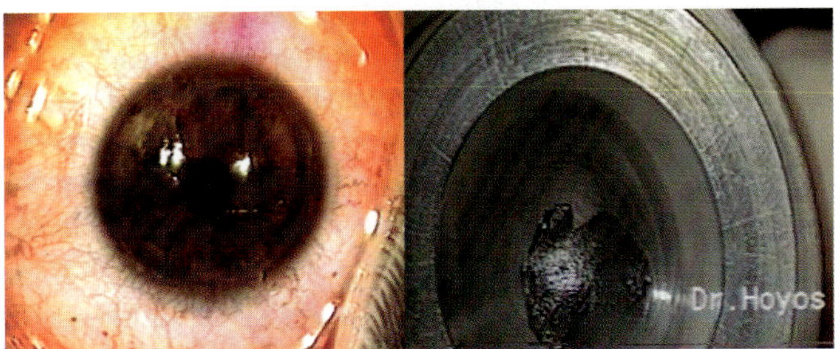

FIGURE 15.4: Lost suction

the pupillary area[1] (Figure 15.4). Most of the new instruments have a protection mechanism to stop cutting when there is a loss in suction pressure. These models at most will give rise to an incomplete flap.

A dull blade creates a thin and perhaps irregular cut.[9] Sometimes, remnants of Bowman's membrane can be

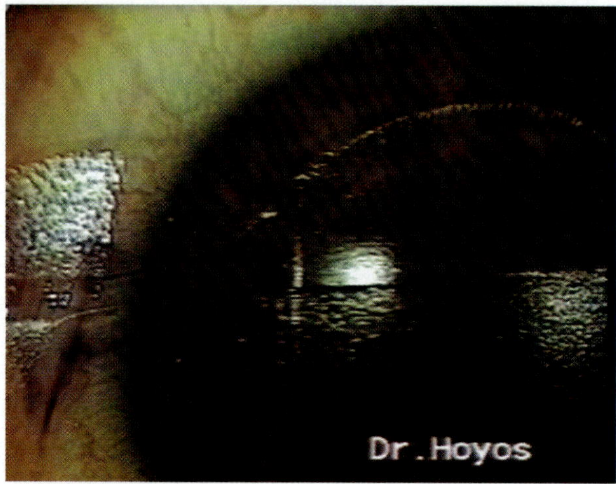

FIGURE 15.5: Thin, irregular flap

seen on the stromal bed (Figure 15.5). Blade quality varies considerably and for this reason it is crucial to check and calibrate the blade in order to reject those with an irregular edge or a small gap (the distance between the blade and plate correlates with the thickness of the keratectomy).[8] Many surgeons reuse the same blade on 4 or 6 eyes. After each pass, the blade looses its sharpness creating a thinner cut each time. We therefore recommend using a new blade for each patient.

Corneal curvatures greater than 46 diopters cause thin and large diameter disks and carry a risk of buttonhole formation due to corneal buckling during the microkeratome pass.[2] In the case of a steep cornea, we recommend the use of a 180 microns plate or a blade with a larger gap.

While performing the keratectomy, the microkeratome should be guided such that it undergoes uniform

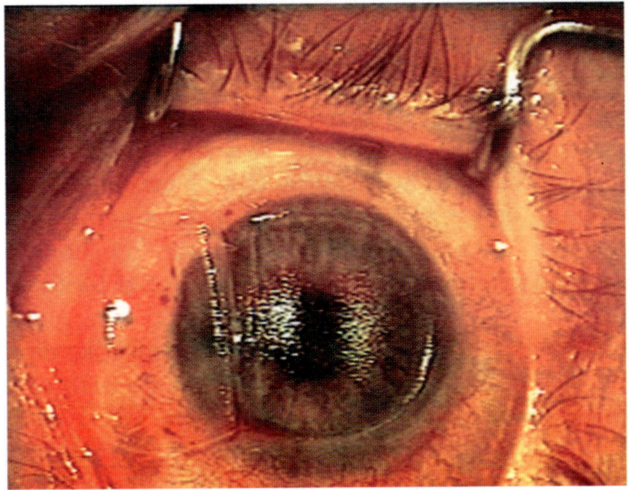

FIGURE 15.6: Irregular cut

movements to achieve a smooth, even corneal bed. Any malfunction of the automatic microkeratome, or slipping of the manual instrument, preventing a uniform stroke can give rise to an irregular resection leading to an uneven stromal bed (Figure 15.6) and thus to irregular astigmatism.

We believe than whenever one of these complications occurs at the time of creating the flap, the best thing is to interrupt the procedure and replace the flap, and then attempt another keratectomy 3 or 6 months later using a thicker plate.

Epithelial Defects

The epithelium of the corneal flap can become damaged during the keratectomy causing late and painful visual recovery. This complication is more common in diabetic or elderly patients or in those with dystrophy of the Bowman's membrane since the corneal epithelium is more fragile.[10] In this subset of patients, both eyes may show epithelial alterations. However, there are also certain intraoperative conditions that will induce damage to epithelial cells such as excessive topical anesthetic, which can be toxic for this delicate layer, or a keratectomy performed on a dry epithelium.[4] Anesthetics should be kept to a minimum and if possible should be free of preservatives. Moreover, the cornea should be moistened at the time of the keratectomy to help the microkeratome slide over the cornea and try to prevent abrasion of the corneal epithelium.

If the corneal epithelium is damaged, we should be careful when handling the flap and should meticulously wash the interface to avoid seeding epithelial cells causing its epithelialization.[2] We prefer to reposition the altered epithelium, but if this is not possible we carefully remove it. To avoid a painful postoperative course, it is best to include a mydriatic in the patient's normal medication and cover the eye or use a therapeutic contact lens until the cornea becomes re-epithelialized. The postoperative course of these cases is usually good, although there are reports of recurrent erosion syndromes,[11] which could be caused by a pre-existing dystrophy of the Bowman's membrane going unnoticed in the preoperative examination. A further possible cause is the transient corneal denervation that occurs after LASIK.

Corneal Bleeding

Corneal bleeding usually occurs in contact lens wearers, who often have more corneal neovessels[4] (Figure 15.7).

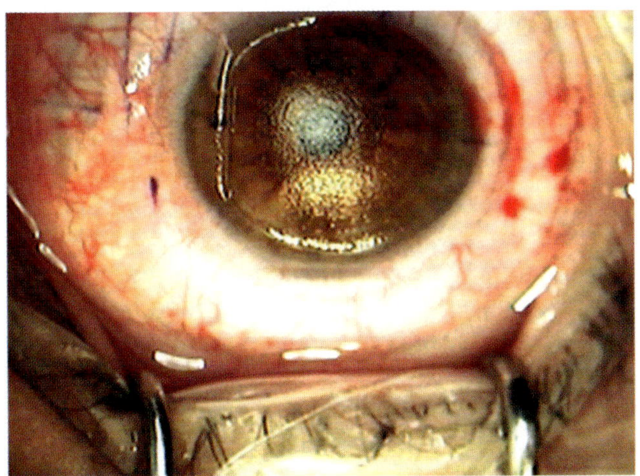

FIGURE 15.7: Corneal bleeding

To prevent corneal bleeding in such cases, the keratectomy may be slightly decentered downwards to avoid cutting neovessels. Bleeding also occurs when the diameter of the corneal flap is excessive and almost practically reaches the limbus.[4] This frequently happens when the cornea is very steep and can sometimes be prevented using a suction ring that yields a smaller flap diameter. This complication is commonly related to the use of certain microkeratomes such as the Hansatome.

Every effort should be made to stop bleeding and we should try to avoid the blood invading the interface during ablation since this might cause uneven ablation. We can wait a few minutes without lifting the flap until the hemorrhage resolves. Compression maneuvers or the use of a sponge with vasoconstrictor over the area of blood loss may be useful.[2] Once ablation is complete, we should make sure we leave no blood remnants at the interface, which should be carefully washed to avoid triggering an inflammation process.

Corneal Perforation

Corneal perforation is the most serious complication related to the use of the microkeratome which occurs when we forget to position the plate in the instrument head or when it is not properly adjusted.[12] Due to an increased intraocular pressure during keratectomy, corneal perforation is usually associated with the partial or total loss of the iris and crystalline lens and even with the loss of eye contents (Figure 15.8). The management of this complication is complex and stressful, but we should try

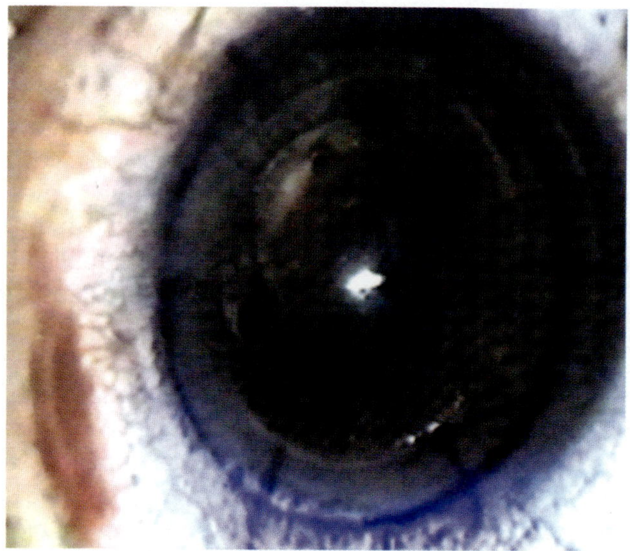

FIGURE 15.8: Corneal perforation

to remain calm and attempt to recompose the globe with the help of viscoelastic, followed by suturing the cornea. At a later date, we will select the best surgical option to restore the patient's vision.

To avoid this devastating complication, new microkeratome models do not have interchangeable plates; their have different heads to obtained different cutting depths.

LASER COMPLICATIONS

Since the first excimer laser was designed in one of IBM's laboratories in 1987, there have been numerous technical advances that have induced the rapid development of laser technology. This has meant a rapidly declining incidence of complications caused by applying the excimer laser on the stromal bed, which are also ever less serious. We propose several therapeutic options for the treatment of these complications.

Decentered Ablation

A decentered ablation may give rise to irregular astigmatism (Figure 15.9) and to symptoms such as glare, ghosting, monocular diplopia, impaired night vision, reduced contrast sensitivity and even loss of best corrected visual acuity.[13] Although small decentrations are usually asymptomatic,[14] symptoms are exacerbated when treatment involves small optical zones or correcting high refractive errors.[15]

The surgeon should first ensure that the laser beam is correctly centered before initiating the laser session and the patient must be correctly positioned under the excimer

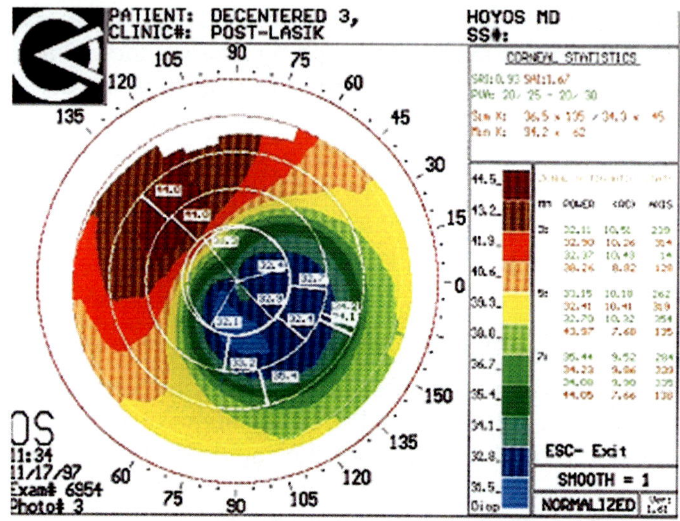

FIGURE 15.9: Decentered ablation

laser. It is helpful to constantly encourage the patient to fix his/her sight on the fixation target. Finally, it is the surgeon's task to adequately center refractive treatment, although there is a lack of consensus concerning the point over which an ablation should be centered: at the corneal reflex or center of the pupil.[16] Most modern lasers have a built-in eye-tracking device which, despite avoiding severe decentration, cannot ensure perfect centering.[17] Several surgical treatments have been proposed for decentered ablations over the last few years. Pallikaris[18] suggests relaxed corneal incisions in the steep zone. Pallikaris[19] and Talamo[20] also advocate smoothing the corneal surface using a viscous solution and performing a phototherapeutic ablation until an even optical surface is achieved. In 1995, Seiler performed an ablation on the opposite side as treatment. The procedure involved establishing the new ablation center by topography and calculating the dioptric power of the new ablation as the topographic difference between the two zones.[21,22] The development of Topolink appeared to be the solution to treating decentered ablations and irregular astigmatism.[23] The technique is based on a topographically-guided ablation using elevation topography and a previously programmed flying spot laser. In this way, the amount of ablation needed at different points on the cornea to achieve a smooth surface is calculated. The final outcome of all these treatment methods has, nevertheless, been highly inconsistent. Customized ablations based on wavefront analysis have recently emerged as the latest treatment option for this complication.

In 1995, we treated a decentered ablation for the first time in a patient who had undergone *in situ* keratomileusis (ALK), by ablating the opposite side by LASIK retreatment.[24] Through elevation topography, we were able to establish the point at which to center treatment and the amount of tissue to be ablated according to the elevation difference in microns indicated in the topographic map. It is currently possible to simulate eccentric ablation treatment using topographic simulation programes that predict the topographic outcome before initiating treatment[25] (Figure 15.10). We presently use the PAR Vision System topographer to measure the elevation and depression in microns at different points on the cornea with respect to a perfect sphere. Thus, points that correspond to a perfect sphere have an elevation of zero. Elevation values in microns are given a plus sign and depression values are indicated with a minus sign. The

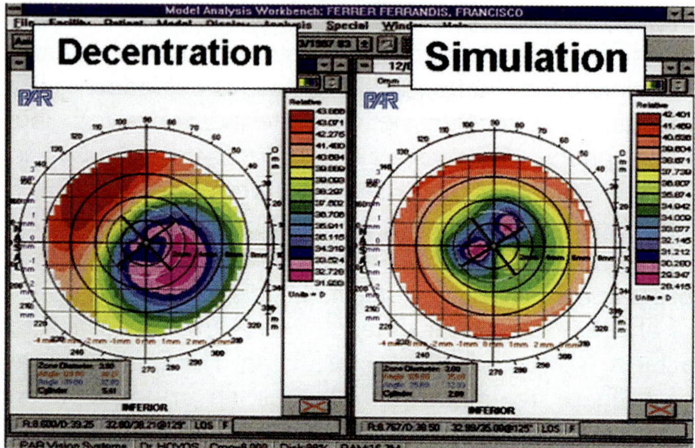

FIGURE 15.10: Treating decentrations by guided topographic simulation: Outcome

topographer determines the center of the decentered ablation and its depression. We use the 1 mm grille topographer tool to measure the distance from the middle of the decentered ablation to the visual axis at "x" and "y" axes. These measures are then used to pinpoint the opposite point ("mirror point") in the topography and the topographer measures the elevation at this point. We then use the simulation software to simulate a new ablation at the mirror point: The depth of the ablation is given by the sum of the elevation and depression calculated beforehand, and the optical zone corresponding to the best simulated topography is selected.

In cases of decentered LASIK, the flap is lifted using the technique normally employed in retreatments. The laser is programmed using the data obtained by guided topographic simulation (optical zone, ablation depth and mirror point). The laser then automatically decenters and focuses on the new ablation center at the established mirror point and the ablation is performed under patient self-fixation. Once treatment achieves a centered topography, the residual refractive error is retreated following a 3 months waiting period.

Central Islands

A central island is a central or paracentral steep area in the topography of 1 to 3 diopters in height and diameter 1 to 3 mm, measured at least 1 month postoperatively[26] (Figure 15.11). Symptoms include monocular diplopia, ghosting of images, fluctuating vision and sometimes loss of lines of corrected visual acuity.[27] Central islands are more frequent when a broad beam laser is used but there

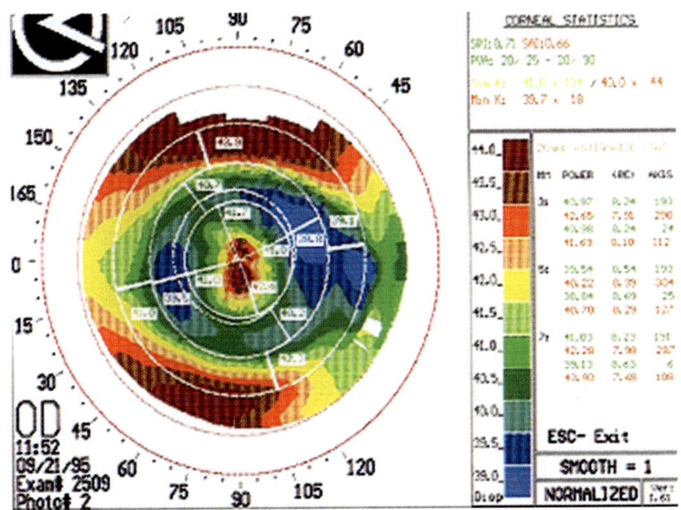

FIGURE 15.11: Central island

are some predisposing factors[28,29] such as a moist cornea during the ablation, large optical zones, high levels of correction, a damaged laser mirror and a laser beam cold in the center. To prevent this complication, we must check the laser mirror and laser beam homogeneity before initiating the laser session, and wipe the bed during the ablation if it is wet. The new broad beam lasers are equipped with anticentral island pretreatment software.

LASIK central islands show modifications during topographical follow-up. Most central islands resolve spontaneously during the first 3 to 4 months and do not require treatment.[30] A variety of surgical treatments have been described to treat elevated central island areas including central reablations,[31] topographically-guided ablations,[32] Healon-assisted PTK[33] and mechanical compression in the center of the cornea (G Avalos-personal communication). We have noted that patients with persisting central islands undergo an improvement in their visual acuity after 3 to 4 months, with a low residual myopic defect left. Three to four months after LASIK surgery, we retreat these patients by lifting the flap and treating the residual myopia with an optical zone 1 mm larger than the diameter of the topographical island.

POSTOPERATIVE COMPLICATIONS

The patient who undergoes LASIK should be subjected to early and frequent follow-up examinations to be able to identify and quickly treat any postoperative complications such as infection, inflammatory or traumatic processes in the corneal flap, as well as problems in the healing process. However, even after the postoperative follow-up period, we should continue to monitor these

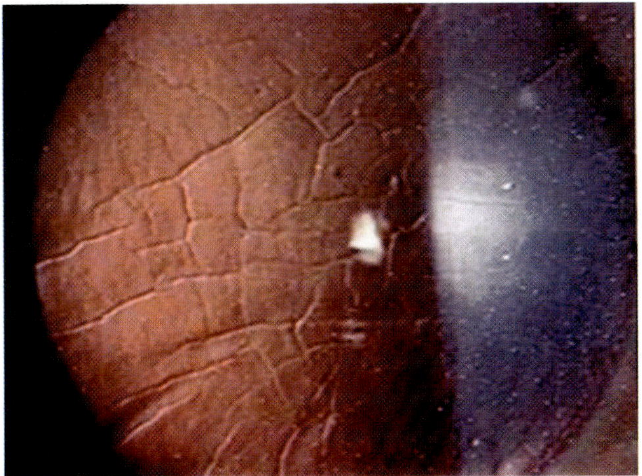

FIGURE 15.12: Flap folds and wrinkles

patients since serious complications can also occur in the longer term. Below we discuss the most common early and late complications of LASIK and options for their treatment.

Flap Folds and Wrinkles

One of the complications of LASIK is the formation of folds or striae in the corneal flap, causing irregular astigmatism and loss of visual acuity (Figure 15.12). Striae may form during surgery due to the incorrect repositioning of the flap over the stromal bed, or in the early postoperative period if the disk is slightly displaced by blinking.[34] In the past it was thought that the nasal flap was a cause of striae formation, since it promoted displacement during blinking in the early postoperative course. Displacement is less common with a superior flap but striae still appear. We generally observe horizontal striae in nasal flaps and vertical striae in superior flaps. In the early days of LASIK, flaps created with large hinges were easily correctly repositioned. Nowadays, however, to perform ablations with large optical zones and peripheral ablations to correct hyperopia, we try to create a flap of minimum hinge. In these cases, it is important to make epithelial reference marks and correctly align these when we reposition the flap over its bed. If the reference marks are misaligned, this means that the flap is wrinkled or slightly displaced leading to the formation of folds and striae. Striae formation is also more common in the case of a thin corneal disk. It is important to check for correct alignment using the slit-lamp, and if this complication is noted, to immediately lift the flap, hydrate it and reposition it by careful alignment.[35]

The LASIK surgeon should be aware of this complication and try to avoid it. If detected, folds and striae need to be rapidly treated. Opinions vary concerning treatment, but these measures are always aimed at rehydrating the disk or de-epithelialization after hydrating old folds.[36] Some years ago we presented a new technique for the treatment of flap striae with good results also for old striae.[37] The technique involves lifting the flap, hydrating, repositioning the flap over the stromal bed and massaging the flap using a spatula over a contact lens. Unlike other methods of treatment, this massaging is effective at removing flap striae as late as one month after surgery.

Flap Loss

Today, whenever LASIK is performed, we use the microkeratome to try to create a corneal flap, since this is considered the safest way of preventing disk displacement and loss. If the microkeratome does not stop at the right moment the cut may result in a free cap. The complication most feared with a free cap is the loss of the disk, such that certain precautions need to be taken before the patient leaves the clinic. First, the eyelids are closed using two crossed adhesive strips for approximately half an hour after surgery. We then check the patient and if we find that the disk has moved, we reposition it and close the lid until the next day. If the disk is found to be in the right position, the patient is sent home wearing only an eye shield and is instructed to follow the general directions for flaps. Due to the risk of losing the disk, we prefer to personally remove the eye shield or patch the next day such that we do not discard any dressing before making sure the disk is adhered to the cornea.

There have been reports of traumatic detachment of a disk despite having the security of a flap, and even cases of surgical amputation of the flap as an attempt to control an infection (Internet forum of the KM Study Group). In both these situations, some of the thickness of the cornea and the Bowman's membrane are lost. The most simple treatment option is to await the re-epithelialization of the cornea and to treat the case as we would treat a PRK to avoid haze.[38] One would think that as corneal tissue was removed, the eye would finish up with tremendous hyperopia, but the results obtain do not show any hyperopic deviations and residual defects are usually slightly irregular myopic astigmatisms.[38] We should not forget that the corneal disk has two parallel sides and therefore has no refractive power of its own. If the final visual outcome is unsatisfactory, we should move onto undertaking a lamellar keratoplasty.

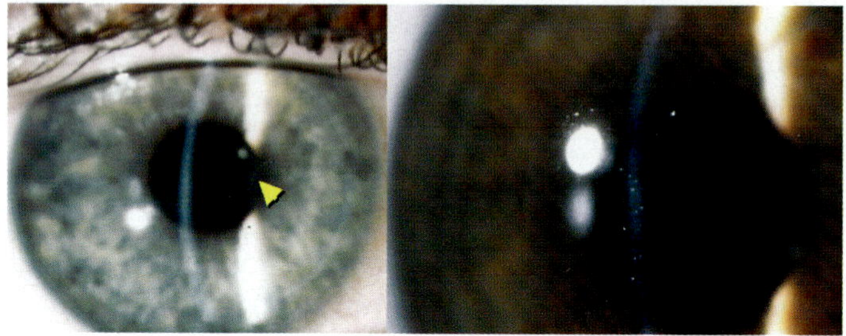

FIGURE 15.13: Interface debris

Interface Debris

On slit-lamp examination, it is sometimes possible to detect small particles at the flap/stromal interface (Figure 15.13). In general, these are of no clinical significance and they do not induce an inflammatory response, but in other cases they could give rise to Sands of the Sahara syndrome.[39] These could be metallic particles[40] from the microkeratome that are difficult to remove during irrigation of the interface. Sometimes, the particles are remnants of cosmetic products, small gauze or cotton threads, talc from the gloves or even secretions that become trapped at the interface when we reposition the flap. To prevent this complication, we should try to keep our surgery free of particles using gloves without talc and avoid the use of gauze, cotton threads or fabrics.[4] Eyelids and lashes should also be meticulously cleaned before surgery and the patient should be asked to avoid the use of eye make-up a few days before surgery. A further important factor is that the stromal side of the bed and flap have to be well cleaned using an irrigation-aspiration system when repositioning the flap. Irrigating the interface with a fine cannula after the flap has been repositioned to remove any trapped particles is also recommended.

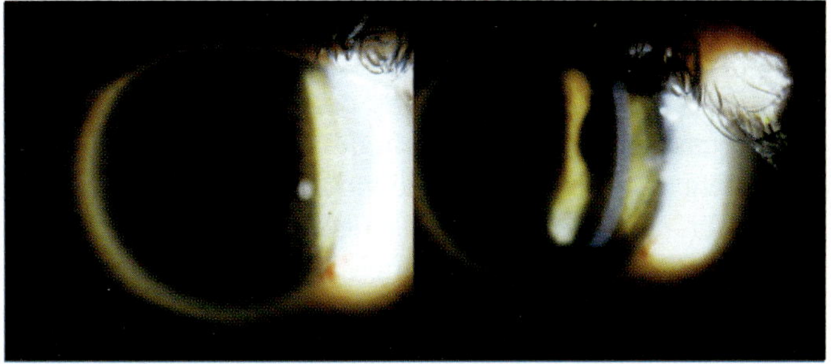

FIGURE 15.14: Sands of the Sahara syndrome

Sands of the Sahara Syndrome

Inflammation of the interface was first described by Robert Maddox who named this phenomenon Sands of the Sahara syndrome, given its desert sand-like appearance[41] (Figure 15.14). This complication is also known as diffuse lamellar keratitis (DLK) and starts within the first 24-48 hours following surgery with the appearance of a diffuse infiltrate at the interface, reduced visual acuity, pain, red eye and topographical irregularity.[39] Microscopy studies have demonstrated the presence of inflammatory cells at the interface.[42] The causes of this inflammation are not clear, but it has been related to the presence of particles at the interface,[39] particles on the microkeratome blades,[41] methods of cleaning the surgical instruments,[43] etc. The risk of this complication is multiplied when there is an epithelial defect[44] and cases have been reported both in primary LASIK surgery and retreatments. Possible causes should be kept in mind to try to avoid this complication in as much as possible.

An early diagnosis and treatment are essential for successfully resolving this complication. Treatment involves increasing topical corticosteroids and in cases of intense inflammation, the flap should be lifted and the interface profusely rinsed to remove the possible toxic substance.[39] These cases are generally effectively resolved with the complete recovery of visual acuity and no sequelae. However, some surgeons describe a greater difficulty in lifting the flap when retreatment is required (Internet forum of the KM Study Group). We should always establish a differential diagnosis from infectious keratitis of the interface.

Epithelial Ingrowth

The proliferation of epithelial cells at the flap/stromal bed interface (Figure 15.15) is a complication that lessens throughout the surgeon's learning curve as the surgical maneuvers aimed at avoiding the introduction of epithelium under the flap improve. This complication is more common in certain situations:

- Retreatments, in which epithelial strands are produced, promoting epithelialization.[45]
- When an epithelial defect is produced during surgery because of an already altered corneal epithelial

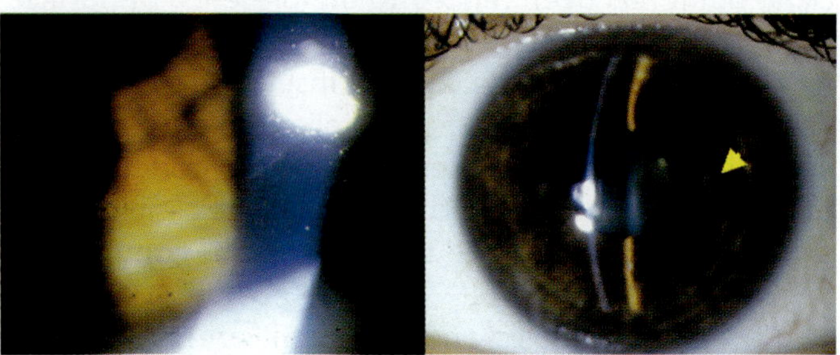

FIGURE 15.15: Epithelial ingrowth

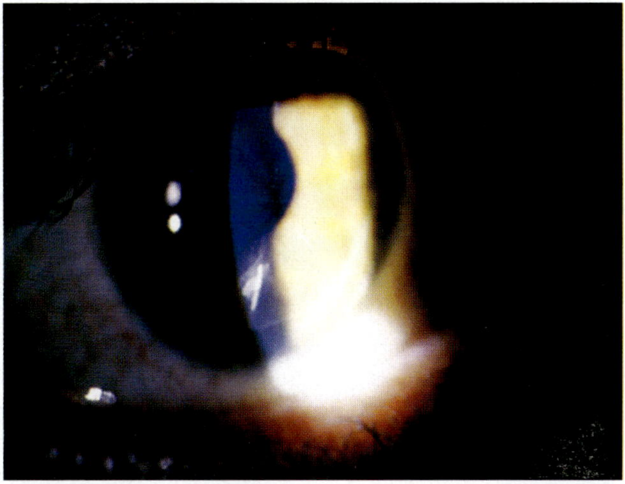

FIGURE 15.16: Epithelial ingrowth through radial keratotomy incisions

basement membrane (elderly or diabetic patients or patients with corneal dystrophy), detached epithelial cells may settle at the interface.[45,46]

- When there is inflammation of the interface causing flap edema this induces peripheral epithelial invasion.[45]
- During hyperopic LASIK, a peripheral ablation will induce the advance of the epithelium from the stromal bed.[47]
- In the case of flaps with radial keratotomy incisions, epithelialization occurs through the insicions[48] (Figure 15.16).

In most cases, epithelial ingrowth occurs as small self-contained peripheral islets observed at 2-3 weeks that do not grow nor cause any symptoms. Thus, no treatment is necessary. However, sometimes epithelial ingrowth

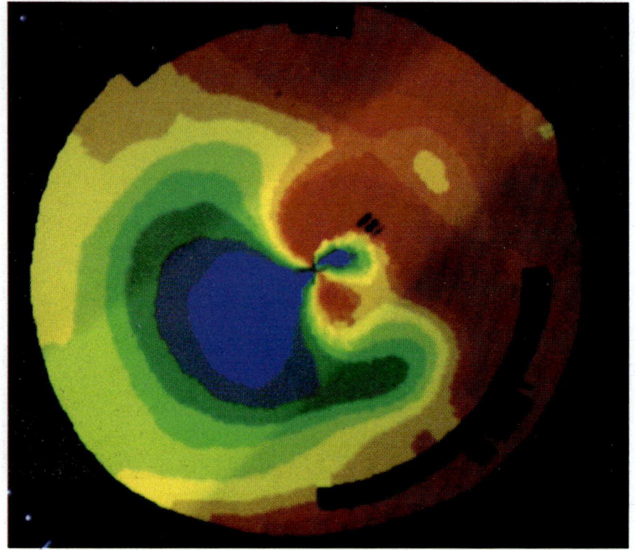

FIGURE 15.17: Epithelial ingrowth causes irregular astigmatism

continues and gives rise to irregular astigmatism and reduced visual acuity such that it needs to be removed[45] (Figure 15.17). There are descriptions of cases of epithelialization causing melting of the flap, attributed to defects in the supply of nutrients to the flap or inflammatory processes secondary to epithelialization.[49] Most cases of melting are peripheral, self-contained and of no clinical significance.

The treatment of epithelial ingrowth is not always definitive and there is always a risk of recurrence. Treatment consists of lifting the flap and scraping the epithelium of the interface. Several surgical treatments have been proposed for recurrences: absolute alcohol, PTK performed on both stromal surfaces, YAG laser treatment and on some occasions, it has even been necessary to amputate the flap and perform a lamellar keratoplasty.[50] We know that during the epithelial healing process of the cornea, epithelium growth from the flap and from the epithelial border of the bed, contacting in the flap border with a risk of recurrence. For this reason we scrape the epithelium of the bed until the limbus and both epithelium growth, contacting near to the limbus and far to the flap border. We should not wait until the epithelium colonises the central zone of the cornea before embarking on treatment, since after removing the ingrowth tissue we are usually left with a leukoma at the interface which could reduce the patient's final visual acuity.

Infection

Infection in uncommon in LASIK surgery since the edge of the flap becomes re-epithelialized a few hours later, thus rapidly restoring the epithelial barrier. However, when this complication arises, its effects are devastating since the focus of infection occurs at the interface and is related to a high risk of corneal perforation and endophthalmitis. Infections can be:

- Intraoperative—due to contamination of the surgical instruments or field of surgery.
- Postoperative—when the patient does not complete the antibiotic prophylaxis regime or exposes him-/herself to a risk of infection in the early postoperative period such as water sports, use of eye make-up, eye trauma, etc.

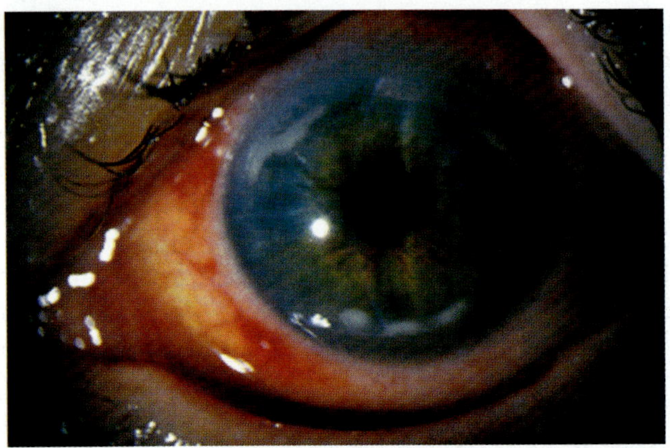

FIGURE 15.18: Infection

Patients with blepharitis are at an increased risk of infection and should be diagnosed and treated before surgery.

The clinical signs of bacterial infection can appear in the first few days but when symptoms appear after several weeks, the causative agent is a fungus, an acanthamoeba or slow-growing bacterium.[51] Patients experience pain, weeping, photophobia and blurred vision, symptoms not pathognomic for diagnosis. A slit-lamp examination reveals conjunctival hyperemia, corneal infiltrates or ulcers (Figure 15.18), flap melting, an inflammatory reaction in the anterior chamber and hypopyon.

When infection is suspected, we should first treat the patient as for a corneal abscess by topical hourly administration of wide-spectrum antibiotics against gram-positive and gram-negative microorganisms. This regime can then be modified according to subsequent culture and antiobiogram results.[51] Some cases require lifting the flap and irrigating the interface with an antibiotic solution.[52] The need for flap amputation[53] or a hot penetrating keratoplasty[54] have also been described. Once the infection is controlled, subsequent surgical measures to improve the visual acuity lost because of the resultant corneal opacity and irregularity will need to be considered.

Dry Eye

Refractive corneal surgery can lead to temporarily reduced tear production lasting weeks or months which appears to be related to the transient corneal denervation that occurs after surgery.[55] As the flap is cut, we also cut the nerve endings of the cornea, causing corneal hypoesthesia that gives rise to reduced tear production, taking months to resolve.[56] The highest density of nerve fibers enters the cornea through the nasal and temporal zones and it is therefore speculated that a superior flap will cause more denervation and greater tear secretion disruption than a nasal flap.[57] Although this complication does not greatly affect the final refractive outcome, over some months, patients complain of visual acuity fluctuations and transient episodes of regression and induced astigmatism which are difficult to correct with spectacles.[58] On slit-lamp examination we can observe a superficial punctate epitheliopathy (Figure 15.19) and the topography shows an irregular cornea.

In our personal experience, these cases benefit from the use of preservative-free artificial tears and blocking the inferior lacrimal punctum. The recommended use of artificial tears during the first postoperative months is general to all patients undergoing corneal refractive surgery

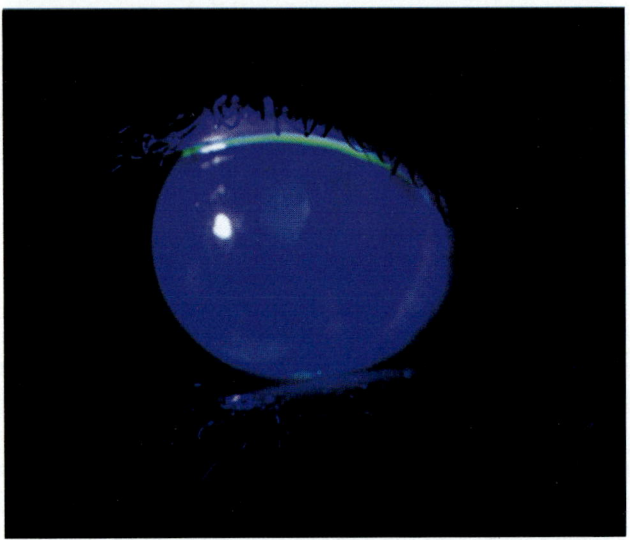

FIGURE 15.19: Superficial punctate epitheliopathy after LASIK

and attempts to avoid visual and refractive fluctuations caused by the reduced tear production. In the preoperative evaluation, we should include the Schirmer test and lacrimal BUT to identify cases of lacrimal hyposecretion that could worsen in the first few weeks after surgery. When preoperative lacrimal hyposecretion is moderate or mild, we should try to improve the quality and quantity of tears before indicating surgery using lacrimal punctum plugs, artificial tears and tear stimulating drugs. We do not recommend corneal surgery in cases of severely impaired tear secretion.

Regression, Undercorrection and Overcorrection

The tissue repair process induced by LASIK surgery is accompanied by a regression of the effect achieved by surgery related to changes in corneal topography.[59] The scarring response varies in each patient precluding any generalizations. Regression has been associated with epithelial hypertrophy.[60] Most regression is thought to occur during the first weeks, and in this period patients describe visual fluctuations as a consequence of topographic and refractive changes.[59-61] Some authors[62] suggest that the length of the stabilizing period depends on the number of diopters corrected and estimate a month for each diopter. Accordingly, if we correct 1 diopter the stabilizing period will be one month, whereas if 10 diopters are corrected the stabilization process will last 10 months. It is true that the greater the correction the longer the period of stabilization.[61] In our routine practice, we usually wait at least a month before assessing refraction for the first time, although in the case of a residual refractive defect we normally wait 3 to 6 months before we make any decision on the possible benefits of retreatment.

Once refractive stability has been reached, there is always the possibility of a remaining refractive defect. Current nomograms have improved the predictability of refractive surgery, but residual refractive defects continue to occur. The gas in the excimer laser is highly unstable and can fluctuate with changes in humidity, pressure and temperature provoking under- and overcorrections. The environmental conditions in the surgery room should be well controlled to avoid laser action fluctuations. Depending on the refractive and visual outcome, the

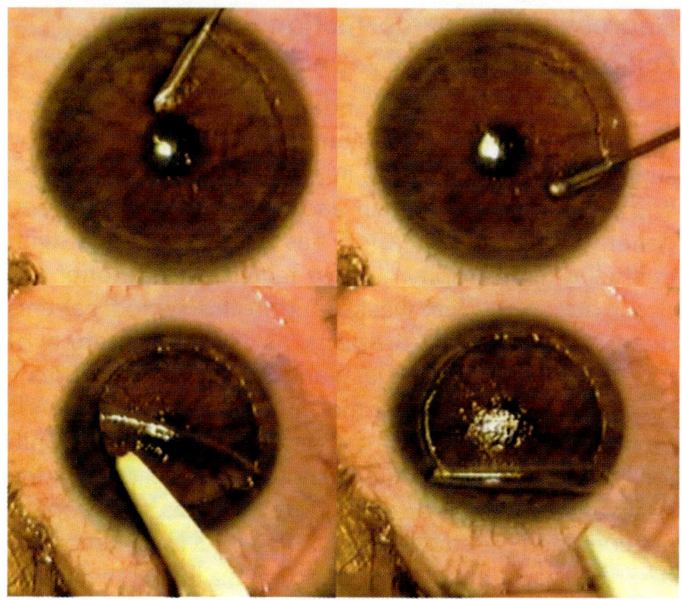

FIGURE 15.20: Lifting the flap

degree of patient satisfaction and the limits of refractive surgery (corneal thickness and curvature), we may want to perform a retreatment. Under- and overcorrections after LASIK can be treated by the same technique, lifting the flap or recutting.[63,64] After eight years of experience in myopic LASIK, we currently try to lift the flap whenever possible (Figure 15.20). This is more difficult after hyperopic LASIK, and we have observed cases in which it was not possible to lift the flap after 2 years. If we create a new flap we should try to make it thicker than the first to avoid loss of tissue which would induce high hyperopia and irregular astigmatism, both being difficult to correct.[6]

However, flap thickness, corneal curvature and repeat refractive surgeries pose a limit to retreatments using corneal techniques, and in some cases, the only surgical treatment option is the implant of an intraocular lens.

Corneal Ectasia

Post-LASIK corneal ectasia manifests as a progressive myopia accompanied by topographic incurving and loss of visual acuity, months or years after the intervention.[65] Topographical analysis is usually the key to detecting this complication.

Since the advent of keratomileusis, there have been descriptions of ectasia related to lamellar techniques, and from the beginning it was established that we should leave a residual stromal bed of 250 microns under the ablation. Some authors prefer a residual bed of 300 microns and others believe we should leave at least 50 percent of the corneal thickness under the ablation.[66] However, we should not forget the extensive range of microkeratome cutting depths, and after making our calculations may find the flap is too thick, highlighting the importance of intraoperative pachymetry.[7,67] Besides leaving a 250 micron residual bed, we try to leave a total corneal thickness of at least 400 microns and never ablate more than 150 microns. We should be particularly careful with retreatment LASIK. First, we should make a differential diagnosis between undercorrection and regression. We should also be aware of the thickness of the cornea so that we do not find ourselves with the surprise of an ectasia after retreating a minimal residual defect.

In some cases there can be a subclinical preoperative keratoconus (Figure 15.21) and LASIK will enhance this

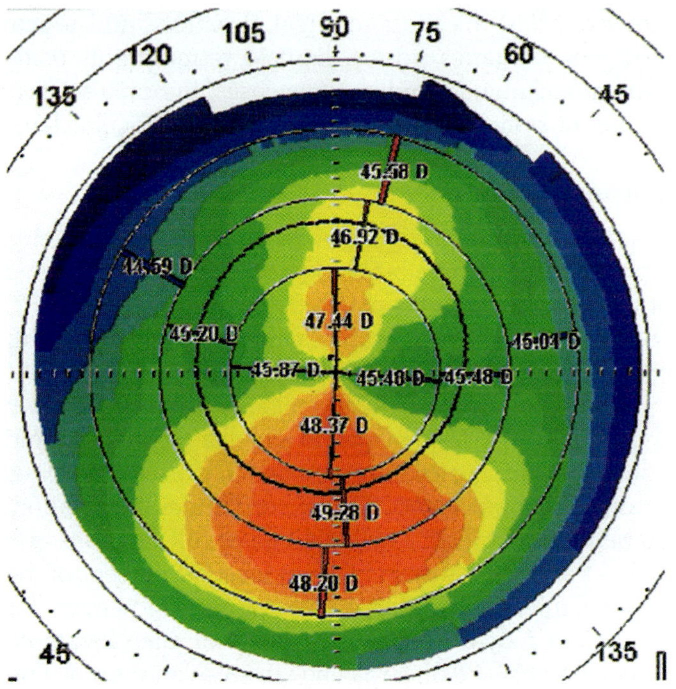

FIGURE 15.21: Sub-clinical keratoconus

corneal degenerative process. This possibility should be kept in mind and corneal surgery discouraged in patients with unstable myopia and a thinned or very steep cornea, especially if they also have some degree of asymmetric astigmatism.[68]

Treatments proposed in cases of ectasia are the use of a contact lens, intracorneal ring segments or penetrating or lamellar keratoplasty.[66,69]

Retinal Complications

There is little agreement among retinal specialists on the risks of LASIK, which include deterioration of the peripheral retina and the posterior pole in myopic patients. We believe that the suction ring used in LASIK to induce an intraocular pressure of 70-160 mmHg, placed 4 mm from the corneoscleral limbus, may produce traction against the anterior vitreous and on the vitreous base provoking stretching of the anterior hyaloid and possibly also of the posterior hyaloid (Figure 15.22). The suction ring time is variable, about 12 seconds, which is the minimum time needed to create the flap, but this time depends on the difficulty of each case, the surgeon's experience and whether suction is applied only during flap cutting or also during the ablation. Suction time is longer in the learning phase of the surgeon and may also vary with the type

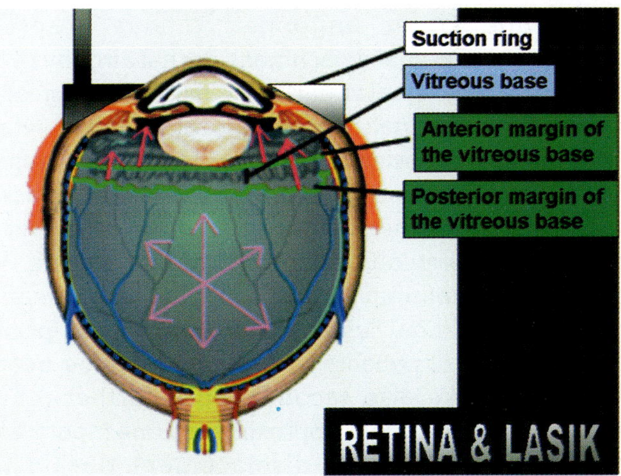

FIGURE 15.22: Suction ring induces vitreous traction

of microkeratome used. We believe the suction time is an important factor in producing changes in vitreous anatomy.[70]

During LASIK, intraocular pressure can be 70-160 mmHg. This hypertension can cause distension of the wall in an already established posterior staphyloma, with lengthening of the choriocapillaris—Bruch's membrane—pigment epithelium complex, producing lacquer cracks which will provoke submacular hemorrhages or subretinal neovascularization in the postoperative period.[71,72]

In a study performed on 755 eyes subjected to LASIK,[70] we detected retinal breaks in quadrants of generally low tear incidence (inferior-nasal sector), an increased intensity of white pressure-free areas, localized retinal detachment, peripheral retinal bleeding, pronounced circumferential folds, posterior extension and enhancement of the oral bays and macular hemorrhages from 12 days to two years post-LASIK. Other surgeons[71-74] have observed regmatogenous retinal detachment, partial atrophy of the optic nerve, paracentral visual field defects, the progression of previous subretinal neovascularization, giant retinal tears, increased posterior vitreous detachment, retinal branch venous occlusion and macular lacquer cracks.

The risk of further lesions post-LASIK is higher in patients with previous peripheral retinal lesions. We recommend examining and prophylactically treating predisposing retinal lesions with argon laser photocoagulation in all patients who are going to be treated with LASIK. We also recommend a further retinal examination post-LASIK, approximately one month later, carefully avoiding flap displacement during the examination.

REFERENCES

1. Jacobs JM, Taravella MJ. Incidence of intraoperative flap complications in laser in situ keratomileusis. J Cataract Refract Surg 2002;28(1):23-28.
2. Slade SG. LASIK complications and their management. Machat JJ (Eds). Excimer Laser Refractive Surgery. Thorofare, NJ: Slack Inc. 1996; 358-400.
3. Cigales M, Hoyos JE J. Free Caps. In: Lucio Buratto, Stephen Brint (Eds). Custom LASIK: Surgical Techniques and Complications. Thorofare-NJ, SLAK Inc. 2003; 226-27.
4. Buratto L, Brint S. Complications of LASIK. In: Buratto L, Brint S (Eds). Custom LASIK: Surgical Techniques and Complications. Thorofare-NJ, SLAK Inc. 2003; 161-224.
5. Holland SP, Srivannaboon S, Reinstein DZ. Avoiding serious corneal complications of laser assisted in situ keratomileusis and photorefractive keratectomy. Ophthalmology 2000; 107(4):640-52.
6. Peters NT, Iskander NG, Gimbel HV. Minimizing the risk of recutting with a Hansatome over an existing Automated Corneal Shaper flap for hyperopic laser in situ keratomileusis enhancement. J Cataract Refract Surg 2001;27(8):1328-32.
7. Gokmen F, Jester JV, Petroll WM, McCulley JP, Cavanagh HD. In vivo confocal microscopy through-focusing to measure corneal flap thickness after laser in situ keratomileusis. J Cataract Refract Surg. 2002;28(6):962-70.
8. Cigales M, Hoyos JE. J. Thin flaps and buttonholes. In: Buratto L, Brint S (Eds). Custom LASIK: Surgical Techniques and Complications. Thorofare-NJ, SLAK Inc. 2003;224-25.
9. Cummings A, Lavery F. Flap complications. In: Agarwal S, Agarwal A, Pallikaris IG, Neuhann TH, Knorz MC, Agarwal A (Eds). Refractive Surgery. New Delhi: Jaypee Brothers Medical Publishers 2000; 329-39.
10. Krüger J. Managing recurrent epithelial ingrowth. In: Buratto L, Brint S (Eds). Custom LASIK: Surgical Techniques and Complications. Thorofare-NJ, SLAK Inc. 2003;233.

11. Ti SE, Tan DT. Recurrent corneal erosion after laser in situ keratomileusis. Cornea. 2001;20(2):156-58.
12. Tabbara KF, El-Sheikh HF, Vera-Cristo CL. Complications of laser in situ keratomileusis (LASIK). Eur J Ophthalmol 2003;13(2):139-46.
13. Mulhern MG, Foley-Nolan A, O'Keefe M, Condon PI. Topographical analysis of ablation centration after excimer laser photorefractive keratectomy and laser in situ keratomileusis for high myopia. J Cataract Refract Surg 1997;23(4):488-94.
14. Verdon W, Bullimore M, Maloney RK. Visual performance after photorefractive keratectomy. Arch Ophthalmol 1996;114:1465-72.
15. Kim WJ, Chung ES, Lee JH. Effect of optic zone size on the outcome of photorefractive keratectomy for myopia. J Cataract Refract Surg 1996;22:197-204.
16. Uozato H, Guyton DL. Centering corneal surgical procedures. Am J Ophthalmol 1987;103:264-70.
17. Tsai YY, Lin JM. Ablation centration after active eye-tracker-assisted photorefractive keratectomy and laser in situ keratomileusis. J Cataract Refract Surg 2000;26(1):28-34.
18. Pallikaris I, Siganos D. LASIK complications management. In: Talamo J, Krueger R (Eds). The Excimer Manual. Boston MA: Little, Brown. 1997; 227-44.
19. Pallikaris I, Panagopoulou S, Katsanevaki V. The PALM technique: Photoablated lenticular modulator. In: Pallikaris I, Siganos D (Eds). LASIK. Thorofare, NJ: SLACK, Inc. 1997; 277-78.
20. Talamo JH, Wagoner MD, Lee SY. Management of ablation decentration following excimer photorefractive keratectomy. Arch Ophthalmol 1995;113:706-07.
21. Seiler T, McDonnell P. Excimer laser photorefractive keratectomy. Surv Ophthalmol 1995;40:89-118.
22. Alkara N, Genth U, Seiler T. Diametral ablation – A technique to manage decentered photorefractive keratectomy for myopia. J Refract Surg 1999;15:436-40.
23. Knorz MC, Jendritza B. Topographically-guided laser in situ keratomileusis to treat corneal irregularities. Ophthalmology 2000;107(6):1138-43.

24. Hoyos JE, Cigales M. Decentration: New approach to manage it (oral presentation). II International Congress KM Study Group. Barcelona-Spain, September 7-9,1995.
25. Hoyos JE, Cigales M, Hoyos-Chacón J. Treating decentered ablations. In: Lucio Buratto, Stephen Brint (Eds). Custom LASIK: Surgical Techniques and Complications. Thorofare-NJ, SLAK Inc. 2003; 249-52.
26. Buratto L, Brint SF. LASIK Principles and techniques. Thorofore, NJ: SLACK Inc. 1998; 127-29.
27. Kang SW, Chung ES, Kim WJ. Clinical analysis of central islands after laser in situ keratomileusis. J Cataract Refract Surg 2000;26:536-42.
28. Schimmick JK, Telfair WB, Munnerlyn DR, et al. Corneal ablation profilometry and steep central islands. J Cataract Refract Surg 1997; 24:899-904.
29. Haw WW, Manche EE. Large optical ablation zone using the VISX S2 Smoothscan excimer laser. J Cataract Refract Surg. 2000; 26:1742-47.
30. Tsai YY, Lin JM. Natural history of central islands after laser in situ keratomileusis. J Cataract Refract Surg 2000; 26:853-58.
31. Manche EE, Maloney RK, Smith RJ. Treatment of topographic central islands following refractive surgery. J Cataract Refract Surg. 1998; 24:464-70.
32. Knorz MC, Jendritza B. Topographically-guided laser in situ keratomileusis to treat corneal irregularities. Ophthalmology 2000; 107:1138-43.
33. Ambrosio R, Wilson SE. Complications of laser in situ keratomileusis: Etiology, prevention and treatment. J Refract Surg 2001; 17:350-79.
34. Carpel EF, Carlson KH, Shannon S. Folds and striae in laser in situ keratomileusis flaps. J Refract Surg 1999;15: 687-90.
35. Gimbel HV, Peters NT, Iskander NG, Penno EA. Laser in situ Keratomileusis Flap Complications and Management. J Refract Surg 2000;16: s223-25.
36. Gutierrez AM. Treatment of flap folds and striae following LASIK. In: Buratto L, Brint SF, (Eds). Custom LASIK: Surgical Techniques and Complications. Thorofare-NJ, SLAK Inc. 2003; 725-27.

37. Hoyos JE, Cigales M, Hoyos-Chacón J. Treatment of flap striae. In: Benjamin F. Boyd, Agarwal S, Agarwal A, Agarwal A (Eds). LASIK and beyond LASIK – Wavefront analysis and customized ablation. Highlights of Ophthalmology Int'l. 2001; 284-86.
38. Eggink FA, Eggink CA, Beekhuis WH. Postoperative management and follow-up after corneal flap loss following laser in situ keratomileusis. J Cataract Refract Surg 2002;28(1):175-79.
39. Chao CW, Azar DT. Lamellar keratitis following laser-assisted in situ keratomileusis. Ophthalmol Clin North Am 2002;15(1):35-40.
40. Perez-Gomez I, Efron N. Confocal microscopic evaluation of particles at the corneal flap interface after myopic laser in situ keratomileusis. J Cataract Refract Surg 2003;29(7):1373-77.
41. Kaufman SC, Maitchouk DY, Chiou AG, Beuerman RW. Interface inflammation after laser in situ keratomileusis. Sands of the Sahara syndrome. J Cataract Refract Surg 1998;24(12):1589-93.
42. Buhren J, Baumeister M, Cichocki M, Kohnen T. Confocal microscopic characteristics of stage 1 to 4 diffuse lamellar keratitis after laser in situ keratomileusis. J Cataract Refract Surg 2002;28(8):1390-99.
43. Sandoval HP, Crosson CE, Holzer MP, Vroman DT, Solomon KD. Residual cleaner after normal cleaning of laser in situ keratomileusis instruments. J Cataract Refract Surg 2003;29(9):1727-32.
44. Shan MN, Misra M. Diffuse lamellar keratitis associated with epithelial defects after laser in situ keratomileusis. J Cataract Refract Surg. 2000;26:1312-18.
45. Asano-Kato N, Toda I, Hori-Komai Y, Takano Y, Tsubota K. Epithelial ingrowth after laser in situ keratomileusis: Clinical features and possible mechanisms. Am J Ophthalmol 2002;134(6):801-07.
46. Sachdev N, McGhee CN, Craig JP, Weed KH, McGhee JJ. Epithelial defect, diffuse lamellar keratitis, and epithelial ingrowth following post-LASIK epithelial toxicity. J Cataract Refract Surg 2002;28(8):1463-66.

47. Ditzen K, Fiedler J, Pieger S. Laser in situ keratomileusis for hyperopia and hyperopic astigmatism using the Meditec MEL 70 spot scanner. J Refract Surg 2002;18(4):430-34.
48. Chung MS, Pepose JS, Manche EE. Management of the corneal flap in laser in situ keratomileusis after previous radial keratotomy. Am J Ophthalmol 2001;132(2):252-53.
49. Perez-Santonja JJ, Ayala MJ, Sakla HF, Ruiz-Moreno JM, Alio JL. Retreatment after laser in situ keratomileusis. Ophthalmology 1999;106(1):21-28.
50. Domniz Y, Comaish IF, Lawless MA, et al. Epithelial ingrowth: Causes, prevention, and treatment in 5 cases. J Cataract Refract Surg 2001; 27(11):1803-11.
51. Karp CL, Tuli SS, Yoo SH, Vroman DT, et al. Infectious keratitis after LASIK. Ophthalmology 2003;110(3):503-10.
52. Pushker N, Dada T, Sony P, Ray M, Agarwal T, Vajpayee RB. Microbial keratitis after laser in situ keratomileusis. J Refract Surg 2002;18(3):280-86.
53. Freitas D, Alvarenga L, Sampaio J, et al. An outbreak of Mycobacterium chelonae infection after LASIK. Ophthalmology 2003;110(2):276-85.
54. Pache M, Schipper I, Flammer J, Meyer P. Unilateral fungal and mycobacterial keratitis after simultaneous laser in situ keratomileusis. Cornea 2003;22(1):72-75.
55. Albietz JM, Lenton LM, McLennan SG. Effect of laser in situ keratomileusis for hyperopia on tear film and ocular surface. J Refract Surg 2002; 18(2):113-23.
56. Benitez-del-Castillo JM, Del-Rio T, Iradier T, et al. Decrease in tear secretion and corneal sensitivity after laser in situ keratomileusis. Cornea 2001; 20(1):30-32.
57. Orfeo V, De Marco R, Loffredo L. Alteration of the tear film following photoablative refractive surgery. In: Buratto L, Brint SF, (Eds). Custom LASIK: Surgical Techniques and Complications. Thorofare-NJ, SLAK Inc. 2003;277-81.
58. Wilson SE, Ambrosio R. Laser in situ keratomileusis-induced (presumed) neurotrophic epitheliopathy. Ophthalmology 2001; 108(6):1082-87.
59. Barker NH, Couper TA, Taylor HR. Changes in corneal topography after laser in situ keratomileusis for myopia. J Refract Surg 1999;15(1):46-52.

60. Spadea L, Fasciani R, Necozione S, Balestrazzi E. Role of the corneal epithelium in refractive changes following laser in situ keratomileusis for high myopia. J Refract Surg 2000;16(2):133-39.
61. Magallanes R, Shah S, Zadok D, Chayet AS, et al. Stability after laser in situ keratomileusis in moderately and extremely myopic eyes. J Cataract Refract Surg 2001;27(7):1007-12.
62. Probst LE. Myopic and hyperopic LASIK enhancements. In: Buratto L, Brint S, (Eds). Custom LASIK: Surgical Techniques and Complications. Thorofare-NJ, SLAK Inc. 2003; 699-708.
63. Gutierrez AM. Reoperations with the excimer laser. In: Buratto L, Brint S, (Eds). LASIK: Principles and Techniques. Thorofare-NJ, SLAK Inc. 1998; 339-50.
64. Domniz Y, Comaish IF, Lawless MA, Rogers CM, Sutton GL. Recutting the cornea versus lifting the flap: Comparison of two enhancement techniques following laser in situ keratomileusis. J Refract Surg 2001; 17(5):505-10.
65. Pallikaris IG, Kymionis GD, Astyrakakis NI. Corneal ectasia induced by laser in situ keratomileusis. J Cataract Refract Surg 2001;27(11):1796-1802.
66. Moncalvi M. Corneal ectasia following LASIK. In: Buratto L, Brint SF, (Eds). Custom LASIK: Surgical Techniques and Complications. Thorofare-NJ, SLAK Inc. 2003; 271-74.
67. Giledi O, Daya SM. Unexpected flap thickness in laser in situ keratomileusis. J Cataract Refract Surg 2003;29(9): 1825-26.
68. Piccoli PM, Gomes AA, Piccoli FV. Corneal ectasia detected 32 months after LASIK for correction of myopia and asymmetric astigmatism. J Cataract Refract Surg 2003; 29(6):1222-25.
69. Lovisolo CF, Fleming JF. Intracorneal ring segments for iatrogenic keratectasia after laser in situ keratomileusis or photorefractive keratectomy. J Refract Surg 2002;18(5): 535-41.
70. R Paradinas R, Cigales M, Hoyos JE. Role of peripheral retina in LASIK. In: Agarwal S, Agarwal A, Apple SJ, Buratto L, Alió JL, Pandey SK, Agarwal A (Eds). Textbook of Ophthalmology. Jaypee Brothers, New Delhi (India). 2002;4:2749-52.

71. Arevalo JF, Ramirez E, Suarez E, et al. Incidence of vitreoretinal pathologic conditions within 24 months after laser in situ keratomileusis. Ophthalmology 2000;107(2): 258-62.
72. Luna JD, et al. Bilateral macular hemorrhage after laser in situ keratomileusis. Graefes Arch Clin Exp Ophthalmol 1999;237(7):611-13.
73. Panozzo G, Parolini B. Relationships between vitreoretinal and refractive surgery. Ophthalmology 2001;108(9):1663-68; discussion 1668-69.
74. Arevalo JF, Ramirez E, Suarez E, Cortez R, Ramirez G, Yepez JB. Retinal detachment in myopic eyes after laser in situ keratomileusis. J Refract Surg 2002;18(6):708-14.

CHAPTER 16

Aberropia: A New Refractive Entity

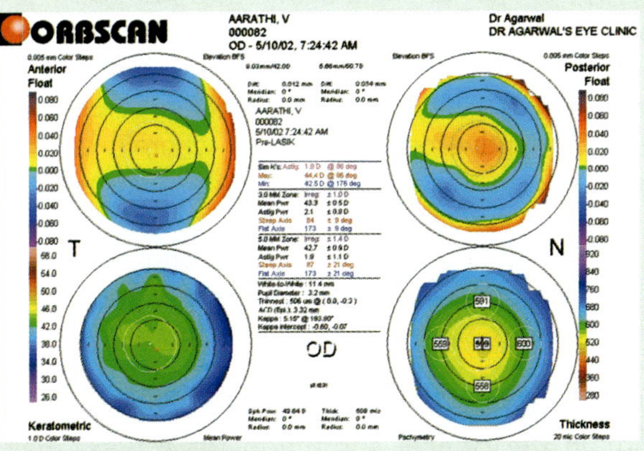

Amar Agarwal
Nilesh Kanjani
Soosan Jacob
Athiya Agarwal
Sunita Agarwal
Tahira Agarwal
Ashok Garg

India

INTRODUCTION

The next evolution to come on to the visual science scene in refractive ocular imaging is the aberrometer, the Orbscan and wavefront analysis. This technology is based on astrophysical principles, which astronomers use to perfect the images impinging on their telescopes. Dr Bille, the Director of the Institute of Applied Physics at the University of Heidelberg first began work in this field while developing this specific technology for astronomy applications in the mid-1970's. For perfect imaging, astrophysicists have to be able to measure and correct the imperfect higher-order aberrations or wavefront distortions that enter their telescopic lens system from the galaxy. To achieve this purpose, adaptive optics are used wherein deformable mirrors reform the distorted wavefront to allow clear visualization of celestial objects. Extrapolating these same principles to the human eye, it was thought that removal of the wavefront aberrations of the eye might finally yield the long awaited and much desired ultimate goal of "super vision".

So far, the only parameters that could be modified to obtain the optical correction for a given patients refractive error were the sphere, cylinder and axis even though this does not give the ideal optical correction many a times. This is because the current modes for correcting the optical aberrations of the eye do not reduce the higher order aberrations. The ideal optical system should be able to correct the optical aberrations in such a way that the spatial resolving ability of the eye is limited only by the limits imposed by the neural retina, i.e. receptor diameter and receptor packing.

Thus, there may be a large group of patients whose best corrected visual acuity (BCVA) may actually improve significantly on removal of the optical aberrations. These optical aberrations are contributed to by the eye's entire optical system, i.e. the cornea, the lens, the vitreous and the retina. This study was conducted to determine the existence of a hitherto unidentified entity which we label as "aberropia" wherein patients with best corrected visual acuity of ≤ 6/9 (0.63), corneal topography not accounting for the lack of improvement in BCVA and with no other known cause for decreased vision improved by ≥ two Snellen lines after refractive correction of their wavefront aberration.

MATERIALS AND METHODS

Sixteen eyes of 10 patients were included in this retrospective study carried out at the Dr Agarwal's Eye Institute, India between May to December 2002. Only patients who had visual acuity less than 6/9 (0.63) prior to the procedure and whose visual acuity improved by more than or equal to two lines after the procedure were included in the study. None of these patients had any other known cause for decreased vision and their corneal topography did not account for the lack of improvement in BCVA. The routine patient evaluation including uncorrected (UCVA) and best corrected (BCVA), slit lamp examination, applanation tonometry, manifest and cycloplegic refractions, Orbscan, aberrometry, corneal pachymetry, corneal diameter, Schirmer test and indirect ophthalmoscopy had been performed for all the patients. Patients wearing contact lenses had been asked to discontinue soft lenses for a minimum of 1 week and rigid gas permeable lenses for a minimum of 2 weeks before the preoperative examination and surgery. Informed consent was obtained form all patients after a thorough explanation of the procedure and its potential benefits and risks.

The Zyoptix procedure was then performed using the Bausch and Lomb Technolas 217 Z machine. The parameters used were: wavelength 193 nm, fluence 130 mJ/cm^2 and ablation zone diameters between 4.8 mm and 6 mm. The Hansatome (Bausch and Lomb) was used in all the eyes. Either the 180 μm or the 160 μm plate was used in all the eyes. The aberrometer and the Orbscan, which checks the corneal topography, are linked and a zylink created. An appropriate software file is created which is then used to generate the laser treatment file.

Postoperatively, the patients underwent complete examination including UCVA, BCVA, slit lamp examination, Orbscan and aberrometry. The mean follow up was 37.5 days.

For statistical analysis, the Snellen acuity was converted to the decimal notation. Continuous variables were described with mean, standard deviation, minimum and maximum values.

RESULTS

Sixteen eyes of 10 patients satisfied the inclusion criteria. The mean age of the patients was 29.43 years (range 22 to 35 years). Six patients were females and 4 were males. The mean preoperative pupil diameter measured on aberrometer was 4.69 mm and mean postoperative pupil diameter measured on aberrometer was 4.53 mm.

The mean preoperative spherical equivalent was – 4.94 D (range –12.50 to –1.5 D). The mean spherical equivalent at 1 month postoperative period was –0.16 ± 0.68 D (range –1.0 to 1.5). Mean preoperative sphere was –4.95 D (range-12.50 to –0.75 D) and the mean postoperative sphere was –0.13 ± 0.68 D (range– to 1.5) at 1 month. The mean preoperative cylinder was –1.34 D (range 0 to –3.50). The mean postoperative cylinder was –0.08 ± 0.24 D (range 0 to –0.75 D) at one month. Postoperatively, at the end of first month, 70 percent of the patients were within ± 0.5D and 90 percent– were within ± 1D of emmetropia (Figure 16.1). Preoperatively mean RMS (Root Mean Square) values (Figure 16.2) were: Z 200 Defocus –9.22, Z 221 Astigmatism 0.12, Z 220 Astigmatism 1.02, Z 311 Coma –0.041, Z 310 Coma –0.04, Z 331 Trefoil 0.23, Z 330 Trefoil 0.016, Z 400 Spherical aberration –0.054, Z 420 Secondary astigmatism 0.103, Z 421 Secondary astigmatism 0.029, Z 440 Quadrafoil –0.103, Z 441 Quadrafoil –0.021, Z 510 Secondary coma 0.025, Z 511 Secondary coma –0.015, Z 530 Secondary trefoil 0.0049, Z 531 Secondary trefoil –0.00219, Z 550 Pentafoil 0.023, Z 551 Pentafoil 0.046. Postoperative mean RMS values were: Z 200 Defocus –0.429, Z 221 Astigmatism 0.07, Z 220 Astigmatism –0.07, Z 311 Coma 0.149, Z 310 Coma –0.079, Z 331 Trefoil –0.102, Z 330 Trefoil –0.004, Z 400 Spherical aberration –0.179, Z 420 Secondary astigmatism 0.015, Z 421 Secondary astigmatism 0.031, Z 440 Quadrafoil 0.019, Z 441 Quadrafoil –0.069, Z 510 Secondary coma –0.008, Z 511 Secondary coma 0.008, Z 530 Secondary Trefoil –0.002, Z 531 Secondary Trefoil –0.014, Z 550 Pentafoil 0.006, Z 551 Pentafoil 0.026.

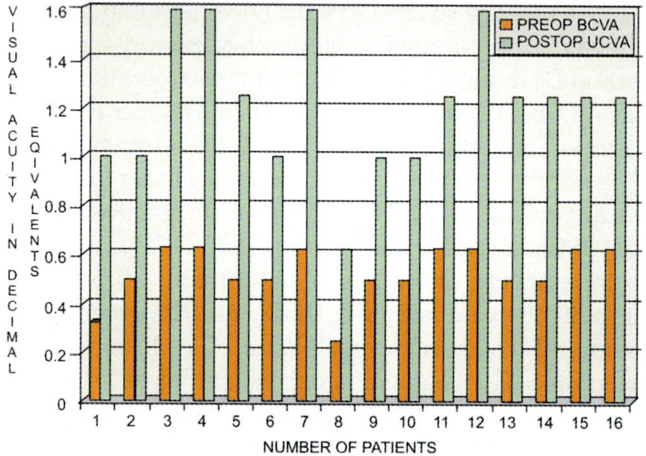

FIGURE 16.1: Preoperative BCVA versus postoperative UCVA

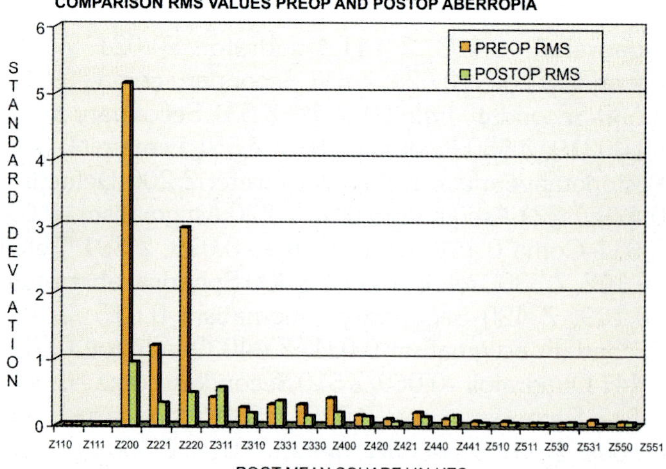

FIGURE 16.2: RMS values preoperative and postoperative

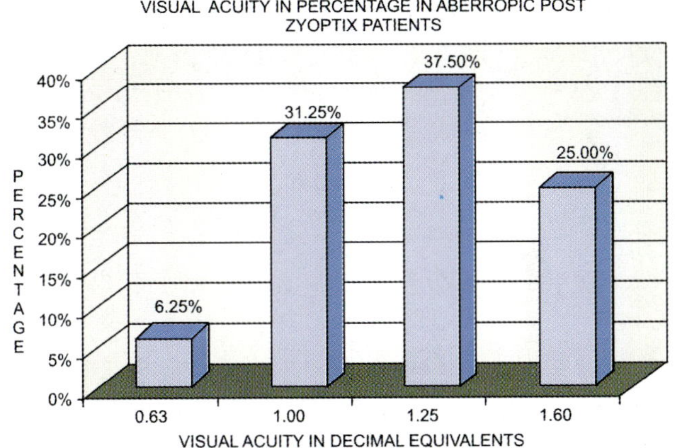

FIGURE 16.3: Percentage values of visual acuity

RMS pre-and postlaser showed a reduction in the higher order aberrations (Tables 16.1 and 16.2). 6.25 percent patients achieved 6/9, 31.25percent patients achieved ≥ 6/6 (1.00), 37.50 percent achieved a BCVA of 6/5 (1.25) and 25 percent achieved a BCVA of 6/4 (1.6) (Figure 16.3). Figure 16.4 shows the preoperative Orbscan picture of a patient showing no abnormality. Figures 16.5 and 16.6 shows the aberrometer maps of the right eye and left eye of a patient in which we can see the aberrations reduced postlaser.

DISCUSSION

Zyoptix is the new generation of excimer laser used for the treatment of refractive disorders. Until recently, refractive disorders were treated with standard techniques, which took into consideration only the subjective

TABLE 16.1: RMS values prelaser

Patient No	Z 110	Z 111	Z 200	Z 221	Z 220	Z 311	Z 310	Z 331	Z 330	Z 400	Z 420	Z 421	Z 440	Z 441	Z 510	Z 511	Z 530	Z 531	Z 550	Z 551	Z 6
1	0	0	-5.77	4.055.	-6.131	0.299	-0.113	0.725	-0.44	0.009	-0.03	0.102	-0.233	0.109	0.131	0.027	-0.048	-0.041	0.052	0.039	-9999
2	0	0	-4.323	-1.719	6.005	-0.273	0.022	-0.353	0.275	0.092	0.092	-0.145	0.199	-0.013	-0.006	0.011	0.034	-0.039	0.042	0.042	-9999
3	0	0	-11.8	-0.088	0.116	0.435	-0.658	-0.444	-0.567	-0.779	-0.089	0.043	-0.202	-0.053	-0.052	-0.057	-0.04	-0.001	0.13	0.111	-9999
4	0	0	-12.46	0.514	-0.155	0.29	-0.006	0.016	0.529	-0.91	0.124	0.124	-0.431	-0.222	0.074	-0.04	0.001	-0.063	-0.141	0.119	-9999
5	0	0	-6.535	-0.123	-0.886	0.156	-0.09	0.094	-0.128	-0.084	-0.072	0.035	-0.009	-0.044	0.001	-0.031	0.01	-0.005	0.001	-0.041	-9999
6	0	0	-7.867	0.185	1.704	-0.02	0.414	0.441	0.197	0.365	0.197	0.107	-0.155	-0.002	0.123	0.026	-0.001	0.049	0.048	0.032	-9999
7	0	0	-4.28	0.167	2.571	0.007	-0.089	0.356	0.125	0.585	0.101	-0.002	-0.17	-0.062	-0.077	0.198	0.001	-0.104	-0.022	0.029	-9999
8	0	0	-10.4	0.502	-0.587	-0.007	-0.331	0.165	-0.126	-0.054	-0.071	0.036	-0.118	-0.128	0.009	0.017	-0.007	-0.026	0.063	-0.052	-9999
9	0	0	-17.15	-0.414	-1.217	0.093	-0.106	0.343	-0.18	-0.254	0.009	0.002	0.001	-0.025	0.007	-0.022	-0.007	-0.042	0.037	0.04	-9999
10	0	0	-16.78	-0.162	-0.637	0.122	-0.159	0.279	0.2	-0.181	0.115	0.007	-0.002	0.042	-0.034	-0.028	0.021	-0.043	-0.006	-0.017	-9999
11	0	0	-4.513	2.916	4.661	-0.634	-0.205	0.477	0.44	0.094	0.377	0.058	-0.201	0.101	0.133	-0.147	0.009	0.011	-0.055	0.118	-9999
12	0	0	-5.736	-1.501	5.195	-1.126	0.32	0.665	-0.254	0.218	0.479	0.122	-0.253	-0.045	0.099	-0.025	0.012	-0.006	-0.05	0.11	-9999
13	0	0	-15.46	1.605	2.754	0.378	0.443	0.208	0.458	0.643	-0.083	0.09	0.407	-0.006	-0.021	0.09	0.033	0.032	0.239	0.149	-9999
14	0	0	-15.26	-0.557	2.865	-0.26	-0.059	0.107	0.122	0.168	0.025	-0.256	-0.003	0.257	0.007	0.051	0.136	-0.061	-0.114	0.124	-9999
15	0	0	-4.955	0.735	0.383	-0.401	0.003	0.62	-0.494	-0.676	0.391	0.163	-0.421	-0.264	0.039	-0.261	-0.079	0.241	0.103	-0.067	-9999
16	0	0	-4.367	-0.195	-0.238	0.28	-0.04	0.021	0.11	-0.112	0.084	-0.022	-0.061	0.013	-0.018	-0.063	0.004	0.063	0.044	0	-9999

TABLE 16.2: RMS values postlaser

Patient No.	Z 110	Z 111	Z 200	Z 221	Z 220	Z 311	Z 310	Z 331	Z 330	Z 400	Z 420	Z 421	Z 440	Z 441	Z 510	Z 511	Z 530	Z 531	Z 550	Z 551	Z 6
1	0	0	-0.022	0.74	-1.294	0.117	-0.067	0.141	0.052	-0.063	-0.076	0.1	0.054	-0.037	-0.028	0.001	0.008	0.007	0.013	0.006	-9999
2	0	0	-0.508	0.12	0.194	-0.085	0.039	-0.12	-0.018	-9999	-9999	-9999	-9999	-9999	-9999	-9999	-9999	-9999	-9999	-9999	-9999
3	0	0	-1.398	-0.606	0.697	-0.558	-0.351	0.841	0.345	-0.39	0.392	0.038	-0.303	-0.038	-0.001	0.103	-0.066	-0.105	-0.021	0.137	-9999
4	0	0	-2.05	-0.499	-0.375	-0.027	-0.269	-0.534	-0.289	-0.58	0.114	0.058	0.236	-0.161	0.034	-0.083	0.004	0.039	0.01	-0.077	-9999
5	0	0	0.229	0.1	-0.123	-9999	-9999	-9999	-9999	-9999	-9999	-9999	-9999	-9999	-9999	-9999	-9999	-9999	-9999	-9999	-9999
6	0	0	-0.036	-0.17	0.425	-0.002	0.069	-0.045	-0.042	-0.342	-0.032	0.094	0.075	-0.05	0.068	0.03	0.064	-0.014	0.012	0.002	-9999
7	0	0	0.687	0.128	-0.028	-0.117	-0.043	0.062	0.088	-0.178	0.179	0.024	-0.045	0.055	0.013	0.016	-0.034	-0.013	-0.013	0.059	-9999
8	0	0	-2.164	0.279	-0.696	-0.25	-0.398	-0.147	-0.128	-0.581	-0.238	0.02	0.032	-0.088	-0.129	0.028	-0.029	0.007	0.089	0.059	-9999
9	0	0	-0.298	0.002	-0.311	0.158	-0.206	0.129	-0.116	-0.105	-0.045	-0.043	-0.1	-0.1	-9999	-9999	-9999	-9999	-9999	-9999	-9999
10	0	0	0.109	0.241	-0.503	0.233	-0.119	-0.16	-0.204	-9999	-9999	-9999	-9999	-9999	-9999	-9999	-9999	-9999	-9999	-9999	-9999
11	0	0	0.034	-0.092	0.076	0.013	-0.03	-0.067	0.003	-9999	-9999	-9999	-9999	-9999	-9999	-9999	-9999	-9999	-9999	-9999	-9999
12	0	0	0.187	0.061	0.004	-0.097	0.015	0.067	0.035	-9999	-9999	-9999	-9999	-9999	-9999	-9999	-9999	-9999	-9999	-9999	-9999
13	0	0	-0.701	0.291	0.598	2.161	0.349	-1.062	-0.201	-0.428	-0.013	0.204	0.258	-0.636	-0.082	0.113	0.069	-0.239	0.062	-9999	-9999
14	0	0	-0.638	0.094	0.391	0.517	-0.328	-0.336	0.188	-0.118	-0.077	0.003	0.157	0.034	-0.006	-0.025	0.004	0.018	-0.066	-9999	-9999
15	0	0	-0.148	0.493	0.017	0.261	0.017	-0.354	0.302	-0.111	0.053	0.07	-0.019	-0.084	-0.007	-0.051	-0.052	0.063	0.011	-9999	-9999
16	0	0	-0.161	-0.038	-0.331	0.072	0.049	-0.05	-0.086	0.025	-0.008	-0.059	-0.028	-9999	-9999	-9999	-9999	-9999	-9999	-9999	-9999

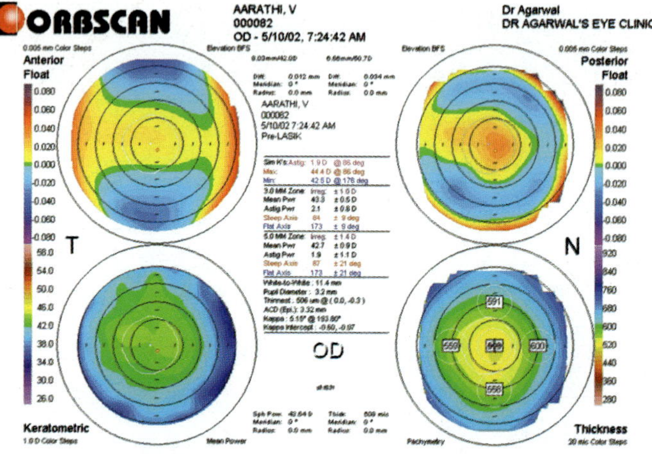

FIGURE 16.4: Preoperative Orbscan

refraction. Zyoptix technique on the other hand, takes into account the patient's subjective refraction, ocular optical aberrations and corneal topography, with the latter not only for the diagnosis, but also for the therapeutic treatment, in order to design a personalized treatment based on the total structure of the eye. The wavefront technology in Zyoptix uses the Hartmann Shack aberrometer based on the Hartmann-Shack principle[1] demonstrated by Liang et al[2] to measure the eye's wave aberration. This wavefront sensor has been improved by increasing the density of samples taken of the wavefront slope in the pupil.[3] All Hartmann-Shack devices are outgoing testing devices in that they evaluate the light being bounced back out through the optical system. A narrow laser beam is focused onto the retina to generate a point source. The out coming light rays which experience

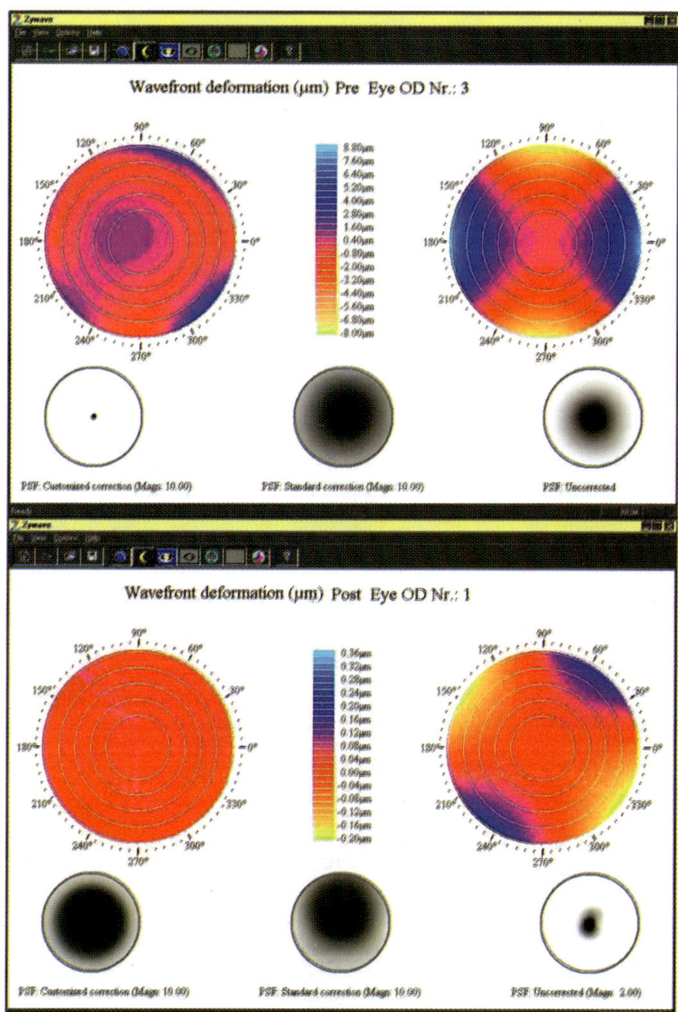
Wavefront deformation (μm) Pre Eye OD Nr.: 3
8.80μm
7.60μm
6.40μm
5.20μm
4.00μm
2.80μm
1.60μm
0.40μm
-0.80μm
-2.00μm
-3.20μm
-4.40μm
-5.60μm
-6.80μm
-8.00μm
PSF: Customized correction (Magn: 10.00)
PSF: Standard correction (Magn: 10.00)
PSF: Uncorrected
Wavefront deformation (μm) Post Eye OD Nr.: 1
0.36μm
0.32μm
0.28μm
0.24μm
0.20μm
0.16μm
0.12μm
0.08μm
0.04μm
0.00μm
-0.04μm
-0.08μm
-0.12μm
-0.16μm
-0.20μm
PSF: Customized correction (Magn: 10.00)
PSF: Standard correction (Magn: 10.00)
PSF: Uncorrected (Magn: 2.00)

FIGURE 16.5

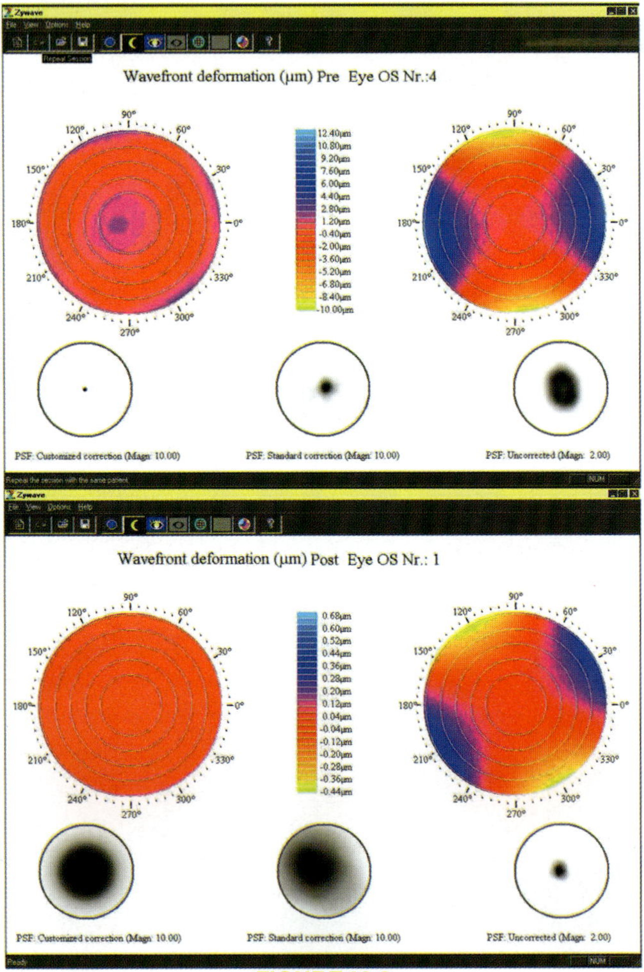

Wavefront deformation (µm) Pre Eye OS Nr.:4

12.40µm
10.80µm
9.20µm
7.60µm
6.00µm
4.40µm
2.80µm
1.20µm
-0.40µm
-2.00µm
-3.60µm
-5.20µm
-6.80µm
-8.40µm
-10.00µm

PSF: Customized correction (Magn: 10.00) PSF: Standard correction (Magn: 10.00) PSF: Uncorrected (Magn: 2.00)

Wavefront deformation (µm) Post Eye OS Nr.: 1

0.68µm
0.60µm
0.52µm
0.44µm
0.36µm
0.28µm
0.20µm
0.12µm
0.04µm
-0.04µm
-0.12µm
-0.20µm
-0.28µm
-0.36µm
-0.44µm

PSF: Customized correction (Magn: 10.00) PSF: Standard correction (Magn: 10.00) PSF: Uncorrected (Magn: 2.00)

FIGURE 16.6

FIGURES 16.5 and 16.6: Pre-and postoperative aberrometry of the right and left eye of the same patient showing removal of higher order aberrations all the aberrations of the eye pass through an array of lenses which detects their deviation. The wavefront deformation is calculated by analyzing the direction of the light rays using this lenslet array. Parallel light beams indicate a good wavefront and non-parallel light beams indicate a wavefront with aberrations, which does not give equidistant focal points. This image is then captured onto a ccd camera and the wavefront is reconstructed. The data is explained mathematically in three dimensions with polynomial functions. Most investigators have chosen the Zernicke method for this analysis although Taylor series can also be used for the same purpose.[4] Data from the wavefront map is presented as a sum of Zernicke polynomials each describing a certain deformation. At any point in the pupil, the wavefront aberration is the optical path difference between the actual image wavefront and the ideal spherical wavefront centered at the image point.[5]

Any refractive error which cannot be corrected by spherocylindrical lens combinations is referred to by physicists as higher order aberrations, i.e. comma, spherical aberration, chromatic aberration. The Zernicke polynomials, which describe ray points, are used to obtain a best fit toric to correct for the refractive error of the eye. The points are described in the x and y coordinates and the third dimension, height, is described in the z-axis. The local refractive correction of each area of the entrance pupil can be determined by calculating from the wavefront polynomial the corresponding local radii of curvature and hence the required spherocylindrical correction.[6] Thus each small region of the entrance pupil has its own three parameters that characterize the local refractive correction: sphere, cylinder and axis.[6] The global aberrations of the entire optical system including the cornea, lens, vitreous and the retina are thus measured. The great advantage of wavefront analysis is that it can describe these other aberrations.

The first order polynomial describes the spherical error or power of the eye. The second order polynomial describes the regular astigmatic component and its orientation or axis. Third order aberrations are considered to be coma and fourth order aberrations are considered to be spherical aberration. Zernicke polynomial descriptions for wavefront analysis typically go up to the tenth order of expression. The first and second orders describe the morphology of a normal straight curve. More local maximum and minimum points require higher orders of the polynomial series to describe the surface. Normal eyes exhibit spherical[7,8] and coma[9,10] aberrations in addition to exhibiting defocus and astigmatism.

Ideally, the difference in the magnitude of the local refractive correction of each area of the entrance pupil should not exceed 0.25 D. Lower spherocylindrical corrections are generally associated with lower wavefront aberrations.[6] These observations regarding variation in local ocular refraction along different meridians are also confirmed by Ivanoff[11] and Jenkins.[12] Van den Brink[13] also commented on the change in refraction across the pupil. Clinically significant changes of at least 0.25 D in one or both components of the spherocylindrical correction might normally be expected for decentrations of about 1 mm. Rayleigh's quarter wavelength rule states that if the wavefront aberration exceeds a quarter of a wavelength, the quality of the retinal image will be impaired significantly.[14] Thus the aberration in eyes starts to become significant when the pupil diameter exceeds 1-2 mm.[6]

Thus it is not possible to correct the entire wavefront aberration with a single spherocylindrical lens. As conventional refractive procedures such as LASIK also reduce only the second order aberrations, the visual acuity will still be limited by aberrations of third and higher order aberrations. These patients are likely to undergo tremendous improvement in their BCVA after correction of their aberrations by Zyoptix.

In the Zyoptix system, the aberrometer and the orbscan, which checks the corneal topography, are linked and a zylink created. An appropriate software file is created which is then used to generate the laser treatment file. The truncated gaussian beam shape used in Zyoptix combines the advantages of the common beam shapes, i.e. flat top beam and the gaussian beam, creating a maximized smoothness and minimized thermal effect. Thus Zyoptix gives a smoother corneal surface, reducing glare and increasing visual acuity. The larger optical zones reduce haloes. Zyoptix also causes a reduction of the ablation depth by 15-20 percent and a reduced enhancement rate.

In a patient with higher order aberrations, LASIK does not remove the higher order aberrations and the point-spread function is a large blur. Zyoptix on the other hand, performs customized ablation and removes the higher order aberrations thus minimizing the wavefront deformation. The point-spread function is therefore a small spot of light.

In our study, the mean preoperative spherical equivalent improved from –4.78 D to –0.16 D ± 0.68 and the mean preoperative cylinder improved from –1.34 D to –0.08 D ± 0.24. The aberrations were reduced drastically in all the eyes and the BCVA improved in all cases by ≥ two lines. Reduction of the aberrations of the eye can thus result in an improved BCVA postoperatively.

Improving the optics of the eye by removing aberrations increases the contrast and spatial detail of the retinal image. Reduction of higher order aberrations may not improve high contrast acuity much more in eyes where spherocylindrical lenses alone improve the BCVA to 6/3 (2.00) or better. In contrast, in otherwise normal eyes where the BCVA is limited to 6/9 (0.50) or 6/6 (1.00) due to optical aberrations, reduction of higher order aberrations should improve visual acuity.

Realization of the best possible unaided visual acuity may be limited at the cortical, retinal and the spectacle, corneal, or implant level. All maculae may not be able to support 6/3 (2.00) vision. Insufficient cone density or sub-optimal orientation of cone receptors or a sub-optimal Stiles-Crawford profile of the macula may make 6/3 (2.00) vision impossible. Clinical or sub-clinical amblyopia may make achievement of super vision impossible. But, in spite of this, there may be a certain patient population who have the potential for an improved BCVA on removal of their wavefront aberrations. The corneal topography does not account for the decreased preoperative visual acuity in these patients, neither do they have any other identifiable cause for the decrease in acuity except for an abnormal wavefront. It is important that this subgroup of patients are identified and their optical aberrations neutralized so that they are not deprived of the opportunity to gain in their BCVA.

Wavefront sensing technology, at present, does not in most cases define the exact locale of the pathology causing the aberration. Hence, clinical examination and other refractive tools, such as corneal topographic mapping, along with sound clinical judgment is required for proper understanding of the eye and its individual refractive status. Also, wavefront aberrations may not remain static. Numerous authors[15-18] have shown that ocular optical aberrations probably remain constant between 20 and 40 years of age but increase after that. Aberrations also change during accommodation [19,20] and may be affected by mydriatics.[21] Thus, the patient should be informed about these possibilities while taking the consent for the procedure. Long-term studies are required to determine the stability of the postoperative refraction, residual aberrations and changes in BCVA if any.

The question of magnification factor improving visual acuity does not arise as these patients preoperatively did not improve with contact lenses. Further the refractive error in some of these patients was not very large.

CONCLUSION

In conclusion, removal of the wavefront aberration may extend the benefit of an improved BCVA to patients with an abnormal wavefront. The subgroup of patients with higher order aberrations, normal corneal topography and no other known cause for decreased vision may thus benefit immensely with wavefront guided refractive surgery. Customized refractive surgery tailor-made for these individual patients, aimed at neutralizing the wavefront aberrations of the eye is safer, more predictable, provides better visual acuities and reduces the incidence of unsatisfactory outcomes. Further studies are required to assess the long-term outcomes.

Till now, when we discuss refractive errors we discuss about spherical and a cylindrical correction. But in todays world we have to think of a third parameter which is the aberrations present in the eye which can be anywhere in the optical media. These can be corrected in the corneal level by the laser treatment.

REFERENCES

1. Platt B, Shack RV. "Lenticular Hartmann screen", Opt Sci Center News (University of Arizona) 1971;5:15-16.
2. Liang J, Grimm B, Goelz S, Bille J. " Objective measurement of the wave aberrations of the human eye with the use of a Hartmann-Shack wavefront sensor". J Opt Soc Am 1994;11:1949-57.
3. Liang J, Williams DR, et al. Aberrations and retinal image quality of the normal human eye. J Opt Soc Am A 1997; 14(11):2873-83.
4. Oshika T, Klyce SD, Applegate RA, et al. Comparison of corneal wavefront aberrations after photorefractive keratectomy and laser in situ keratomileusis. Am J Ophthalmol 1999; 127:1-7.
5. Fincham WHA, Freeman MH. Optics. 9th ed. London: Butterworths, 1980. Born M, Wolf E. Principles of Optics. 2nd ed. New York: Macmillan, 1964;203-32.
6. Charman WN, Walsh G. Variations in the local refractive correction of the eye across its entrance pupil. Optometry and Vision Science 1989 Jan;66(1)34-40.
7. Rosenblum WM, Christensen JL. "Objective and subjective spherical aberration measurement of the human eye." In: Wolf E (Ed): Progress in Optics, (North-Holland, Amsterdam) 1976;13:69-91.
8. Campbell MC, Harrison EM, Simonet P. "Psychophysical measurement of the blur on the retina due to optical aberrations of the eye." Vision Res 1990;30:1587-1602.

9. Howland HC, Howland B. "A subjective method for the measurement of monochromatic aberrations of the eye. J Opt Soc Am. 1977;67:1508-18.
10. Walsh G, Charman WN, Howland HC. "Objective technique for the determination of monochromatic aberrations of the human eye". J Opt Soc Am A1, 1984;987-92.
11. Ivanoff A. About the spherical aberration of the eye. J Opt Soc Am 1956;46:901-03.
12. Jenkins TCA. Aberrations of the eye and their effects on vision. Part 1. Br J Physiol Opt 1963; 20: 59-91.
13. Van den Brink G. Measurements of the geometric aberrations of the eye. Vision Res. 1962; 2: 233-44.
14. Born M, Wolf E. Principles of Optics. 2nd ed. New York: Macmillan, 1964:203-32.
15. Kaemerrer M, Mrochen M, Mierdel P, et al. Optical aberrations of the human eye. Nature Medicine (in press)
16. Oshika T, Klyce SD, Applegate RA, et al. Changes in corneal wavefront aberration with aging. Invest Ophthalmol Vis Sci 1999; 40: 1351-55.
17. Calver RI, Cox MJ, Elliot DB. Effect of aging on the monochromatic aberrations of the human eye. J Opt Soc Am A 1999;16: 2069-78.
18. Guirao A, Gonzalez C, Redondo M, et al. Average optical performance of the human eye as a function of age in a normal population. Invest Ophthalmol Vis Sci 1999;40: 203-13.
19. Krueger R, Kaemerrer M, Mrochen M, et al. Understanding refraction and accommodation through "ingoing optics" aberrometry: A case report. Ophthalmology (in press).
20. He JC, Burns SA, Marcos S. Monochromatic aberrations in the accommodated human eye. Vis Res 2000; 40:41-48.
21. Fankhauser F, Kaemerrer M, Mrochen M, et al. The effect of accommodation, mydriasis, and cycloplegia on aberrometry. ARVO abstract 2248. Invest Ophthalmol Vis Sci 2000; 41; S461.

CHAPTER 17

Epi-LASIK: An Advanced Surface Ablation Procedure

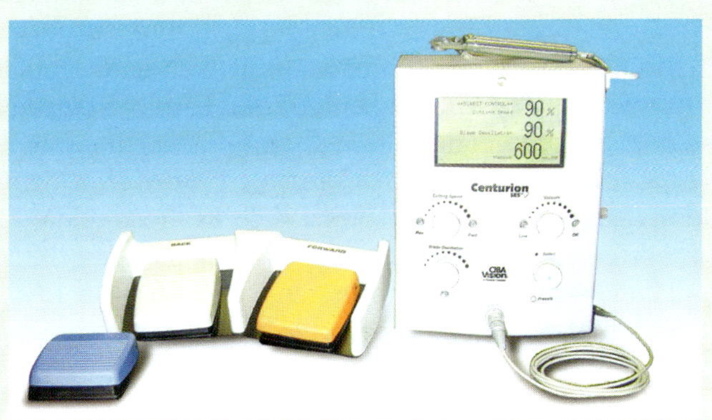

Vikentia J Katsanevaki
Maria I Kalyvianaki
Ioannis G Pallikaris

(Greece)

INTRODUCTION

Since the introduction of excimer lasers for photorefractive corrections the surgical trends are continuously changing in order to achieve the best possible clinical results with minimal complications. Photorefractive Keratectomy (PRK) initially introduced in the beginning of 90s[1,2] was the first technique to be used for photo refractive corrections. Despite its encouraging results for low and moderate myopia, during the evolvement of refractive surgery PRK was partially abandoned mostly due to the postoperative pain of the treated patients as well as the risk of corneal postoperative haze. Laser *in situ* keratomileusis (LASIK),[3,4] which involves the ablation deeper in the stroma after the creation of a corneal flap, soon became popular among refractive surgeons. Providing fast visual rehabilitation as well as the ability to correct higher degrees of ametropias LASIK is currently the undisputable leader within photorefractive treatments. However, LASIK is not without complications. Complications unique to LASIK such as those related to the use of the microkeratome,[5,6] LASIK induced diffuse lamellar keratitis[7] and the increasing reports of LASIK patients that developed corneal ectasia;[8] have set the stage for the revival of surface treatments.

Laser subepithelial keratomileusis[9] (LASEK) was the first attempt to modify surface treatments in order to control the major drawbacks of PRK, i.e. the postoperative pain and the risk of haze formation. The modification of the surgical technique as compared to the conventional PRK, was the separation of corneal epithelium as a sheet rather than its scrapping prior to the photo ablation. This epithelial sheet which is separated en toto and is replaced onto the ablated cornea, is thought to act as a natural contact lens on the operative eye[10] is expected to control the epithelial healing and thus provide better postoperative results as compared to PRK.

EPI-LASIK: AN EVOLVING TECHNIQUE

The separation of the epithelial sheet in LASEK as described by Camellin, requires the preparation of the cornea with a short-term exposure to a diluted (18-20%) alcohol solution. In order to avoid the probable toxic effect of alcohol on the epithelium and the underlying stroma,[13, 14] Pallikaris described Epi- LASIK.[11,12] With this modality, the epithelial sheet is separated mechanically with the use of a customized device (Centurion Epiedge Epikeratome, Ciba Vision Surgical, GA) without the need of prior corneal preparation with alcohol. This device has recently granted CE mark and 510K aproval for clinical use and is commercially available. Epi-LASIK,[11, 12] is currently the treatment of choice for low myopia in the University of Crete and up to now has been performed in more than 400 eyes worldwide (Figure 17.1). Its name is derived from the Greek word "epipolis" that means superficial and LASIK.

HISTOLOGICAL FINDINGS OF MECHANICALLY SEPARATED EPITHELIAL SHEETS

Transmission electron microscopy of harvested epithelial sheets in eyes that the treatments were reversed to PRK demonstrated that the cleavage plane of mechanical

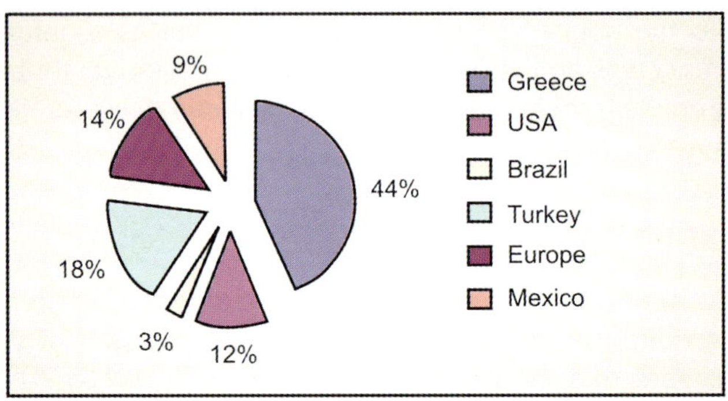

FIGURE 17.1: Epi-LASIK: Experience around the globe (N-402)

separation was located under the level of the basement membrane.[11] Basal epithelial cells had normal morphology with minimal evidence of trauma and edema and rested upon the prominent basal lamina, which consisted of an apparently structure less lamina lucida and an electron-dense lamina densa. Under the basal lamina an upper part on Bowman layer was evident in the epithelial sheets (Figure 17.2). Intracellular organelles and intercellular desmosomal connections, as well as hemidesmosomal connections with the basement membrane appeared close to normal with only focal disruptions.

Alcohol assisted epithelial separations are reported to take place within the basement membrane thus affecting its integrity.[11,15,16] The presence of an intact basement membrane has been shown to be important in the control of epithelial wound healing[17] minimizing the fibrotic activation of keratocytes. Even though alcohol solutions are not reported toxic in the specific concentrations and exposure times that are advocated for epithelial separations

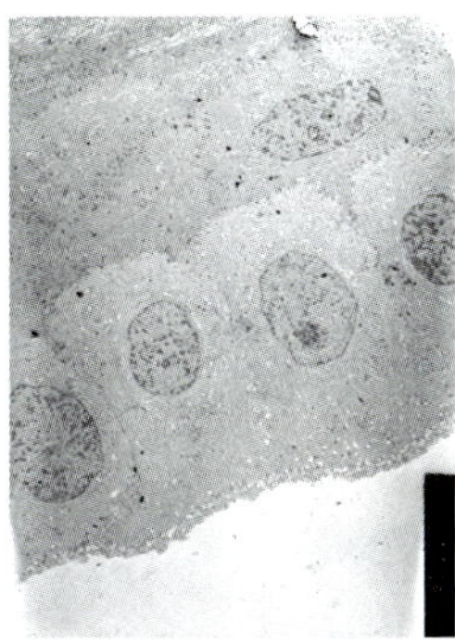

FIGURE 17.2: Transmit ion electron microscopy of a mechanically assisted separated sheet harvested from the operative eye immediately after the separation

in LASEK,[18, 19] mechanical separation appears to have the advantage of a deeper cleavage plane over alcohol assisted separations thus being expected to provide better control of corneal healing within the first postoperative days.

EPI-LASIK: THE SURGICAL PROCEDURE

The operative eye is prepared with three drops of topical tetracaine hydrochloride 0.5 percent (applied every 5 minutes before the procedure) and povidone-iodine and is covered with a sterile drape. Before the epithelial separation the cornea is marked with a customized Epi-LASIK marker (Epi-LASIK marker, Duckworth & Kent, Baldock, UK). This marker features two concentric circles crossed by 8 radial arms. Upon the replacement of the

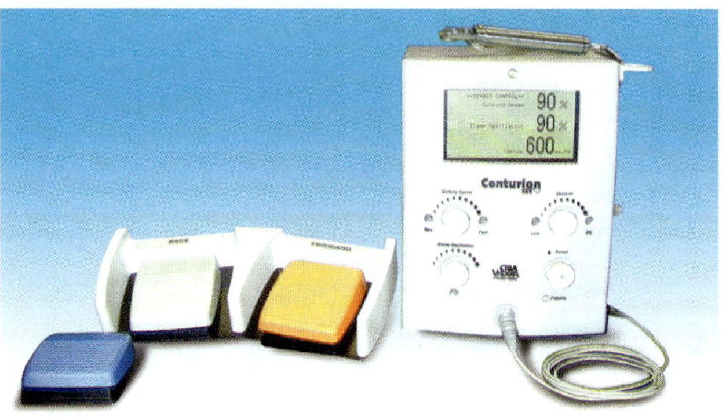

FIGURE 17.3: The Centurion subepithelial epikeratome

epithelial sheet, any deformity of the preoperative marks dictates its proper repositioning.

The Centurion EpiEdge Epikeratome is an electrically powered device (Figure 17.3) that operates under low suction similarly to a conventional microkeratome. Instead of a blade it features a disposable, oscillating polymethylmethacrylate (PMMA) separator with an advance speed of 3.5 mm/sec. The resulting separated epithelial sheet has a nasal hinge and a diameter of 9.5 to 10 mm. Any manipulations of the epithelial sheet both for its reflection and replacement, are performed with the use of a moistened sponge. The replacement of the separated epithelial sheet is often achieved with a single movement. Any inward or outward folds of its edges can be restored with the use of an anterior chamber irrigation cannula under constant irrigation. Once the epithelial sheet is stuck to the underlying stroma, a therapeutic contact lens is applied onto the operative eye.

POSTOPERATIVE TREATMENT

Postoperative treatment includes eyedrops of Diclofenac sodium 0.1 percent qid for two days and combined eyedrops of tobramycin-dexamethasone qid until the removal of the therapeutic lens. After the removal of the lens all treated eyes receive fluorometholone eyedrops qid for five weeks in a tapered dose. Artificial tears are prescribed to be used at the patients' discretion.

EARLY POSTOPERATIVE COURSE

At the end of the surgery, the replaced epithelial sheet often overlays its initial gutter probably due to the intra-operative mechanical stretch on the epithelial sheet upon separation. Immediately after the operation the epithelial sheet is transparent. During the healing process of the surface, slit lamp biomicroscopy reveals the borderline between the migrating epithelium and the remnants of the separated sheet. The migrating cells gradually replace the separated epithelial sheet, which is subsequently constricted in the central area. Starting from its peripheral part around the edges on the first postoperative day the sheet becomes hazy in its total area until about the third day after the treatment. At that time the hazy area measures about the central 1 to 2 mm whereas a front of newly synthesized, transparent epithelium migrates from the corneal periphery towards the center of the corneal surface. After that stage, the transparency of the corneal epithelium is restored within 24 to 48 hours and the therapeutic contact lens is removed. The time of epithelial healing ranges from 3 to 5 days between the treated eyes.

CLINICAL RESULTS

Up-to-date we have performed 183 mechanically assisted epithelial separations in the University of Crete. Seventy-six eyes were left to heal as Epi-LASIK whereas the rest of the separated sheets underwent histological evaluation and the treatments were reversed to PRK. The preoperative spherical equivalent of the treated eyes was up to -7.75 D, with cylinder up to -2.25 D.

Postoperative pain of the treated patients was assessed subjectively with a use of a questionnaire that graded pain in a scale from 0 to 4. The patients graded postoperative pain in two-hour intervals on the operative day and once daily in the following days. No patient reported pain after the operative day.On the operative day, the mean scores remained below the threshold of pain in the reported series of eyes (Figure 17.4). Similarly as after LASEK,[25,26] epi-LASIK was not proved a totally pain-free procedure. We observed that discomfort or pain was mainly reported within the first postoperative hours. In order to deal with this finding we included intraoperative corneal cooling in the standard treatment of the last 20 eyes. We cooled the cornea immediately before the separation and after the ablation with the instillation of pre-freezed balanced salt solution. After this alteration of the technique, the reported discomfort was below the threshold of pain in all patients even in the first postoperative hours.

During the early postoperative course, the mean uncorrected visual acuity (UCVA) of the treated eyes corresponded well with the progress of the epithelial healing and the transparency of the replaced epithelial sheet. More particularly, UCVA was better on the first postoperative day, when the epithelial sheet was transparent, to decrease

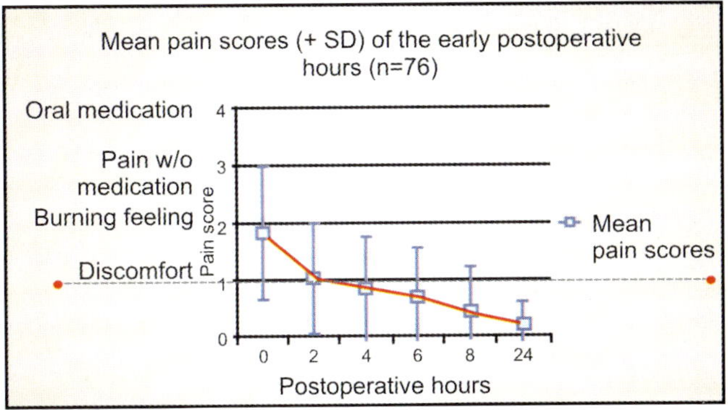

FIGURE 17.4: The mean pain scores remained below the threshold of burning feeling in the reported series of eyes

around the third postoperative day, as the epithelial sheet became hazy, and, finally rise again, when the epithelial healing was complete (Figure 17.5). On the sixth month interval 94 percent of eyes had visual acuity of 20/25 or better whereas 48 percent of eyes have gained one or two (8%) Snellen lines of best-corrected visual acuity.

The vast majority of Epi-LASIK eyes had clear corneas or trace haze at three (96%) and six month's (100%) postoperative intervals.

CONCLUSIONS

Histological findings of mechanically separated epithelial sheets have shown that mechanical separation preserves the epithelial cell viability, the stratification of the sheet and the integrity of the epithelial basement membrane. In contrast to the varying solution dilutions and exposure times required for alcohol assisted separations[20-22] the epikeratome can achieve mechanically assisted separations

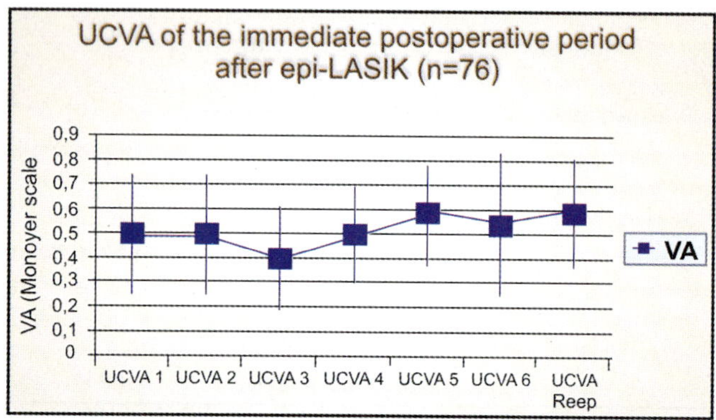

FIGURE 17.5: Early postoperative course

in a repetitive and fully automated way with a short learning curve for experienced LASIK surgeons. Preliminary clinical results are comparable to that of LASEK[15, 21,23,24] and suggest epi-LASIK as an efficient and safe alternative surgical modality for low myopia. Given the preliminary encouraging results for low myopia the next goal will be to apply this technique for higher myopic corrections. Intraoperative corneal cooling has an additive effect to the retained epithelial sheet minimizing discomfort below the threshold of pain in all the treated eyes. Future randomized comparative studies between epi-LASIK and PRK are expected to prove the advantages of the retained epithelial sheet in surface treatments.

REFERENCES

1. Seiler T, Wollensak J. Myopic photorefractive keratectomy with excimer laser; one-year follow up. Ophthalmology 1991; 98:1156-63.

2. Epstein D, Fagerholm P, Hamberg-Nystroem H, Tengroth B. Twenty four-month follow up of excimer laser photorefractive keratectomy for myopia; refractive and visual outcome results. Ophthalmology 1994;101:1558-63.
3. Pallikaris IG, Papatzanaki ME, Siganos DS, Tsilimbaris MK. A corneal flap technique for laser in situ keratomileusis. Human studies. Arch Ophthalmol 1991; 109(12): 1699-1702.
4. Hersh PS, Brint SF, Maloney RK, et al. Photorefractive keratectomy versus laser in situ keratomileusis for moderate to high myopia; a randomized prospective study. Ophthalmology 1998;105:1512-22.
5. Pallikaris IG, Katsanevaki VJ, Panagopoulou SI. Laser in situ keratomileusis intraoperative complications using one type of microkeratome. Ophthalmology 2002;109(1):57-63.
6. Melki SA, Azar DT. LASIK complications: Etiology, management, and prevention. Surv Ophthalmol 2001(2); 46:95-116.
7. Smith RJ, Maloney RK. Diffuse lamellar keratitis. A new syndrome in lamellar refractive surgery. Ophthalmology 1998; 105(9):1721-26.
8. Pallikaris IG, Kymionis GD, Astyrakakis NI. Corneal ectasia induced by laser in situ keratomileusis. J Cataract Refract Surg 2001;27(11):1796-1802.
9. Camellin M, Cimberle M. LASEK technique promising after 1 year of experience. Ocular Surg News 2000; 18 (1): 14-17.
10. Lee JB, Seong GJ, Lee JH, Seo KY, Lee YG, Kim EK. Comparison of laser epithelial keratomileusis and photorefractive keratectomy for low to moderate myopia. J Cataract Refract Surg 2001;27(4):565-70.
11. Pallikaris IG, Naoumidi II, Kalyvianaki MI, Katsanevaki VJ. Epi-LASIK: Comparative histological evaluation of mechanical and alcohol-assisted epithelial separation. J Cataract Refract Surg 2003; 29(8):1496-1501.
12. Pallikaris IG, Katsanevaki VJ, Kalyvianaki MI, Naoumidi II. Advances in subepithelial excimer refractive surgery techniques: Epi-LASIK. Curr Opin Ophthalmol 2003; 14(4):207-12.

13. Kamm O. The relation between structure and physiological action of the alcohols. J Am Pharmaceutical Association 1921; 10:87-92.
14. Kim SY, Sah WJ, Lim YW, Hahn TW. Twenty percent alcohol toxicity on rabbit corneal epithelial cells: Electron microscopic study. Cornea 2002;21(4):388-92.
15. Azar DT, Ang RT, Lee JB, Kato T, Chen CC, Jain S, Gabison E, Abad JC. Laser subepithelial keratomileusis: Electron microscopy and visual outcomes of photorefractive keratectomy. Curr Opin Ophthalmol 2001; 12(4): 323-28.
16. Espana EM, Gruetereich M, Mateo A, Romano AC, Yee SB, Yee RW, Tseng SCG. Cleavage plane of corneal basement membrane components by ethanol exposure in laser-assisted subepithelial keratectomy. J Cataract Refract Surg 2003;29:1192-97.
17. Stramer BM, Zieske JD, Jung JC, Austin JS, Fini ME. Molecular mechanisms controlling the fibrotic repair phenotype in cornea: Implications for surgical outcomes. Invest Ophthalmol Vis Sci 2003;44(10):4237-46.
18. Chen CC, Chang JH, Lee JB, Javier J, Azar DT. Human corneal epithelial cell viability and morphology after dilute alcohol exposure. Invest Ophthalmol Vis Sci 2002;43(8): 2593-2602.
19. Gabler B, Winkler von Mohrenfelds C, Dreiss AK, Marshall J, Lohmann CP. Vitality of epithelial cells after alcohol exposure during laser-assisted subepithelial keratectomy flap preparation. J Cataract Refract Surg 2002;28:1841-46.
20. Camellin M. Laser epithelial keratomileusis for myopia. J Refract Surg 2003;19:666-70.
21. Chalita MR, Tekwani NH, Krueger RR. Laser epithelial keratomileusis: Outcome of initial cases performed by an experienced surgeon. J Refract Surg 2003;19:412-15.
22. Litwak S, Zadok D, Garcia-de Quevedo V, Robledo N, Chayet AS. Laser-assisted subepithelial keratectomy versus photorefractive keratectomy for the correction of myopia. A prospective comparative study. J Cataract Refract Surg 2002; 28:1330-33.

23. Anderson NJ, Beran RF, Schneider TL. Epi-LASEK for the correction of myopia and myopic astigmatism. J Cataract Refract Surg 2002;28:1343-47.
24. Claringbold VT. Laser-assisted subepithelial keratectomy for the correction of myopia. J Cataract Refract Surg 2002; 28:18-22.
25. Shahinian L. Laser-assisted subepithelial keratectomy for low to high myopia and astigmatism. J Cataract Refract Surg 2002;28:1334-42.
26. Rouweyha RM, Chuang AZ, Mitra S, Phillips CB,Yee RW. Laser Epithelial Keratomileusis for myopia with the Autonomous Laser. J Refract Surg 2002;18:217-24.

CHAPTER 18

Excimer Laser Subepithelial Ablation (ELSA) or LASEK Offers Return to Surface Ablation

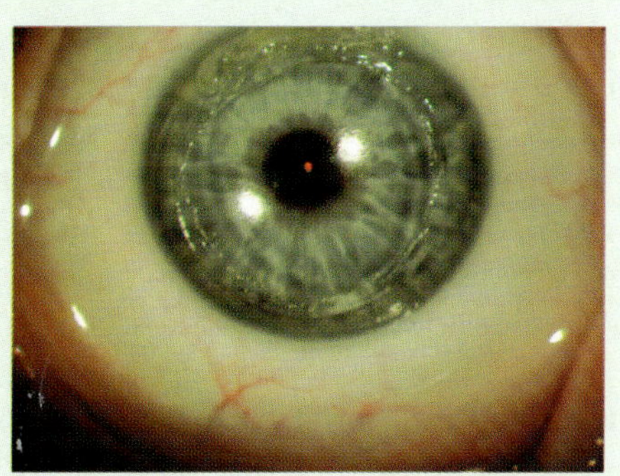

Chris P Lohmann (Germany)

INTRODUCTION

Refractive surgery is a field that is constantly changing with new technologies being developed and introduced routinely. Currently excimer laser photorefractive keratectomy (PRK) and excimer laser in situ keratomileusis (LASIK) are the surgical procedures most commonly been used to treat myopia. PRK makes changes in the corneal curvature by ablating part of Bowman's layer and anterior corneal stroma tissue after removing the epithelium. In contrast, LASIK does not remove the epithelium, Bowman's layer, or anterior stroma tissue but does remove deep stromal tissue after making a cut into the cornea stroma at approximately 160 micron using a microkeratome. Various peer reviewed studies have shown that the refractive results and long time visual outcomes are good and similar for PRK and LASIK in low to moderate myopia up to – 8 diopters (D).

A new keratorefractive technique, laser assisted subepithelial keratectomy (LASEK), was introduced by Massimo Camellin in 1999. LASEK is based on the detachment of the epithelium using an alcohol solution, creating an epithelial flap that is then repositioned after the laser ablation. The epithelium regenerates itself within a few days and in the meantime the existing flap protects the ablated corneal surface. This technique has the potential to eliminate or reduce many disadvantages of PRK (i.e. postoperative pain, slow visual recovery and corneal haze) and LASIK (i.e. flap complications, interface problems and possibly attenuated long time biomechanical stability of the cornea) and combine their advantages. Early studies suggest that refractive and visual results, stability and safety of LASEK are comparable to those of PRK and LASIK, but haze levels and pain seem to be lower than PRK. Visual recovery seems to be relatively faster after LASEK; approximately two third of the treated eyes have an uncorrected visual acuity (UCVA) of 20/40 or better at day three.

As there is some degree of similarity in pronouncing the names LASEK and LASIK and therefore confuse both the ophthalmic community and the patients we have re-named this procedure to ELSA (**E**xcimer **L**aser **S**ubepithelial **A**blation).

THE SURGICAL PROCEDURE

Although various types of LASEK procedures have been described the majority of surgeons are using the alcohol assisted classical Camellin technique which is illustrated in Figure 18.1. The surgery is performed under topical anesthesia. After a lid speculum is applied to the patients eye the surgery consists of the following steps:

1. An incision of the corneal epithelium is performed using a 8.0 mm cornea trephine with a 70 micron depth calibrated blade. The trephine is designed to create a 280-degree epithelial incision leaving a blunt section of 80 degrees at the 12-o'clock position for the formation of a hinge. The trephine is placed centrally on the papillary axis and downward pressure of the trephine is evenly applied to the blade and slight rotation of the blade (approximately 5 degrees in both directions) is used to create the incision.
2. An 8.5 mm LASEK alcohol cone is placed on the corneal surface encircling the epithelial incision. This

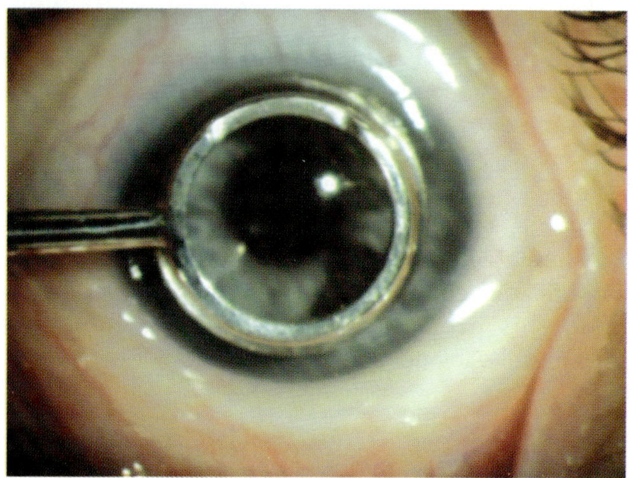

FIGURE 18.1A: Trepanation of the epithelium

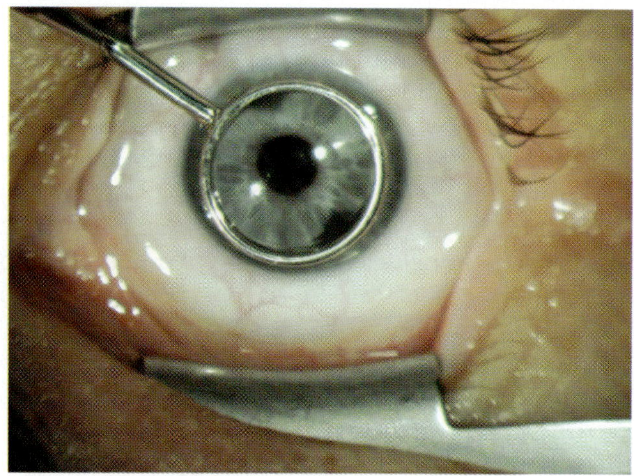

FIGURE 18.1B: 30 sec alcohol

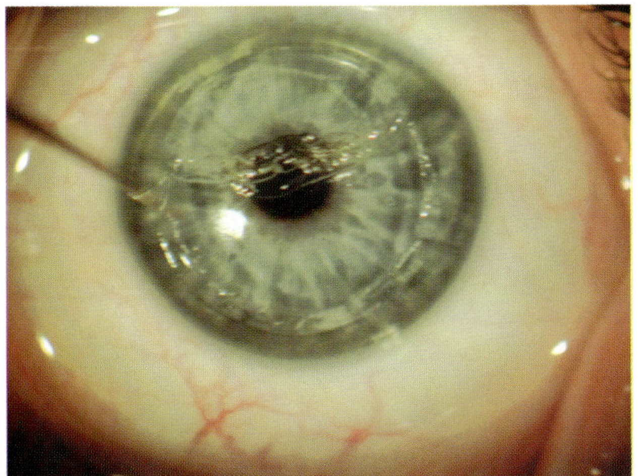

FIGURE 18.1C: Mobilization of the epithelium

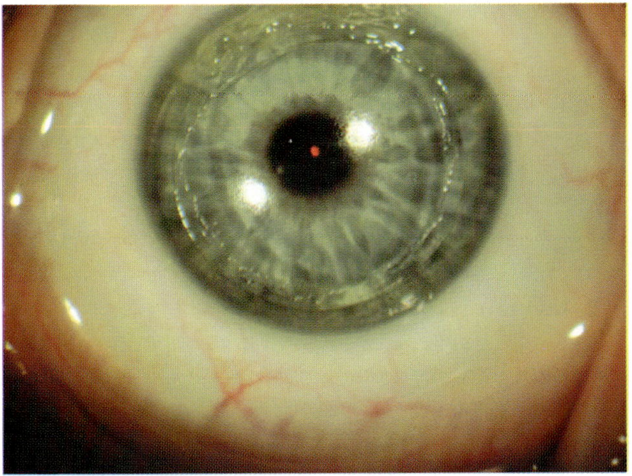

FIGURE 18.1D: Excimer laser ablation

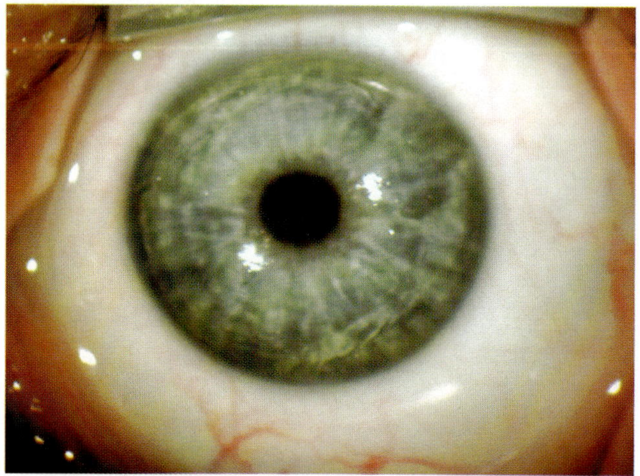

FIGURE 18.1E: Re-positioning of the epithelium

FIGURES 18.1A to E: The LASEK procedure (Camellin's technique)

cone is filled with 20 percent ethanol (in distilled water) and left for 30 seconds. After this time the alcohol is absorbed with a small sponge, the alcohol cone is removed and the cornea is thoroughly washed with BSS to remove all remaining alcohol. The area of epithelial incision is then dried with a small sponge.

3. To create the epithelial flap the pre-cut margin of the epithelium is lifted using the sharp side of a special epithelial peeler, starting at the edges of the epithelial incision and the epithelial flap is gently detached and folded-up at the 12-o'clock position using the blunt side of the epi-peeler.
4. If the epithelium shows strong adherence, the corneal surface is re-exposed to the alcohol for additional 10 to 15 seconds.

5. Then the laser ablation is performed and we are using the normal LASIK normograms.
6. After the laser ablation the cornea is flooded with BSS and the flap is repositioned with the blunt side of the epithelial peeler. A 14.0 mm soft bandage contact lens (we recommend Pure Vision Bausch and Lomb or Ciba Vision daily focus) is applied for protection of the epithelial flap for 3 days.

SURGICAL INSTRUMENTS

Almost all ophthalmic instrument companies have LASEK instruments in their portfolio. The original ones were from Janach (Como, Italy) which are shown in Figure 18.1. The set of instruments usually consists of a epithelial trephine and alcohol cone, and a peeler or microhoe to mobilize and push back the epithelium.

For astigmatic correction there are elliptical instruments distributed by Geuder (Heidelberg, Germany) which are shown in Figure 18.2.

Just recently they have been disposable instruments introduced to the ophthalmic community. These are also been distributed by Geuder (Heidelberg, Germany) and are shown in Figure 18.3. The main advantage of these disposable instruments that they are disposable and therefore reduces the risk of infection. There is no need for sterilization which maybe of importance for high volume clinic. You will always have an ultrasharp trephine for a good quality of the epithelial incision. This is of importance for a reduced rate of postoperative pain and haze.

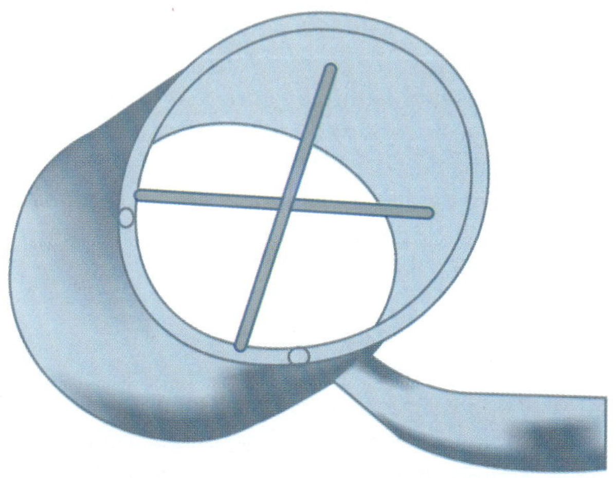

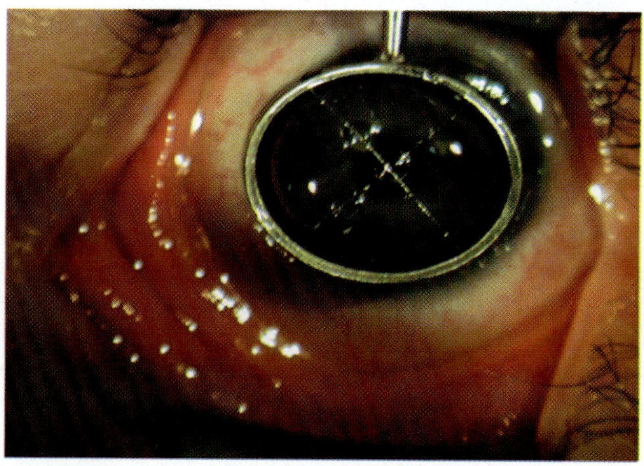

FIGURE 18.2: Elliptical LASEK instrument for astigmatic corrections

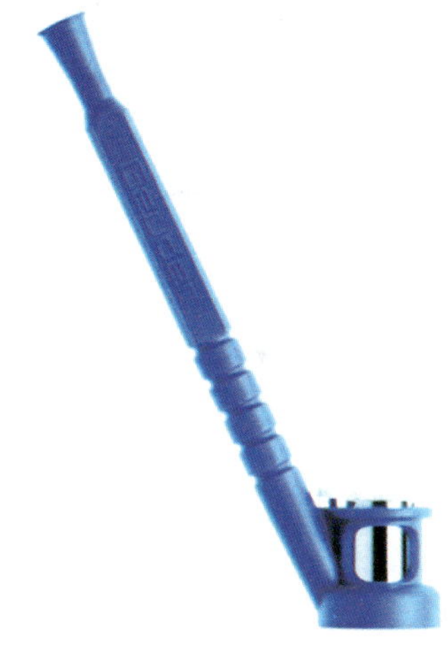

18.3A

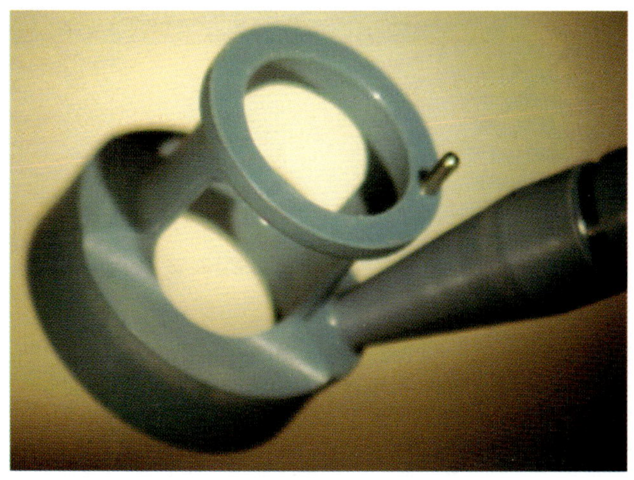

18.3B

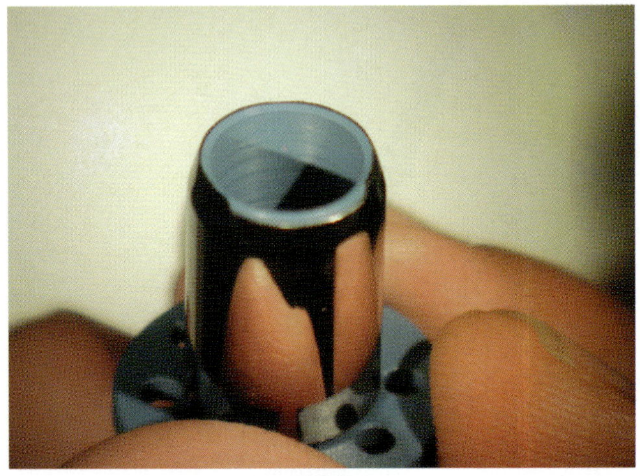

18.3C

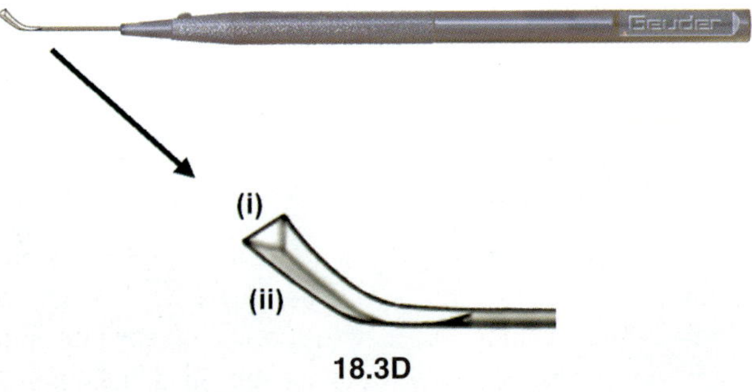

18.3D

FIGURE 18.3: Disposable LASEK instruments (a) the combined instrument, (b) alcohol well, (c) the trephine, (d) disposable epi-peeler—(i) sharp part to mobilize the epithelium, (ii) blunt part to push back the epithelium

POSTOPERATIVE MEDICATION

A bandage soft contact lens is of critical importance to keep the epithelium in place after the surgery. This contact lens should not be removed before the third postoperative day. Until the removal of the bandage contact lens the postoperative therapy should consist of a topical antibiotic agent and a corticosteroid 4 times daily and lubrication (we prefer carbomer 2.0 mg) 5 to 8 times a day. As there is a contact lens on the eye we recommend the use of nonpreserved eye drops. After the removal of the contact lens the eyes should be treated with carbomer 2.0 mg 4 times daily and with topical corticosteroids 4 times daily for 2 weeks and twice a day for 2 weeks. All medications should be withdrawn after 4 weeks.

CLINICAL RESULTS

So far there have been very few clinical studies published in peer-reviewed journals. In the following we have summarized the results.

Myopia

Up to a myopic correction of 8 D (spherical equivalent, SE) between 81 and 97percent are within +/– 0.5 D after 6 months. Uncorrected visual acuity of 20/20 are between 73 and 92 percent of the treated eyes, and between 96 and 100 percent are within 20/40. None of the eyes have lost more than 1 line of Snellen visual acuity.

Astigmatism

Today there is only one larger studies of the treatment of astigmatism. This have been performed by our group.

We have treated 60 eyes with a myopic astigmatism between –1 and – 4.5 D with a follow up of 12 months. All of these eyes were postoperatively within +/- 0.75 D of SE with an astigmatic correction with less than 0.5 D. None of the eyes lost more than 1 line of visual acuity, in contrast 39 percent gained 1 or 2 lines of visual acuity. No significant haze of greater 0.5 was seem in these eyes.

Hyperopia

So far no studies have been published in peer-reviewed journals on the treatment of hyperopia using LASEK.

ADVANTAGES AND DISADVANTAGES OF LASEK

LASEK or ELSA is not as comfortable as LASIK but much less painful than PRK. In our experience 17 percent of our treated eyes have some kind of pain within the first 4 hours which there after disappears. Visual rehabilitation is faster in LASIK than in LASEK or ELSA. But it seems to us, that using the new LASEK microkeratom from Ciba or Gebauer (the procedure called Epi-LASIK) postoperative visual recovery is not much slower than in LASIK. The main advantage of LASEK or ELSA is that it does need a cut in the stroma as with LASIK. Therefore the LASIK flap related complications like diffuse lamellar keratitis, free flaps, button holes, incomplete flap, flap wrinkles, epithelial ingrowth, microbiological infections, biomechanical problems, and an increase in higher order aberrations are excluded with LASEK or ELSA. In particular we think of customized ablation just like wavefront- or topography-guided ablations LASEK or ELSA is obviously superior than LASIK.

CONCLUSIONS

LASEK or ELSA is a very good alternative for LASIK corrections for myopia up to – 8.0 D and astigmatism up to – 5.0 D. In particular for customized ablations it is superior to LASIK.

CHAPTER 19

Presbyopic Multifocal LASIK (PML): A New Approach in Corneal Refractive Surgery

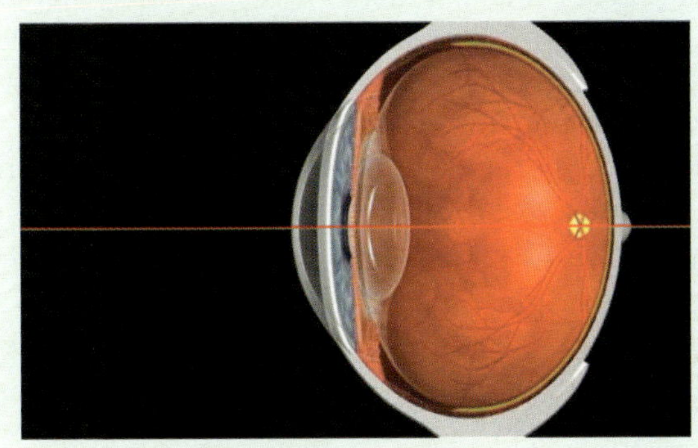

Roberto Pinelli (Italy)

INTRODUCTION

In all refractive surgery, our goal has been to surgically correct the visual defects, i.e. myopia, hyperopia, astigmatism, and presbyopia. Correction of these defects is possible through corneal surgical procedures or lenticular surgery.

Of all the visual defects, presbyopia has been the most challenging to correct, partly because the mechanisms of accommodation and the causes of presbyopia are complex and not fully understood. Thus far, it has largely been managed through the use of progressively stronger spectacles, which gradually take over the near focus work of the crystalline lens. Presbyopia is also unique in that it is the only refractive error that is considered to be progressive in nature. Although our management and most of our experience seems to point to the progressive nature of presbyopia, in truth, we don't know for sure that it truly progresses. It may be that in our "prosthetic culture" we have merely become unnecessarily dependent on our glasses and contacts.

In any case, a surgical alternative to the correction of presbyopia is appealing because of the enormous pool of presbyopic patients with a desire for good uncorrected vision. Mild hyperopes and emmetropes who have never worn glasses are particularly uncomfortable with presbyopia and its associated inconveniences.

APPROACHES TO THE SURGICAL CORRECTION OF PRESBYOPIA

The mission of presbyopic surgery as with all other refractive surgeries should be to eliminate the symptoms of the refractive error, rather than to correct the anatomical defect itself. For this reason, I think an approach that provides pseudoaccommodation is natural and appropriate. If we can provide patients with good functional vision at multiple distances, it is not necessary to restore true accommodative function in the form of a dynamically adjusting optical power of the eye.

There are several potential sites for correction of presbyopia. The cornea is probably the most common target, as it is the area refractive surgeons are most comfortable operating on. Theoretically, the anterior chamber provides another site for the correction of presbyopia, but this is as yet theoretical and would likely prove extremely difficult in reality. The human crystalline lens can be replaced with a multifocal or accommodative intraocular lens, of which many different styles are now under development and coming to market. Finally, a number of scleral implant or ciliary muscle surgical procedures have been developed. This approach, however, is complicated, largely untested, and seems "more surgical" than is necessary.

As a familiar corneal procedure, LASIK has been the most popular and easiest surgical approach. In addition to the surgeon comfort level with the procedure, patients in the presbyopic baby boomer generation are also familiar with and accepting of the procedure. In addition, LASIK can be performed bilaterally on the same day, is relatively quick and painless, and has proven to be quite safe.

Even with LASIK, we have several options for addressing presbyopia. Most conventionally, we have taken a monofocal approach with surgically-induced monovision, but bifocal and multifocal approaches are increasing. LASIK is ideal for presbyopia because of the absence of haze and its associated refractive complications, the absence of regression, and the presence of a regular and, hopefully, thin flap that can protect the multifocality created in the stroma.

In designing a multifocal LASIK procedure, we must take advantage of some of the lessons learned from current and past procedures. Some myopes treated with radial keratotomy have retained good near and distance vision well into the presbyopic age range. Why is that? Similarly, some hyperopic LASIK patients also have retained their pseudoaccommodative function well into their older years. Again, why would that be? The secret lies in the asphericity of the cornea. A prolate cornea seems to have the capability to focus both far and near better than an oblate cornea. We have seen that again recently with conductive keratoplasty, which I perform and have been involved in studying in Italy. CK is an excellent technique for correcting hyperopia and restoring near vision. It appears to provide some degree of multifocality because eyes corrected for near visual acuity with CK typically have much better distance visual acuity than would be expected. This may be due to the prolateness of the post-CK cornea. In any case, the "blended vision" of CK permits the presbyopic patient to read by treating just the non-dominant eye.

In the past three years, my purpose has been to create a truly multifocal corneal procedure that can be performed bilaterally if necessary, and that will work for any eye, regardless of preoperative refractive error. Intuitively, we know that many zones should do a better job of mimicking natural vision than just two zones, but obtaining a gradual but effective multifocality is nonetheless challenging. The ultimate presbyopic LASIK procedure must also be easy to perform, with standardized nomograms that any surgeon can use as a basis for successful surgery.

THE PML™ PROCEDURE

With the above goals in mind, I developed and have been investigating at ILMO a patented procedure which we call PML™ (Presbyopic Multifocal LASIK). This procedure can be performed on presbyopic myopes, hyperopes, astigmats, and emmetropes. Multifocality on the cornea is created using a multi-step treatment in which several independently calculated ablations are performed at various optical zones. Depending on the patient's refractive error, there may be anywhere from three to

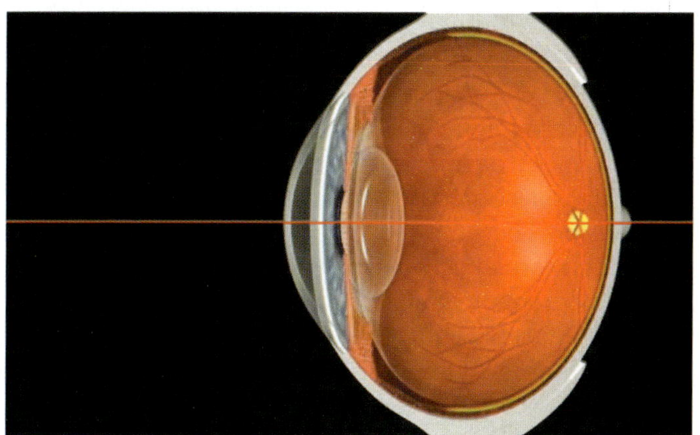

FIGURE 19.1: Central area of the cornea: Focus on the retina

eight different concentric zones. In all cases, the goal is to treat the central cornea for distance vision, with a multifocal peripheral cornea that is able to provide functional near vision. Some other multifocal LASIK procedures take the opposite approach, with the near correction in the center. However, the central cornea provides an excellent site for distance vision because it is relatively aberration-free, while peripheral aberrations may actually be useful for near focusing.

In this multi-step process, we first treat astigmatism in the classic manner, as if we were doing a purely astigmatic laser correction. Next we treat the distance defect in a zone on the central cornea. Then, we treat the near defect in a larger optical zone. Finally, other zones may be created to ensure that the overall power of the cornea is emmetropic, even though there are varying powers in the different optical zones. It is a procedure that is highly customizable for each patient's optical needs.

I began doing this procedure in 2002, starting cautiously by treating 10 patients in only their non-dominant eyes. One year postoperatively, five of these patients were happy with their outcomes; the other five required retreatment. These unilateral patients experienced some of the benefits and problems of monovision. I became convinced that a bilateral approach would be more effective, and began to adjust and refine the nomograms towards this end.

For our first bilateral study cohort, we treated 100 eyes of 50 patients with. Our studies so far have been performed with the Technolas 217 Z (Bausch and Lomb) and the Lasitome microkeratome (Gebauer). However, the procedure is technology-independent and was designed to work with any keratome and laser combination.

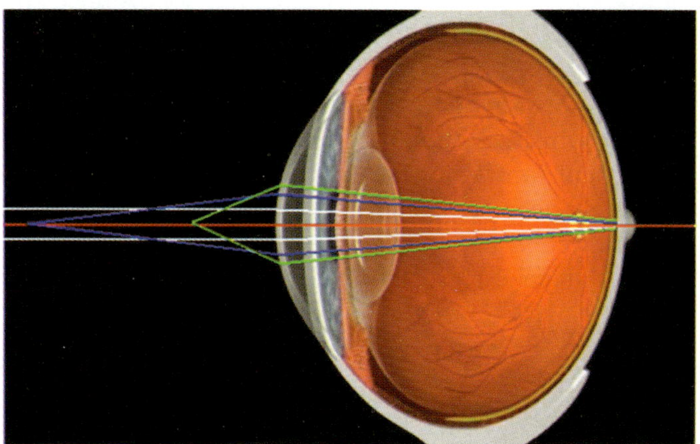

FIGURE 19.2: Multifocality permits to focus both far and near objects on macula (pseudo-accommodation)

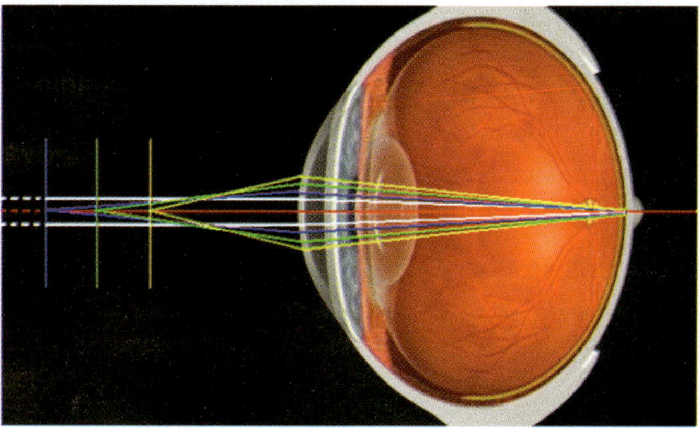

FIGURE 19.3: Effects of a completely multifocal cornea

RESULTS

All 50 patients were seeing at least 20/25 for distance and at least J3 for near. Eighty percent had bilateral uncorrected vision of 20/20 or better for distance and J2 or better for near. Another 10 percent were 20/25 and J2, while the remaining 10 percent were 20/25 and J3. Patient satisfaction levels have been very high, and there have been no retreatments thus far. Typically, patients experience a myopic shift during the first month postoperatively, then stabilize at plano.

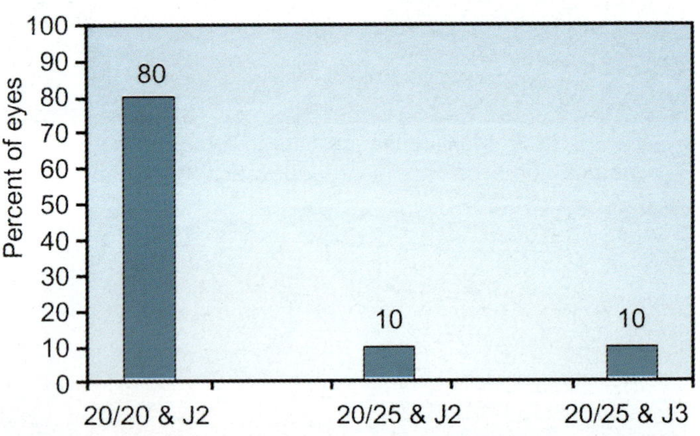

FIGURE 19.4: Fifty patients eyes postoperative results

A few cases illustrate well the potential of this procedure. The first example is a 50-year-old female who was a -6.0 D myope with a +1.5 D add for reading. We treated the cornea in six different zones: a -1.5 D correction in each of the following optical zones: 4.8, 5.2, 5.4, 5.6, and 6.0 mm; and a +2.00 D correction at the 6.5 mm optical zone. Six months postoperative, her uncorrected vision is 20/20 and J2 in both eyes.

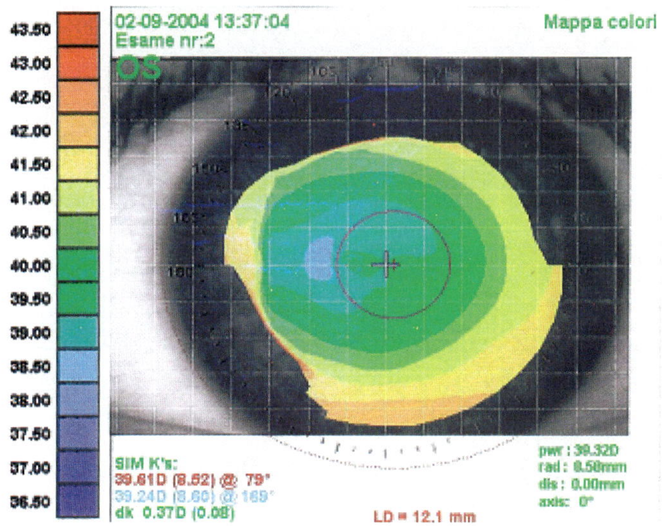

FIGURE 19.5: A prolate cornea after PML™ case # 1

The second case is a 54-year-old patient who was plano in both eyes preoperatively but using a +1.5 D add for near vision. We performed two treatment rings for near vision, each +0.75 D, at the 6.0 and 6.5 mm optical zones. In addition, I did three treatment rings for distance vision, ablating a –0.50 D spherical correction at the 5.0, 5.2, and 5.4 mm optical zones. After a myopic reaction initially, the eyes are now emmetropic, and six months postoperative, this patient's uncorrected visual acuity is 20/20 and J2 in both eyes. Ultimately, my goal is to be able to correct emmetropes like this as soon as they start experiencing presbyopic symptoms at age 45 or 50.

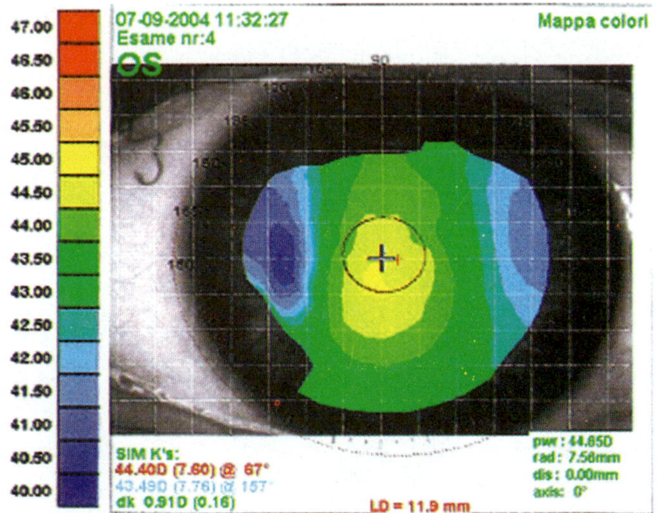

FIGURE 19.6: An oblate cornea after PML™ case # 2

PEARLS AND LESSONS LEARNED

We have found that it is better to overcorrect hyperopia and to undercorrect myopia, and that astigmatism must be fully corrected for a satisfactory outcome. In some cases (hyperopes and emmetropes), the cornea becomes more prolate; in other cases (primarily myopes) it actually becomes more oblate. Pupil size is not an important factor in determining outcomes from this procedure. We have not had to manage patients with especially large pupils any differently than we would with a monofocal LASIK procedure.

The PML™ technique uses the same or less tissue as other laser vision correction procedures, so although pachymetry is important, it is no more a factor than in monofocal LASIK. Keratometry is very important, as it is essential to keep the pre- and postoperative K values constant.

Patients must be willing to participate in training their eyes to learn how to see at near with the multifocal correction. Our patients are instructed not to use reading glasses after the procedure at all and to do visual exercises (for which we provide instruction) in order to maintain the eye's focusing power with age.

In our experience so far, is a very successful procedure that has been well-accepted by patients and is in high demand at our center. Currently, about 30 percent of our patients are PML™ candidates. The procedure and the excellent results experienced by patients have enhanced the reputation of our center and generated many referrals. Ongoing research is required to determine whether and when regression might occur.

CHAPTER 20

Solid-state Lasers for Refractive Surgery

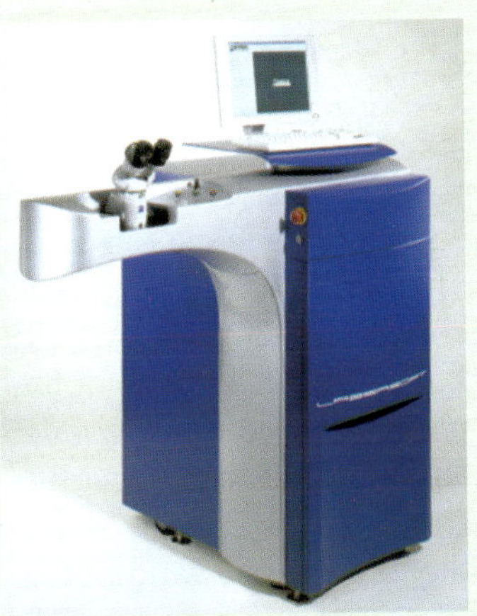

Matteo Piovella
Fabrizio I Camesasca
Barbara Kusa

(Italy)

INTRODUCTION

Laser technology for refractive surgery advanced with unrelentless pace during the past 20 years. The introduction of concepts such as wavefront analysis and customized ablation required manifold developments dealing with an increased, outmost precision of treatment.

Solid-state lasers in ophthalmic surgery have meant increased energy efficiency, as well as reduced size and costs. Presently, a new generation of UV-generating solid-state lasers is becoming available even for refractive surgery, including lasers such as the LaserSoft and the CustomVis.[1, 2]

KATANA, SOLID-STATE UV LASER FOR REFRACTIVE SURGERY SINCE 2003

A good example of solid-state laser for refractive surgery, LaserSoft, is a continuous wave diode-pumped all-solid-state UV laser for refractive surgery recently introduced by Katana Technologies GmbH. A solid-state is not an excimer laser, since the UV laser ablation radiation is generated by nonlinear frequency conversion of infrared laser light in a laser crystal. A sequential frequency conversion with nonlinear crystals shifts the wavelength of the laser radiation into the range of 208-210 nm. The resonator structure and the beam delivery ensure an emission of the laser radiation with a TEM_{00} transversal mode, as well as an emission of laser radiation with a true Gaussian beam. The continuous wave-diode pumping provides a very stable shot-to-shot UV output with impressive long-term stability.

A Gaussian beam means excellent UV light spot distribution on the cornea. In fact, differently from the usual excimer laser, the solid-state laser does not need beam-forming elements – i.e., mirrors - in the beam path. Thus, energy at the corneal surface – fluency – is very stable. The laser beam is highly collimated, providing an increased beam precision and the technical features adequate to a fast scanning. Furthermore, the ablation pattern utilized in LaserSoft ensures an extremely homogenous cornea surface due to the accurate overlap made possible by true Gaussian spots.

Differently from an excimer laser, in a solid-state laser there is no gas exchange and gas discharge involved, with the related instabilities in output radiation, due to the physical nature of the discharge process. The solid-state approach reduces the requirements for maintenance and costs, providing high stability and long lifetime.

This device generates a flying spot of 0.2 mm in diameter, operating at repetition rate of 1 kHz. Thanks to this high repetition rate, the energy per pulse is lower then in standard excimer treatments. Ablation has strongly reduced shock waves, and to no audible sound due to ablation or laser firing. The whole procedure takes place in a silent environment, much reassuring to the patient, without the risk of noise-induced abrupt motion.

To fully exploit the opportunities provided by custom ablation, a very fast laser like LaserSoft requires a fast eye-tracker. The LaserSoft eye-tracker has a latency of 1 ms and controls ablation cent ration at very high repetition rates. This very fast eye-tracker ensures a reliable, high repetition cent ration of ablation on the x-y axes as well as well as the ocular rotation.

All these features makes the solid-state laser an ideal device for accurate custom ablation (Figures 20.1 and 20.2).

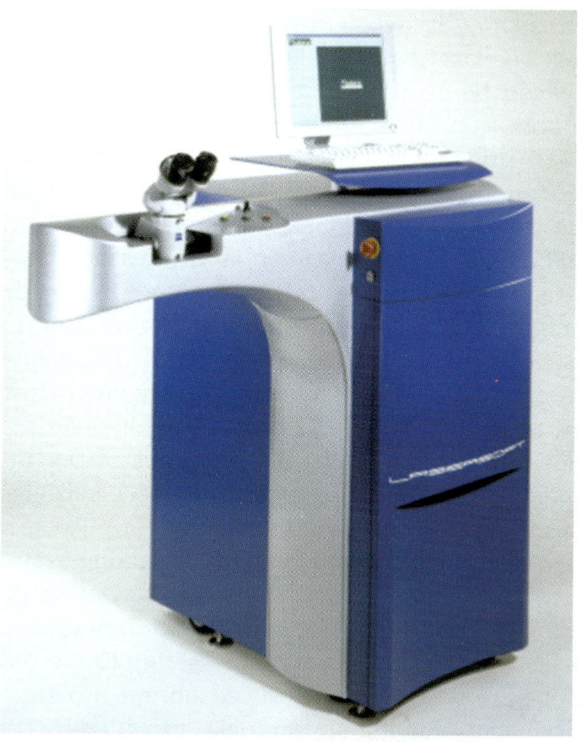

FIGURE 20.1: LaserSoft solid-state laser

The ablation profiles currently adopted by this laser are designed to preserve the strongly aspherical physiological corneal curvature, as well as to minimize the induced spherical aberration.

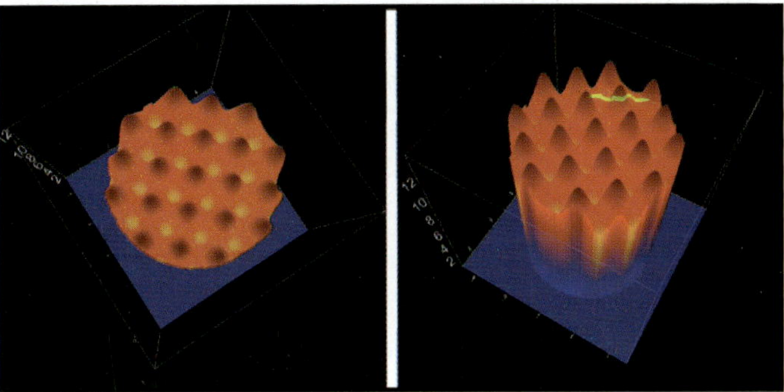

FIGURE 20.2: Experimental model, possibilities for custom ablation offered by small spot size. Views of the attempted profile

Different reflection losses and fluence values for different angles of incidence of the ablating laser radiation during surgery are also taken into account in the ablation algorithm.

CLINICAL EXPERIENCE

We hereafter illustrate our clinical experience with a solid-state laser. Patients were treated at two different centers: Messina (PRK) and Campobasso (LASIK), Italy. The results were gathered after one year and were analyzed with the software Datagraph, using graphs recommended by G. O. Waring III.[3, 4] After signing a specific informed consent, 37 eyes, were treated with LASIK and PRK procedures with LaserSoft ablation. Preoperative refractive data are reported in Table 20.1. Preoperative BSCVA of all eyes was between 0.3 and 1.0. LASIK was performed with the Hansatome microkeratome, choosing a flap

TABLE 20.1: Preoperative vs one-month data, 37 eyes

	SE refractive defect (mean ± SD)	*Sphere (mean ± SD)*	*Cylinder (mean ± SD)*	*SE refractive defect, range*	*BSCVA*
Preoperative	-1.71 D ± 3.71 D	-1.46 D ± 3.32 D	-0.51 D ± 1.97 D	-8.00 D to +6.75 D	0.80 ± 0.23
One year	-0.03 D ± 0.13 D	-0.03 D ± 0.19 D	-0.01 D ± 0.19 D	-0.50 D to +0.25 D	0.83 ± 0.23

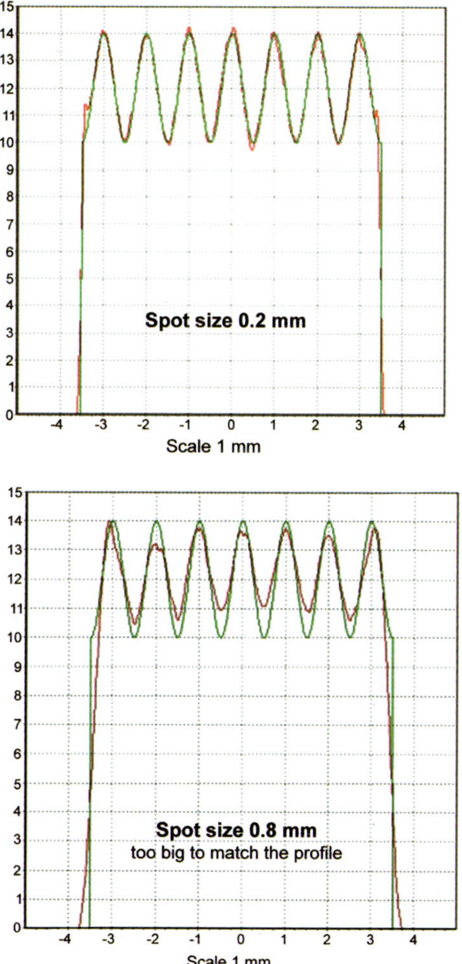

FIGURE 20.3: Experimental model, small spot size and custom ablation. Views of the attempted profile with a 0.2 spot size solid-state laser vs. that of a 0.8 mm spot size

thickness of 180 micrometer. Treatment diameters ranged between 6 and 7 mm, and transition zones between 8 and 9 mm.

One-year results were well within the current standards provided by normal excimer lasers (Table 20.1). Figure 20.3 shows the scattergram of the attempted versus the achieved refractive change for each eye. Figure 20.4 shows the spherical equivalent refractive outcome with the corresponding numbers. At one year, 100 percent of the eyes were in the so called happiness zone of +- 1D, 94 percent were within +- 0.5 D, and 87 percent were within +- 0.25 D. Figure 20.5 shows stability of refraction. The mean achieved change of spherical equivalent with time is also given. Table 20.2 provides the refractive and BSCVA results at one-year.

Efficacy consists of two components: component 1 is the spectacle corrected visual acuity at baseline (BSCVA);

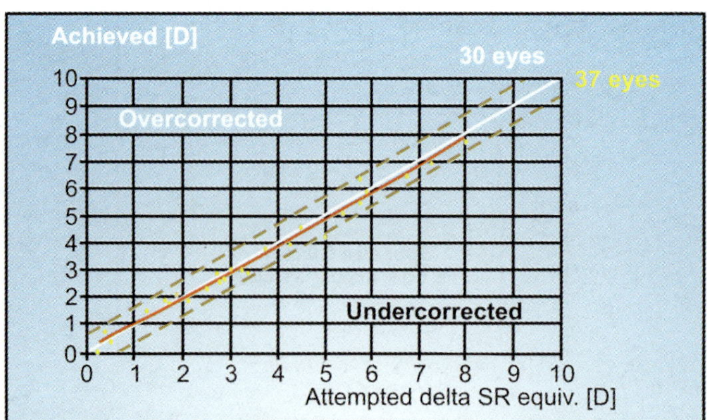

FIGURE 20.4: Show the scattergram and therefore an impression of the spread of cases of the attempted versus the achieved refractive change for each eye for LASIK

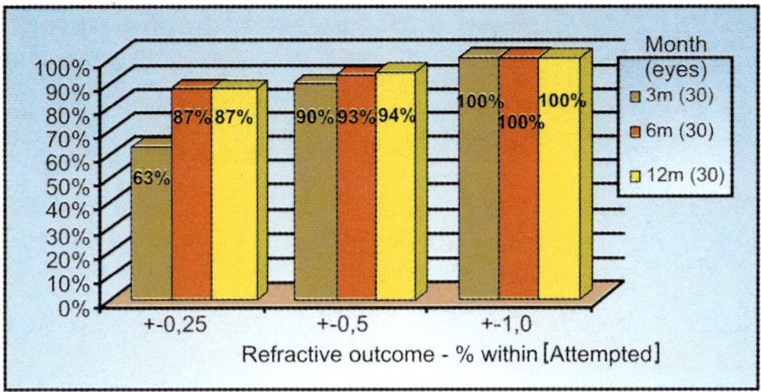

FIGURE 20.5: Spherical equivalent refractive outcome at one year. Of all eyes, 100 % are in the so-called happiness zone of +- 1D, 94% are within +- 0.5 D, and 87% are within +- 0.25 D

TABLE 20.2: Refractive and BSCVA results at one-year follow up, 37 eyes

SE refractive defect, Attempted vs Obtained	*BSCVA Preoperative vs One-year*
-0.03 D ± 0.20 D	0.0 ± 0.2

component 2 is the cumulative graph of uncorrected visual acuities after refractive surgery (UCVA). In our study, 45 percent of the eyes show a postoperative UCVA better then 20/20 from a cohort with 41 percent being preoperatively at 20/20 with best correction. The preoperative BSCVA of all eyes was between 1.0 and 0.3.

Solid-State Lasers vs. Excimer Lasers

Table 20.3 presents the differences between common excimer lasers and solid-state laser. Presently, solid-state laser

TABLE 20.3: Excimer vs. Solid-state lasers for refractive surgery

	Common excimer laser	*LaserSoft solid-state laser*
Spot size (mm)	0.8 – 1.0	0.2
Beam quality	Multimode (additional optics for clearing the excimer beam)	Single mode (Gaussian)
Repetition rate	50 –500 Hz	1 kHz
Eye-tracker speed	Approximately 150 Hz	More than 1 kHz

presents several significant examples of technical evolution in refractive surgery lasers. The solid-state laser features a tiny flying spot with a diameter of 0.2 mm and it operates at repetition rate of 1 kHz. Its very small spot size fits the present requirements for effective custom ablation.

The vast majority of excimer lasers commonly available on the market features a 1-mm flying spot, and they never have spots smaller than 0.65 mm, thus with a much wider spot ablation area than a solid-state laser (Figure 20.6). There is a technical limit in decreasing the spot size of an excimer laser, as smaller spots would have a less homogeneous beam. Utilizing the usual excimer laser repetition rates, a 0.2 spot size would mean a very long treatment time, with the entire precision problem related to eye motion. To maintain ablation time within acceptable limits, and thanks to its technical features, the repetition rate of a solid-state laser is much higher in the solid-state than in excimer lasers.

The mirrors in a solid-state laser transmit the UV light without further elaborating it, unlike an excimer laser. This thanks to the true Gaussian profile of the beam.

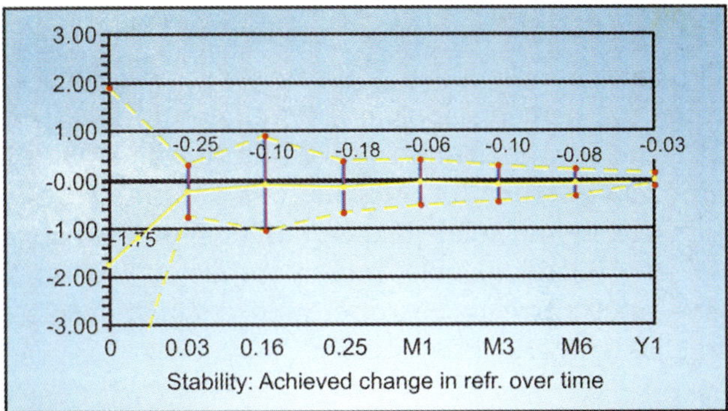

FIGURE 20.6: Refractive stability of the study group, at one year

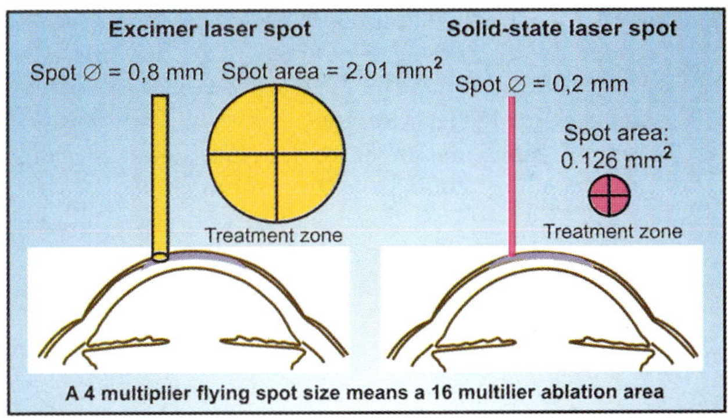

FIGURE 20.7: Solid-state vs. excimer laser spot size

Solid-state lasers appear to be easier to use lasers for refractive surgery, requiring less maintenance.

The fast eyetracking ensures a reliable cent ration of ablation for x-y directions as well as the rotation of the eye at high repetition rates.

CONCLUSION

Solid-state lasers appear to be a promising solution for a refractive surgery, applying less energy to the cornea and using a small flying spot of 0.2 mm, thus with the theoretical potential of inducing less scarring.

LaserSoft and solid-state UV lasers in general appear as a safe, reliable, stable, more compact as well as less costly alternative to gas-operating excimer lasers for refractive surgery.

REFERENCES

1. Personal Communications, 2003 Meeting of the ISRS/AAO, November 14-15, 2003, Anaheim, CA. Syllabus, 289.
2. Personal Communication, 2004 Meeting of the ISRS/AAO, October 22-23, 2004, New Orleans, LA. Syllabus, 10.
3. Datagraph med (Medical Data Analysis Software) Ingenieurbüro Pieger, Germany.
4. Waring G., Standard Graphs for Reporting Refractive Surgery. J. Refract. Surg. 2000;16:459.

CHAPTER 21

The Femtosecond Laser: A New Tool in Corneal Surgery

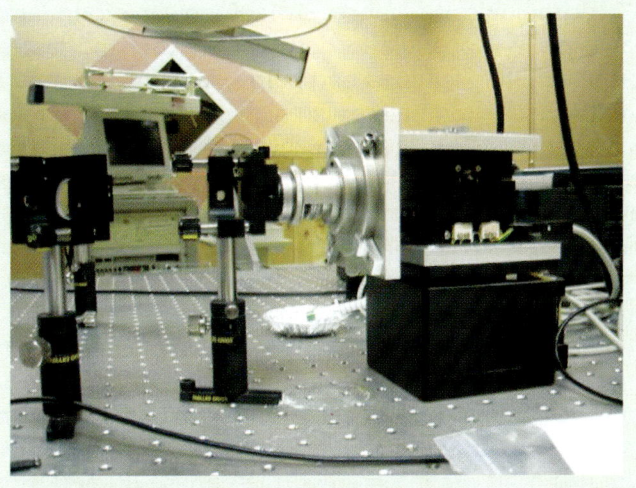

Jean-Marc Legeais (France)

INTRODUCTION

Research into ways of using lasers for corneal ablation has been carried out with the aim of providing completely automated surgical procedures.[1] The goal was to carry out fully reproducible surgical procedures without any contact with the patient. The initial trials were carried out using Excimer lasers, but this was succeeded by the infrared nanosecond laser,[2] and then by the picosecond laser.[3] Excimer lasers can only be used for surface treatments (PRK) or full-thickness incisions, but are not as suitable as ultrafast lasers for use within the thickness of structures. The nano- and picosecond lasers proved to be rather unsuitable for corneal surgery,[4] because of the heat-related effects they produce.

Technological advances in high-power diode lasers have made it possible to develop femtosecond lasers.[5] Lasers emitting femtosecond pulses have the property of emitting ultrashort pulses with high crest power from low energy pulses. The development of the femtosecond laser was mainly dependent on titanium:sapphire lasers.[6] These lasers were very expensive and cumbersome, because of the pumping system they required, and so were not suitable for medical applications. Femtosecond technology was only very recently been mastered with the invention of neodymium:glass lasers. Various laboratories, including the CUOS laboratory at Michigan University (USA), have recently developed lasers of this type that are now being used in eye surgery. Their first application is the LASIK.[7] The first trials are in progress (FDA phase III) and more than 50,000 eyes have been operated on to date. The applications of the femtosecond laser arise from the fact that it makes it possible to focus the beam very accurately (to within the order of a micrometer) in a transparent medium, and to produce the local destruction of material without producing any heat damage in the surrounding tissue.[8]

These lasers produce the destruction of the material by photodisruption.[9] This occurs when the density of the crest power produced at the focal point is sufficiently great to produce plasma out of the material. This high-density gas (a mixture of electrons and ions) produces a cavitation bubble.[10] When the laser impacts are juxtaposed, the bubbles of gas merge and produce the ablation. The minimum energy threshold required to produce plasma is known as the plasma or optical burst threshold. If more energy is supplied than is necessary to produce the plasma, collateral damage will occur. This collateral damage consists mainly of heat damage, but also an acoustic shock wave and an increase in the size of the cavitation bubble.[5] The emission of plasma with short pulses depends on a deterministic multiphoton regime,[11] which implies that once the output of the laser reaches or exceeds the threshold, plasma is always produced. This means that in theory at least, it is possible to carry out incisions near the threshold value, and so to induce little or no damage. It is therefore very difficult to assess these collateral effects, and this has only been attempted by destructive methods: transmission electron microscopy (TEM) and scanning electron microscopy (SEM). These methods have the drawback of denaturing the samples, which can result in artifacts and mask changes in the ultrastructure of the cornea, and of making it impossible to carry out a real-time analysis. It is necessary to compare the non-destructive imaging methods[12-16] and destructive imaging methods for determining the plasma threshold, and determine the collateral damage produced by a femtosecond laser source on the cornea in order to understand the kinetics of the cavitation production to develop firing algorithms that take into account the quantity of tissue photoablated. It is still difficult to assess this, which currently restricts the procedures to use for a LASIK flap.

FEMTOSECOND LASER

How is a femtosecond laser constructed, and what are its various constituents?

The Oscillator

The femtosecond laser system used consists of a laser oscillator that delivers femtosecond pulses ($1fs=10^{-15}s$) followed by an amplifier providing the energy necessary for the ablation in transparent biological tissues. The laser oscillator consists of a glass matrix spiked with neodymium, and a Z-shaped linear optical resonance. The femtosecond pulses are obtained by phase blocking the laser modes. The fluorescence band is centered on 1.065 µm. The pumping is carried out by a laser diode with an emission wavelength (900 nm) that is centered on the absorption peak of neodymium. The pulse that emerges from the oscillator lasts about a hundred femtoseconds, and has an energy of the order of a nano Joule. It is, therefore, very short but of low intensity.

The CPA System (Chirped Pulse Amplification)

Short laser pulses, such as the femtosecond pulses, are characterized by a wide spectrum (Heisenberg uncertainty principle). The spectrum of the laser is centered on 1.065 nm, and has a width of a few tens of nanometers. The CPA system makes it possible to stretch the pulse by linear retardation of the frequencies that constitute the spectrum of the laser, so as to spread the energy of each pulse over a time of several tens of picoseconds. In this way, the energy density in the amplifying medium is reduced, which makes it possible to produce greater amplification without any risk of damaging the medium. To achieve this frequency stretching, the optical pathway followed by each frequency in the spectrum of the pulse must be altered. To do this, a diffraction network is used that can separate the various frequencies. In our case, we used the same network to stretch?? spread?? the pulse in time and then, after amplification, to re-compress it to its original duration. The amplifying medium, like the oscillator consists of neodymium:glass and is pumped by a diode. When it emerges from the compressor system, each pulse lasts about 500 fs and its energy was found to be 60 μ joules for a repetition rate of 10 KHz. The stability of the amplified pulses was excellent, with fluctuations between different peaks of less than 1 percent. The pulse repetition rate of 10 KHz provides high-speed incision. By reducing the output to a single pulse, it is possible to investigate the effects of a single pulse and thus to separate the effects of the pulse from the cumulative effects. The beam has a Gaussian TEM_{00} shape. The density of the crest power obtained is of the order of $10^{15} W/cm^2$.

The Delivery System

The commercial systems that are currently available cannot be adjusted by the surgeon; the assessment of these lasers calls for evaluation systems that will allow physicists and physicians to alter the parameters of the system. In the system currently under development at the Hôtel-Dieu Hospital in Paris [France] the laser beam is channeled through to the samples via a series of mirrors and lenses. This system makes it possible adjust the horizontal and vertical alignments of the beam and to obtain a focal distance of about 5 cm, with a focal spot of about 4 μm. The beam delivery system is currently fixed so as to yield the best possible optical quality, to ensure a fixed size of the focal point for the performance of our experiments, and to ensure that it is reproducible. For the incisions, it is the samples that are moved in front of the laser beam (Figure 21.1).

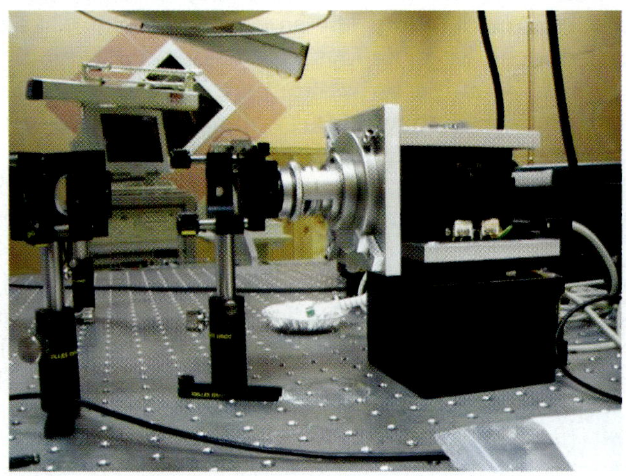

FIGURE 21.1: Experimental system for corneal investigation. Artificial chamber and delivery system

The samples are fixed in a front chamber and which is moved by a micrometric mobilized system. Movement along all three axes is controlled by an IT system that ensures that the incisions are completely reproducible. The energy of the laser is controlled by a calibrated photodiode.

The Anterior Chamber

This is linked to a system infusing a physiological solution (BSS). This continuous irrigation maintains constant hydration and pressure during the laser treatment. The cornea displays anterior convexity, and so to be able to produce an incision to a constant deph it is necessary to have a flattening system. A glass slide held by a ring attached to the anterior chamber flattens the cornea and delivers impacts in the same plane. This solution is much simpler that attempting to set the movement of the beam in all three dimensions, which would make it necessary to modulate the geometry of the displacement on the basis of the keratometric characteristics of the cornea.

Various factors are involved at the laser/tissue interface. The energy and the plasma threshold both depend in part on the degree of hydration and the transparency of the cornea. Controls and real-time assessment systems are required to determine these various aspects (Figure 21.2 and 21.3).

Samples of "silicone dioxide" are used to calibrate the laser, to check the incisions performed and to carry out the initial imaging experiments. These samples have the advantage of having constant transparency and hydration (Figure 21.4).

Indeed, in the case of corneas, it is necessary to check the degree of hydration and transparency. These two

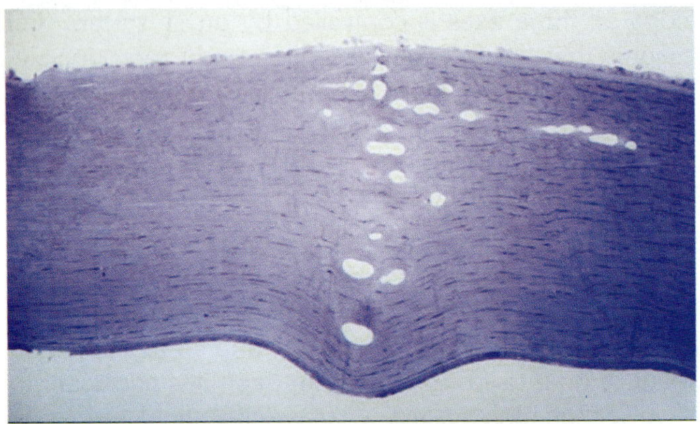

FIGURE 21.2: Maximum incident energy: Intrastromal cavitation bubbles. No thermal damage

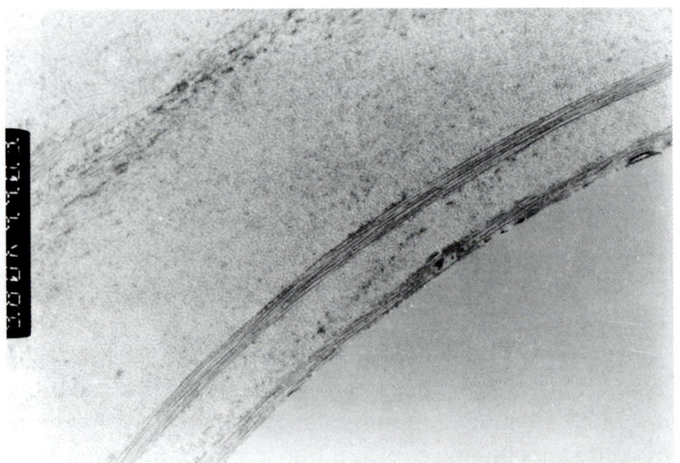

FIGURE 21.3: Transmission electron microscopy. Human cornea providing by the French Eye Bank. Eye cavitation bubbles. Intrastromal interface. No thermal damage

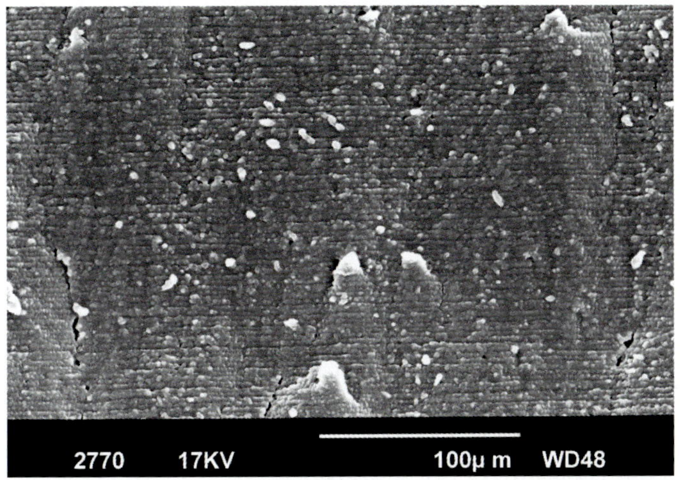

FIGURE 21.4: Silicon dioxide sample. Maximum incident energy. High quality interface by scan microscopy

characteristics are intimately linked, and can affect the effects of the laser.[16]

High-frequency ultrasound, confocal microscopy and two-photon microscopy are imaging techniques known to be nondestructive and that can be used to assess the direct effects of the laser on the tissue of the cornea because, unlike conventional transmission or scanning electron microscopy it does not affect its characteristics. The samples do not need any preparation before analysis.

The Plasma Threshold

The plasma threshold is determined using samples that have undergone horizontal incisions at decreasing?? energy levels. It is determined at the surface of the sample and at various depths. For the non-destructive imaging techniques (conventional optical microscopy, confocal microscopy and two-photon microscopy), the assessment criterion is the presence of laser impacts or cavitation bubbles.

Thermal and Mechanical Damage

The analysis of the mechanical and thermal damage in the thickness of the sample is carried out on samples subjected to horizontal incisions at increasing energy levels.

They are assessed using ultrasound, confocal microscopy, two-photon microscopy and by the reference method, transmission electron microscopy (TEM).

The Regularity of Incision

The regularity of incision is determined on flap ablations. The energy, the spacing of shots, and the depth of the treatment are the variables investigated. At present, flap ablations are carried out by means of a linear scan starting at one end of the plane. After this flap ablation, the second stage consists of juxtaposing circles from the bottom up towards the surface in order to complete the trepanation.

The analysis is carried out by the reference method, using SEM, for which the assessment criterion is subjective, and compared to the high-frequency ultrasound assessment, for which the assessment criterion is the quantification of the coefficient of reflection.

Kinetics of the Cavitation Bubble

The kinetics of the cavitation bubble is determined from samples that have undergone shots at distances of a few microns into their thickness. This can only be assessed by means of nondestructive examinations: confocal microscopy and two-photon microscopy. The size of the cavitation bubble is measured as a function of time for various laser energy levels and firing depths.

DISCUSSION

Different sorts of lasers are used to produce the photodisruption of materials: the nanosecond lasers ($1ns=10^{-9}s$), the best known of which is the Nd:Yag laser, the picosecond lasers ($1ps=10^{-12}s$) and recently, the femtosecond lasers ($1fs=10^{-15}s$). In all these lasers, the wavelength is close to that of the visible spectrum. This means that they can be focused in the thickness of the cornea with very little absorption or diffusion. The incision can be made through the full thickness without damaging the material through which it passes before it is focused. The main difference between these lasers is the duration of the pulse. When a laser pulse is focused in the thickness of a medium and if it has enough energy, photodisruption of the material occurs, and it is converted into a gas, a mixture of ions and high-density electrons, known as plasma. As a result, the medium becomes absorbent, and the additional energy deposited in the medium induces collateral damage. This collateral damage consists mainly of an acoustic shock wave, an increase in the local temperature, which may burn the surrounding tissues, and an increase in the volume of the plasma in the form of a cavitation bubble. We have not investigated the consequences of the acoustic shock wave. This phenomenon travels very fast (about 1500 m/s), and we do not have any instruments capable of measuring it.

However, this phenomenon has been described in the literature, and does not seem to have any effect on the ultrastructure of the cornea.

The optical burst threshold and the energy threshold at which plasma appears in the material can be determined in several ways. A photodiode is commonly used, which can be used to measure the luminescence of the plasma.[19] It is also possible to determine the threshold by microscopic examination of laser impacts on the surface of a sample.[2,18] The surface threshold is usually found to be between 0.5 and 3 J/cm^2, regardless of the material involved. For the two imaging methods that we have been able to test, scanning electron microcopy and optical microscopy, we found a threshold of about 10 j/cm^2 at the surface.

The threshold rises virtually linearly with the thickness of the cornea crossed. A cornea with normal transparency transmits more than 85 percent of the incident light for wavelengths of between 300 and 2500 nm. Some of the incident light is therefore lost by scatter, reflection and absorption. It has been shown that about 10 percent of the incident energy is lost for every 100 microns.

In theory, the advantage of using short pulses, lasting a few hundred femtoseconds, is that they provide only the amount of energy required to produce plasma and therefore minimize the thermal effects.

Indeed, transmission electron microscopy shows that the ultrastructural changes produced are limited to a distance of about one micron if the energy used is close to the plasma threshold.[20,21]

Long pulses (nanosecond or picosecond) carry a lot more energy into the medium than is required to create the plasma, and as a result the heat damage is considerable and the cavitation bubble is relatively large.[18, 21] For pulses of 500 fs, the plasma threshold is stable, because it depends on a determinist regime of the interaction between the laser and the material. Indeed for short pulses, ionization is the consequence of multi-photon photo-ionization rather than of an avalanche of random electronic interactions, as in the case of longer pulses. Thus, for longer pulses, the cavitation bubbles are big and irregular in size, which makes it impossible to carry out a regular and accurate ablation.[22] In contrast, for femtosecond pulses, the cavitation bubbles are small and are all of the same size.[23] Consequently, when several pulses are juxtaposed, the cavitation bubbles merge to produce a regular incision without damaging the surrounding tissues. The regularity of the incision therefore depends on the spacing of shots. If the gap between two successive shots is too big, bridges of tissue will remain between the impacts. Conversely, if the distance between them is not big enough, there is a cumulative effect that increases the collateral effects (including the size of the cavitation bubble), leading to an irregular incision.

This is why it is important to know the exact kinetics of this cavitation bubble. Knowing the instantaneous?? size of the bubble would make it possible to shift the next pulse to the optimum distance away. In the literature, the analysis of this kinetic process has been carried out in water or in porcine corneas.[23] The size of the bubble was measured on successive photographs of the surface.

CONCLUSION

The femtosecond laser is currently being developed for applications in ophthalmologic surgery. Corneal surgery is one of its main applications. This laser has the theoretical advantage of not inducing collateral damage, notably heat-induced damage, around the impact zone. These lasers are currently on sale in the USA, and will become available in Europe within a few months. For the moment, they can only be used to carry out ablations in the thickness of the cornea and to free the surgeon from mechanical microkeratomes. They have very promising prospects for future development in eye surgery. Suture-free grafts, surgery for glaucoma may be their applications of tomorrow.

REFERENCES

1. Sletten KR, Yen KG, Sayegh S, et al. An in vivo model of femtosecond laser intrastromal refractive surgery. Ophthalmic Surg Lasers 1999;30:742-49.
2. Stern D, Schoenlein RW, Puliafito CA, Dobi ET, Birngruber R, Fujimoto JG. Corneal ablation by nanosecond, picosecond, and femtosecond lasers at 532 and 625 nm. Arch Ophthalmol 1989;107:587-92.
3. Krueger RR, Juhasz T, Gualano A, Marchi V. The picosecond laser for nonmechanical laser in situ keratomileusis. J Refract Surg 1998;14:467-69.
4. Vogel A, Capon MR, Asiyo-Vogel MN, Birngruber R. Intraocular photodisruption with picosecond and nanosecond laser pulses: tissue effects in cornea, lens, and retina. Invest Ophthalmol Vis Sci 1994;35:3032-44.
5. Kurtz RM, Horvath C, Liu HH, Krueger RR, Juhasz T. Lamellar refractive surgery with scanned intrastromal picosecond and femtosecond laser pulses in animal eyes. J Refract Surg 1998;14:541-48.
6. Stern D, Lin WZ, Puliafito CA, Fujimoto JG. Femtosecond optical ranging of corneal incision depth. Invest Ophthalmol Vis Sci 1989;30:99-104.

7. Nordan LT, Slade SG, Baker RN, Suarez C, Juhasz T, Kurtz R. Femtosecond laser flap creation for laser in situ keratomileusis: six- month follow-up of initial U.S. clinical series. J Refract Surg 2003;19:8-14.
8. Roach WP, Rogers ME, Rockwell BA, Boppart SA, Stein CD, Bramlette CM. Ultrashort laser pulse effects in ocular and related media. Aviat Space Environ Med 1994;65:A100-07.
9. Lubatschowski H, Maatz G, Heisterkamp A, et al. Application of ultrashort laser pulses for intrastromal refractive surgery. Graefes Arch Clin Exp Ophthalmol 2000;238:33-39.
10. Jungnickel K, Rein S, Vogel A. [Plasma formation in Nd:YAG laser surgery]. Ophthalmologe 1992;89:283-87.
11. An-Chun Tien, Sterling Backus, Henry Kapteyn, Margaret Murmane, and Gérard Mourou. Short-Pulse Laser Damage in Transparent Materials as a Function of Pulse Duration. Physical review letters. 1999; 19:3883-86.
12. Vesaluoma M, Perez-Santonja J, Petroll WM, Linna T, Alio J, Tervo T. Corneal stromal changes induced by myopic LASIK. Invest Ophthalmol Vis Sci 2000;41:369-76.
13. Allemann N, Chamon W, Silverman RH, et al. High-frequency ultrasound quantitative analyses of corneal scarring following excimer laser keratectomy. Arch Ophthalmol 1993;111:968-73.
14. Reinstein DZ, Aslanides IM, Silverman RH, Asbell PA, Coleman DJ. High-frequency ultrasound corneal pachymetry in the assessment of corneal scars for therapeutic planning. Clao J 1994;20:198-203.
15. Silverman RH, Reinstein DZ, Raevsky T, Coleman DJ. Improved system for sonographic imaging and biometry of the cornea. J Ultrasound Med 1997;16:117-24.
16. Silverman RH, Lizzi FL, Ursea BG, et al. Safety levels for exposure of cornea and lens to very high-frequency ultrasound. J Ultrasound Med 2001;20:979-86.
17. March WF, Bauer NJ. Non-invasive measurement of corneal hydration. J Refract Surg 2001;17:S205-11.
18. Kurtz RM, Liu X, Elner VM, Squier JA, Du D, Mourou GA. Photodisruption in the human cornea as a function of laser pulse width. J Refract Surg 1997;13:653-58.

19. Pronko PP, VanRompay PA, Horvath C, Loesel F, Juhasz T, Liu X, Mourou G. Avalanche ionisation and dielectric breakdown in silicon with ultrafast laser pulses. Physical review 1998;5:2387-90.
20. Ratkay-Traub I, Juhasz T, Horvath C, et al. Ultra-short pulse (femtosecond) laser surgery: initial use in LASIK flap creation. Ophthalmol Clin North Am 2001;14:347-55, viii-ix.
21. Heisterkamp A, Ripken T, Lutkefels E, et al. [Optimizing laser parameters for intrastromal incision with ultra-short laser pulses]. Ophthalmologe 2001;98:623-28.
22. Juhasz T, Hu XH, Turi L, Bor Z. Dynamics of shock waves and cavitation bubbles generated by picosecond laser pulses in corneal tissue and water. Lasers Surg Med 1994;15: 91-98.
23. Juhasz T, Kastis GA, Suarez C, Bor Z, Bron WE. Time-resolved observations of shock waves and cavitation bubbles generated by femtosecond laser pulses in corneal tissue and water. Lasers Surg Med 1996;19:23-31.
24. Donate D, Albert O, Colliac JP,Tubelis P,Sabatier P, Mourou G, Burillon C, Pouliquen Y, Legeais JM. Femtosecond laser–: incident energy theresholds and corneal hydration. Invest Vis Sci 2004;4:S175.

Chapter 22

Conductive Keratoplasty

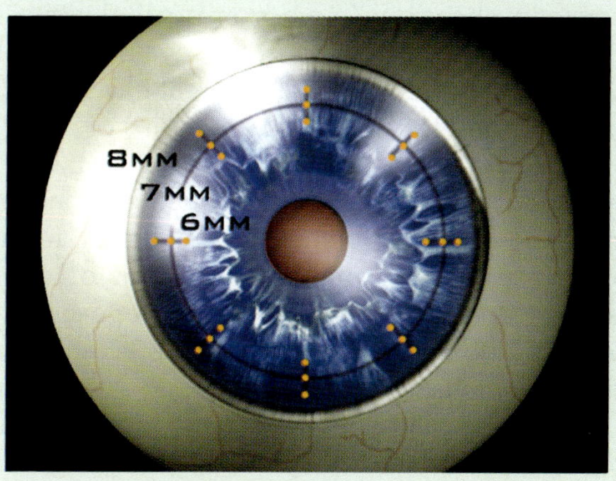

Roberto Pinelli (Italy)

INTRODUCTION

Conductive Keratoplasty (CK) with the ViewPoint System from Refractec, Inc. (Irvine, California) is a non-laser, radiofrequency-based procedure for treating presbyopia that avoids LASIK-associated complications, as well as many of the disadvantages of traditional monovision. High frequency (350 KHz) energy is delivered into the stroma with a specially designed contact probe. The temperature and duration of the radiofrequency energy applied by the probe is optimal for collagen shrinkage without necrosis.

Conductive keratoplasty requires no ablation or incisions, does not invade the central cornea, cause flap-related complications, compromise the integrity or structure of the cornea, or cause dry eye or central haze.

CK has been used primarily to treat low to moderate hyperopia[1-3] and to reduce the symptoms of presbyopia in presbyopic hyperopes (+1.00 to +2.25 D) or emmetropes through induction of mild myopia in the non-dominant eye.[4] Other potential uses of the CK technique under investigation include treatment of over- or undercorrections following LASIK or other excimer laser procedures, enhancing outcomes of cataract surgery, and treating astigmatism.

This chapter will briefly review the history of the CK procedure, explain how the system works and the surgical technique and procedures used by this author, and review the US clinical trial results for the treatment of presbyopia.

HISTORY OF CONDUCTIVE KERATOPLASTY

Thermokeratoplasty techniques aim to change corneal curvature through the application of heat, which shrinks corneal collagen. There were several attempts in the 1980s to use thermokeratoplasty to change corneal refraction in humans, but these were largely unsuccessful.[5-12]

Following the 1990 report by Seiler and associates of stable corneal steepening achieved in blind eyes with a pulsed holmium:YAG laser used in the contact mode,[13] Sunrise Technologies of Fremont, California, began to develop a noncontact method of holmium:YAG laser treatment for hyperopia. US clinical studies with two-year follow-up were published in 1996 and 1997[14-15] and the device was ultimately approved for use in the US in 2000, based on a study cohort of 612 eyes, with 80 percent available for analysis at 12 months and only 12 percent at 24 months postoperatively.[16]

Over time, LTK became unpopular because it lacked predictability and stability. The manufacturer went out of business and the Hyperion device is no longer manufactured.

Also in the 1990s, Antonio Mendez, MD, studied radiofrequency as an alternative to procedures that applied heat directly to the corneal surface.[17] His success in denaturing collagen and steepening the cornea led to the development of Refractec's ViewPoint CK System.

Unlike previous thermokeratoplasty methods that used a laser to generate heat intrastromally, conductive keratoplasty with the ViewPoint CK System uses radiofrequency energy to shrink corneal collagen.

A precise amount of radiofrequency energy is applied through a 450 × 90 µm contact probe inserted into the peripheral corneal stroma. Treatment is applied in a ring pattern outside of the visual axis at a defined number of treatment spots, with a greater number of spots applied to achieve a greater effect.

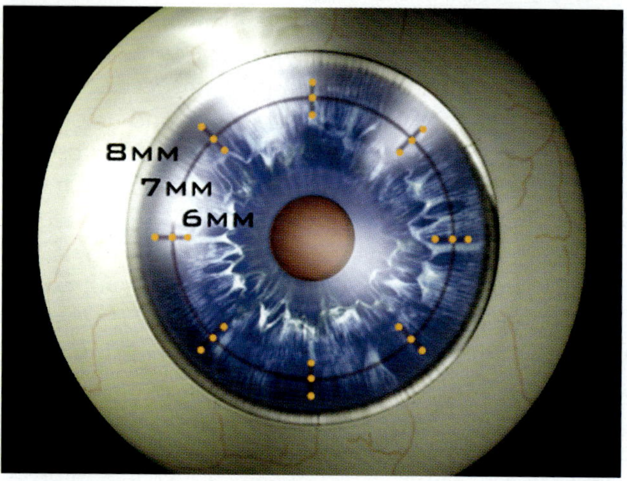

FIGURE 22.1: Shows the optical zone marks made by the marker to guide the surgeon in placement of the treatment spots. A circular mark is made on the 7 mm optical zone with the CK marker. An inner hatch mark lies on the 6 mm and an outer hatch mark on the 8 mm optical zone

A full circle of treatment spots acts like a belt tightening the cornea in the periphery so that the central cornea steepens.

During conductive keratoplasty treatment, corneal tissue is exposed to the same temperature at the bottom of the probe as at the corneal surface. The footprint after conductive keratoplasty is cylindrical and extends deep into the stroma to approximately 80 percent depth. This is in contrast to the conical stromal footprint made with the LTK technique.

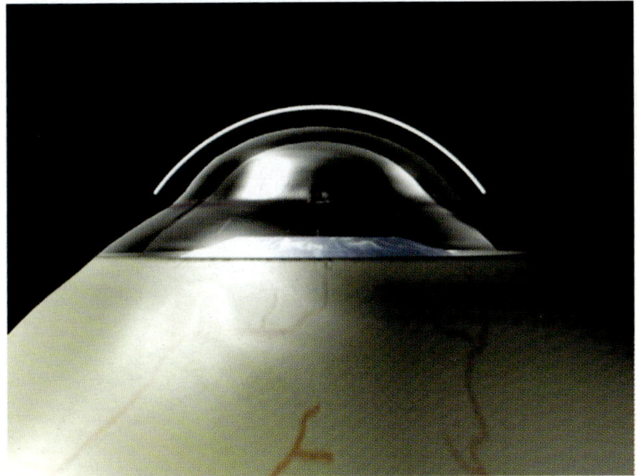

FIGURE 22.2: The conductive keratoplasty technique cinches the peripheral cornea which increases the curvature of the central cornea

The CK System

The ViewPoint CK System (Figure 22.3) used to perform the CK procedure consists of a radiofrequency energy-generating console, a reusable, pen-shaped handpiece attached by a removable cable and connector, a foot pedal that controls the release of energy, a corneal marker, and a speculum that provides a large surface for an electrical return path.

Attached to the probe is a single-use, disposable, stainless-steel, Keratoplast tip, 90 µm in diameter and 450 µm long, that delivers the current directly to the corneal stroma (Figure 22.4). The tip has a proximal bend of 45° and a distal bend of 90° to allow access to the cornea

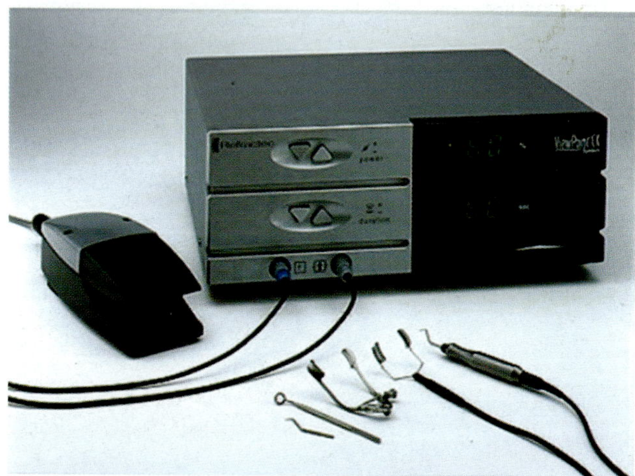

FIGURE 22.3: ViewPoint™ CK System. The ViewPointä CK system from Refractec, Inc. consists of a portable console, a corneal marker, choice of lid specula, a handpiece that holds the KeratoplastÔ Tip, and a foot pedal

over the patient's brow and nasal regions. At the very distal portion of the tip is an insulated stainless-steel stop (cuff) that controls depth of penetration.

Treatment application of 0.6 seconds per spot causes the surrounding tissue to undergo a temperature increase. As the heated tissue dehydrates, its resistance to radiofrequency current increases. Since current seeks the path of least resistance, the current path moves up the shaft of the Keratoplast Tip. Tissue heating progresses from bottom (approximately 80% of the depth of the stroma) to top (corneal surface), and creates a thermal lesion that is uniformly cylindrical. (Figure 22.5).

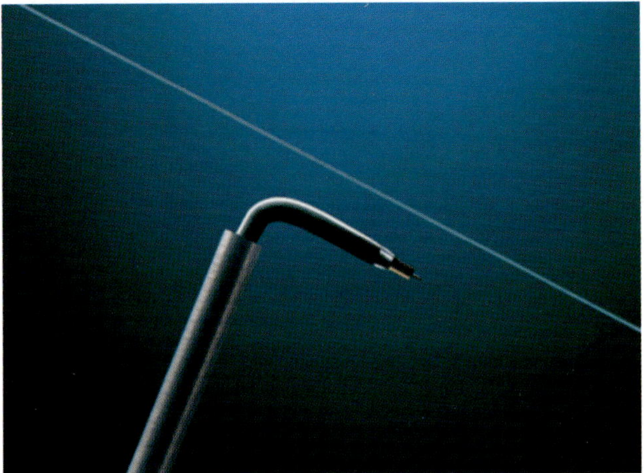

FIGURE 22.4: Keratoplast™ Tip: The Keratoplast™ Tip, (shown next to a 7-0 suture). The tip is 450 μm long and 90 μm wide and is used to deliver radiofrequency energy into the corneal stroma at the marked treatment points. A cuff on the probe assures correct depth of penetration

THE NEAR VISION CK PROCEDURE

Conductive keratoplasty for presbyopic correction is often referred to as NearVision CK. For this procedure, patients should be 40 years old or older and presbyopic. Preoperative testing includes slit lamp examination, keratometry, pachymetry, corneal topography, dominance assessment, near and distance vision assessment, and monovision tolerance assessment.

Vision should be correctable to 20/40 or better, and there should be no more than 0.75 D of refractive astigmatism, as determined by cycloplegic refraction. Contact lens wearers should have a stable refraction and should

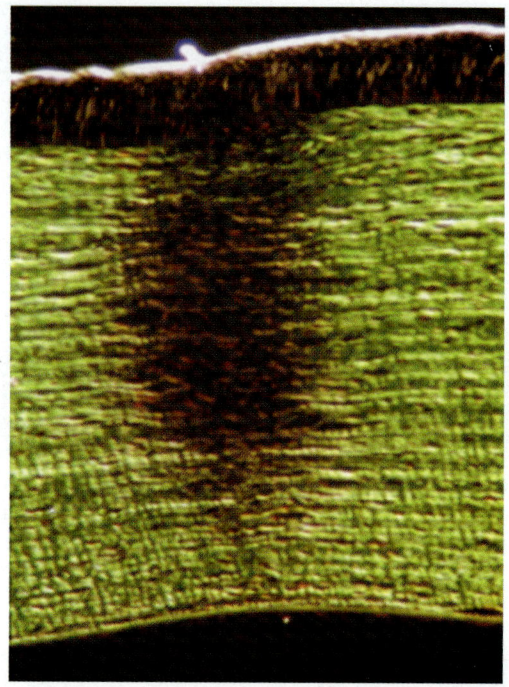

FIGURE 22.5: CK footprint. A polarized light micrograph of a histological section from a pig cornea, seven days after CK treatment. The footprint (dark region) is cylindrical and approximately 80 percent of corneal depth. Deep treatment penetration contributes to permanence of effect

discontinue lens use for two (soft) to three (hard or gas permeable) weeks before the procedure. Evidence of monovision success from previous contact lens monovision, a contact lens trial, the loose-lens test, or other preoperative testing is an important factor in patient selection.

For near vision correction in presbyopic emmetropes and hyperopes, the goal is to overcorrect the non-dominant eye by inducing slight to moderate myopia, –1.0 to –2.0 D (myopic endpoint) through the application of 8 to 24 CK treatment spots. If the dominant eye is significantly hyperopic, it can be targeted for a distance correction of +0.50 to –0.25 D. Treated patients display a reduction of symptoms of presbyopia without compromising binocular functional distance vision.

At the Institute, we begin on the day of surgery by verifying that the patient's pachymetry measurement is at least 560 μm at the 6 mm optical zone. After checking the device settings, the Keratoplast tip is interested into the handpiece and inspected under a microscope. I use foamed alcohol on my hands before performing CK; I do not use gloves for this procedure.

Preoperatively, we administer one drop of Tobradex followed by one drop of topical anesthetic (Proparacaine) three times at five-minute intervals. A lid speculum is placed in the eye to obtain maximal exposure and provide the electrical return path. To ensure direct contact of the speculum with the lids, we do not drape.

With the patient fixating under the excimer laser microscope, the surgeon should center carefully on the pupil and mark the eye. Proper centration is critical to avoiding the induction of astigmatism. We use gentian-violet ink and the standard CK marker, although there is also a newer 24-point marker developed by Dr. Strauss. The marker should be applied straight down and then lifted straight up after a short pause to obtain clear marking. After marking, the surgeon dries the corneal surface and then uses a dry fiber-free sponge to remove any excess ink.

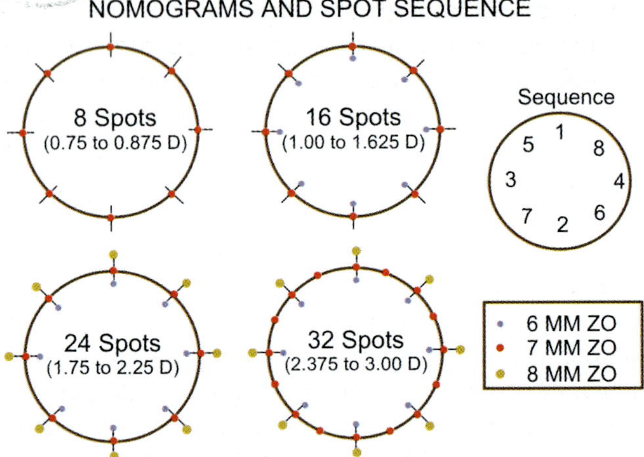

FIGURE 22.6: Nomogram. According to the nomogram in use at the ILMO, most patients need 8-16 spots for presbyopic correction

The surgeon then inserts the Keratoplast tip into the stroma at defined spots in a ring pattern around the peripheral cornea. At the Institute, we use the nomogram and sequence shown in Figure 22.6. The handpiece should be held in the dominant hand in a relaxed position, with the index finger of the opposite hand used to steady it, if necessary. At the marked treatment spot, tip the body of the handpiece approximately tangential to the optical zone mark. The Keratoplast tip should be perpendicular to the corneal surface to ensure full depth of penetration. The cuff around the probe, which settles perpendicular to the cornea, helps to achieve perpendicular placement. We apply uniform downward pressure until the tip penetrates the stroma. Then, energy is applied by depressing the foot pedal. During treatment, the amount of pressure applied is very important. Recent studies have shown that a Light Touch or neutral pressure technique, in which the cornea is indented and the ring light displaced as little as possible, is ideal for most primary treatments.

Spots should be applied smoothly and evenly. Begin treatment at the 12 o'clock position and continue, following the sequence in Figure 22.6, until the full ring of spots has been completed for that optical zone. Each spot should be applied parallel to the others in that ring and to those in the other optical zones. When applying a second or third ring of treatment, aim for precise radial alignment of treatment spots so that the spots in each ring just barely touch each other. Any tissue debris that accumulates on the tip can be removed with a fiber-free sponge.

If the ring light indicates that any cylinder has been induced during the procedure, a balancing spot can be placed intraoperatively. In total, the CK procedure takes only a few minutes to complete.

Postoperatively, we follow the same regimen that we use for LASIK: One drop of Tobradex four times daily for one week and artificial tears as needed for one month. At the first followup visit (Day 1), patients may experience mild foreign body sensation, possibly with photophobia. This usually resolves in 24 to 48 hours. There may also be some edema, which may persist through the next followup visit, at one to two weeks postop. At this point, the patient's visual acuity is generally good, although there will be further improvement. The patient may need reassurance that it will continue to get better. If there is any late-developing astigmatism, a balancing spot can be added. By the four- to six-week follow-up visit, patients should have no discomfort or edema, and good near and distance visual acuity. In fact, vision is often better than would be expected with the measured refraction. Enhancement can be discussed at this visit, if necessary.

CLINICAL RESULTS

The FDA clinical study for approval of NearVision CK for the correction of presbyopia was conducted at five sites in the United States. A total of 150 presbyopic patients (188 eyes) were enrolled and treated with CK. One hundred twelve patients were treated unilaterally for near vision correction; 38 patients were treated bilaterally for distance correction in one eye and near in the other. The average age was 53 years old; 96 percent of all patients were Caucasian, and 61 percent were female. The mean intended correction for eyes treated for near was +2.03 D ± 0.63 D (range +0.75 D to 3.00 D).

Visual Acuity

Of the eyes treated for near, 81 percent had J2 or better binocular UCVA-Near at six months; 77 percent at 12 months. For UCVA-Near of J3 or better, the percentage was 90 and 89 percent, compared with only (15%) that had this uncorrected binocular near acuity pre-operatively (Figure 22.7).

Binocular UCVA-Distance results showed 95 and 97 percent with 20/20 or better acuity at six and 12 months, respectively, 100 and 98 percent with 20/25 or better, and 100 percent with 20/32 or better (Figure 22.8).

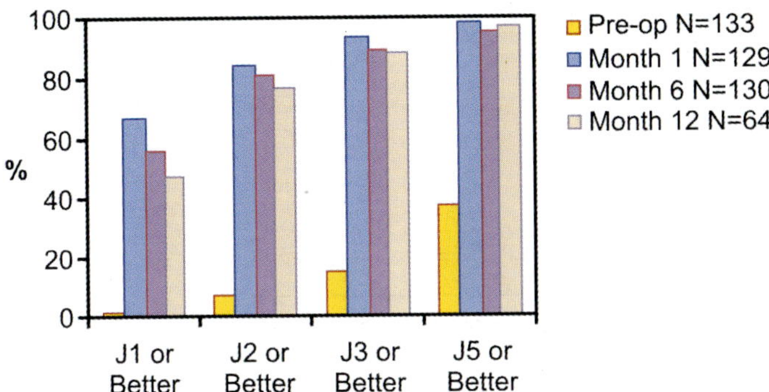

FIGURE 22.7: Binocular UCVA-Near following CK Presbyopia Treatment

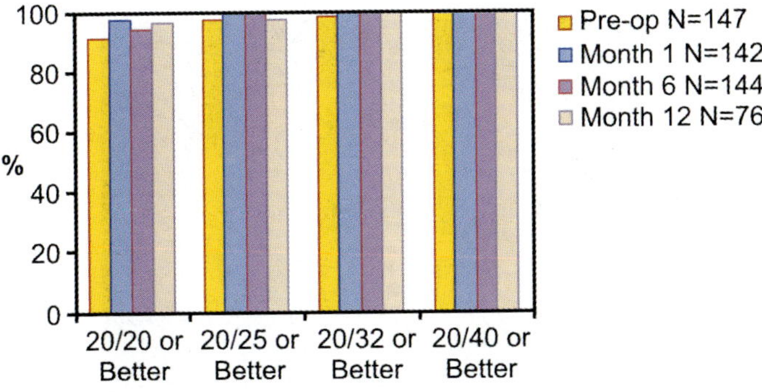

FIGURE 22.8: Binocular UCVA-Distance following CK Presbyopia Treatment

The combination of binocular UCVA-Distance of 20/20 or better with UCVA-Near of J2 or better was achieved by 100 of 130 eyes (77%) at six months and 48 of 64 eyes (75%) at 12 months. Approximately 90 percent of patients could see binocularly 20/20 or better distance and J3 or better near uncorrected (Figure 22.9).

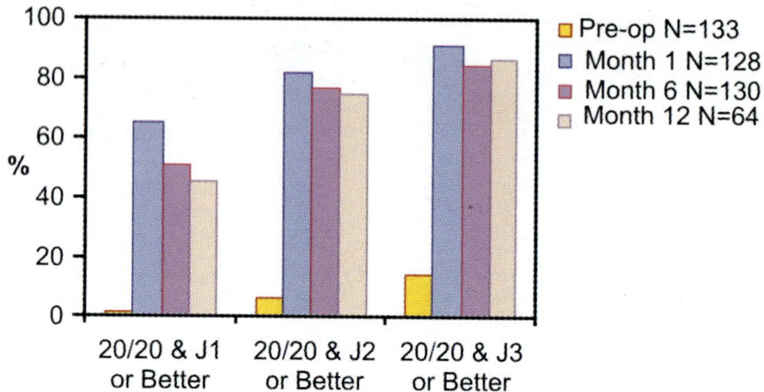

FIGURE 22.9: Binocular Combined UCVA-Distance and Near following CK Presbyopia Treatment

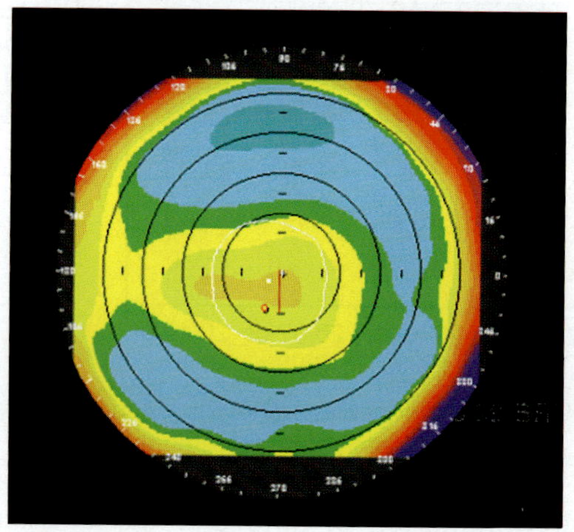

FIGURE 22.10: Preop topography

Safety

At one month, 2 percent of the treated eyes showed a loss of more than two lines of BSCVA-Distance; this

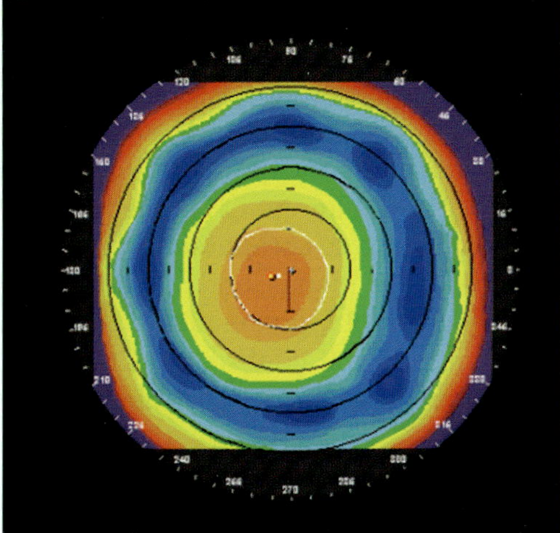

FIGURE 22.11: Post-op topography

incidence fell to 0 percent for all subsequent months. There were no cases of BSCVA worse than 20/40, increases of =2.00 D of cylinder, or eyes that had 20/20 or better BSCVA preoperatively that had worse than 20/25 postoperatively. Postoperative increases in absolute cylinder were generally 1.50 D or less and decreased with time. No intraoperative complications or adverse events occurred during any of the surgeries.

Vision Quality and Patient Satisfaction

Of the patients who had eyes treated for near, 97 percent reported improvement in quality of vision at one month; 98 percent at 12 months. At these time periods, a total of 85 and 84 percent reported being satisfied or very satisfied with their outcome. All patients reported fair to excellent quality of depth perception. Mesopic contrast sensitivity testing with and without glare showed that contrast sensitivity was maintained following CK.

A patient questionnaire about spectacle use following the CK procedure showed that most patients had significantly reduced their dependence on spectacles for common daily tasks. After the CK procedure, 90 percent of patients could use a computer without spectacles, 86 percent could read menus, and 86 percent could read newspaper-sized print (approximately J5 or 8-point font size). This reinforces the goal of the CK procedure, to allow the patient to perform most daily tasks without spectacles.

SUMMARY

Conductive keratoplasty is a non-laser procedure for changing corneal curvature to treat presbyopia, low to moderate spherical hyperopia, and other refractive conditions. The largest potential population for CK appears to be the presbyopes, many of whom are interested in a non-laser procedure that can extend the period of spectacle-free near vision.

The US FDA multicenter study showed that CK was safe and effective for improving near vision in presbyopic patients, and the clinical results at our Institute have been similarly excellent.

Importantly, none of the disadvantages typically associated with monovision seem to occur with NearVision CK. Depth perception is maintained, binocular corrected distance acuity is generally better than preoperative levels, and there is no loss of contrast sensitivity (quality of vision) from preoperative levels. Patient satisfaction is very high, and the vast majority of patients have binocular visual acuity of 20/20 or better at distance and J3 or better at near, for good functional vision without glasses.

NearVision CK is a safe, effective, and well-established approach to treating presbyopia and/or hyperopia. It also has the potential for treating other conditions. At the Institute, for example, we are treating keratoconus and astigmatism in post-cataract surgery patients by placing treatment spots on specifically chosen locations on the cornea. However, the surgeon must be highly experienced with conventional CK procedures before undertaking such procedures.

REFERENCES

1. McDonald MB, Davidorf J, Maloney RK, Manche EE, Hersh P. Conductive keratoplasty for the correction of low to moderate hyperopia: 1-year results on the first 54 eyes. Ophthalmology 2002;109:637-49.
2. McDonald MB, Hersh PS, Manche EE, Maloney RK, Davidorf J, Sabry M, Conductive keratoplasty for the correction of low to moderate hyperopia: U.S. clinical trial 1-year results on 355 eyes. Ophthalmology. 2002; 109: 1978-89.
3. Asbell PA, Maloney RK, Davidorf J, Hersh P, McDonald M, Manche E; Conductive Keratoplasty Study Group. Conductive keratoplasty for the correction of hyperopia. Trans Am Ophthalmol Soc. 2001;99:79-84.
4. McDonald, MB, Durrie DS, Asbell PA, Maloney R, Nichamin L. Treatment of presbyopia with conductive keratoplasty: six-month results of the 1-year United States FDA clinical trial. Cornea. 2004;23:661-68.
5. Caster AI. The Fyodorov technique of hyperopia correction by thermal coagulation: A preliminary report. J Refract Surg 1988;4:105-08.
6. Neumann A, Sanders D, Salz J. Radial thermokeratoplasty for hyperopia. J Refract Corneal Surg 1989;5:50-54.

7. Neumann A, Fyodorov S, Sanders D. Radial thermo-keratoplasty for the correction of hyperopia. J Refract Corneal Surg 1990;6:404-12.
8. Neumann A, Sanders D, Raanan M, DeLuca M. Hyperopic thermokeratoplasty: clinical evaluation. J Cataract Refract Surg 1991;17:830-38.
9. Feldman S, Ellis W, Frucht-Pery J, et al. Regression of effect following radial thermokeratoplasty in humans. J Refract Surg 1995;18:288-91.
10. Rowsey JJ, Doss JD. Preliminary report of Los Alamos keratoplasty techniques. Ophthalmology 1981;88:755-760.
11. Rowsey JJ, Gaylor JR, Dahlstrom R, et al. Contact Intraocul Lens Med J 1980;6:1-12.
12. Rowsey JJ. Electrosurgical keratoplasty: Update and retraction. Invest Ophthalmol Vis Sci 1987;28 (suppl):224.
13. Seiler T, Matallana M, Bende T. Laser thermokeratoplasty by means of a pulsed holmium:YAG laser for hyperopic correction. Refract Corneal Surg1990;6:355-59.
14. Koch DD, Abarca A, Villareal R, et al. Hyperopia correction by non-contact holmium:YAG laser thermokeratoplasty; clinical study with two-year follow-up.
15. Koch D, Kohnen T, McDonnell P, et al. Hyperopia correction by noncontact holmium:YAG laser thermal keratoplasty. U.S. Phase IIA Clinical Study with 2-year follow-up. Ophthalmology 1997; 104:1938-47.
16. United States FDA PMA P990078. Hyperion LTK System Device Labeling, Sunrise Technologies, Fremont, California, May 2000.
17. Mendez A, Mendez Noble A. Conductive keratoplasty for the correction of hyperopia. In: Sher N. (Ed). Surgery for Hyperopia and Presbyopia. Philadelphia: Williams and Wilkins: 1997;163-71.

CHAPTER 23

VisioDynamics Theory: A Biomechanical Application for the Aging Eye and LaserACE™ Natural Vision Restoration

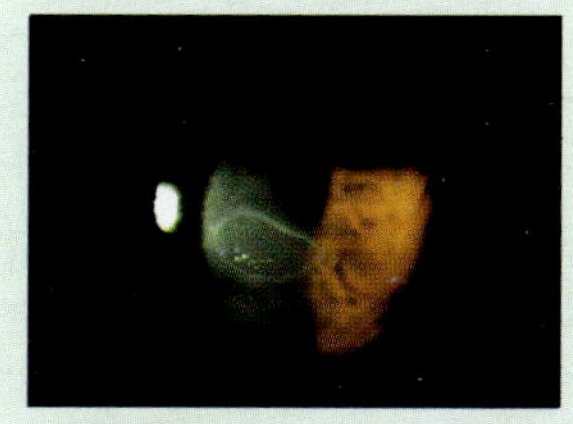

AnnMarie Hipsley (USA)
Dimitrii Dementiev (Italy)

VISIODYNAMICS: BIOMECHANICAL MODEL FOR THE AGING OCULAR ORGAN

The defining concept of VisioDynamic Theory is that *presbyopia is NOT a refractive error or simply the loss in the ability to focus on near objects, rather it is an AGING DISEASE* whereas the age-related consequences on connective tissue as they occur throughout the body produce significant but reversible impact on biomechanical efficiency of ocular function which includes visual function, ocular biotransport, and ocular metabolic efficiency among other ocular organ functions.[1] The limiting factors for eye function throughout development and during aging can be broken down into *three* basic categories:

- Structural/Mechanical
- Physiological
- Extracellular and Intracellar

Connective Tissues (CT) can change their strength depending on the forces applied to them. Without force acting on them, the chemical structures and property of the tissues change, and therefore the fibers and mechanical properties of the tissue change. In muscle tissue this is called atrophy; in other supporting CT this is called hysteresis.[2] The SAID (Specific Adaptation to Imposed Demands) principle applies here, whereas the internal design of CT works as a feedback loop which is responsive to force, mass and gravity.[3] The opposite can happen if a CT begins to receive a persistent stress. If you do something to stress the CT, it will gradually add new CT at the point of stress, this is called hypertrophy.

The *internal design of* CT also responds to organismal experience such as environmental stress, biological stress, chemical stress which can manifest itself into various disease processes or traumas if the cycle is not broken. CT remodels itself in order to accommodate the new stress.[4] Chronic stress which exceeds the threshold of tissue healing can produce a low grade chronic inflammatory process which triggers a cycle of cell damage ultimately resulting in cell death and/or irreversible tissue changes which affect homeostatic equilibrium—this is 'aging'.[5] Despite the normal loss of elastin, collagen and dehydration of tissue, tissue morphology is limited by genetic predisposition, cultural (race) and environmental (altitude/ sunlight) impact and inherent structural characteristics of health.[6] In the VisioDynamic Theory, the loss of accommodation in presbyopia is due to age-related changes of the eye which affect its normal biomechanical and therefore physiological function.[7] Biomechanical dysfunction leads to increased mechanical load, shear stress and consequential tissue strain. Tissue strain and deformation has effects on micro tissue layer interactions, collagenous integral structure/remodelling and ultimately extracellular matrix chemical and nutrient balance and efficiency.[8] Tissue properties and architecture are critical considerations when determining the impact of the pathophysiology of age-related changes (Figure 23.1).[9] The cornea is responsible for two-thirds of the eye's total focusing power, while the crystalline lens accounts for the remaining one-third. The focusing power of the cornea is fixed, whereas focusing power of lens complex is not fixed and depends largely on the mechanical efficiency of accommodation mechanism which is dependent upon the biomechanical relationships of the structures of the eye. Therefore, any surgical solution implemented for an

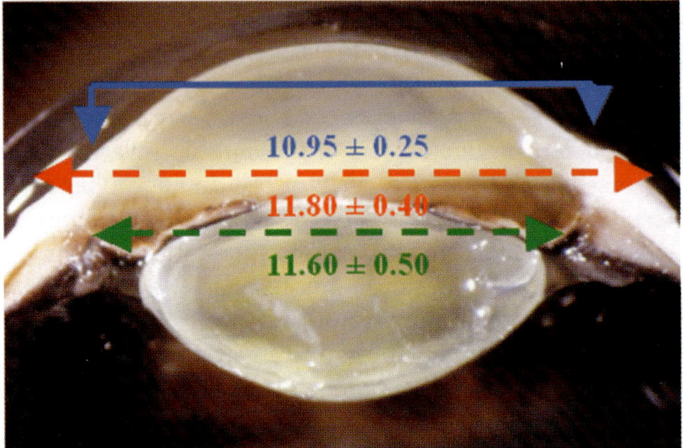

FIGURE 23.1: Biomechanical relationship of ocular structures *in vivo.* White-to-white, Anterior chamber diameter, ciliary sulcus diameter

aging ocular organ would be enhanced by restoring biomechanical balance in the structures included in the *Kinematic chain* of the *Oculociliary Complex.*

BIOMECHANICAL IMPACT OF AGE-RELATED CHANGES IN OCULAR TISSUE

Biomechanical Dysfunction Hypothesis

The *Biomechanical Dysfunction Hypothesis* postulates there is a highly structured inter-relationship in terms of the homeostatic stimuli which are shared in common by different ocular tissues as suggested by the close anatomic and functional relationship which they have evolved from.[1] Biomechanical efficiency relys on: *or* $ME = W \times 100/E - e$ *where E is the gross energy output, e is the resting metabolic rate, and W is the external work performed.* Optimal positive work or mechanical efficiency of ocular organ function occurs when this equation is balanced.[10] Every joint has a particular biomechanical arrangement with its associated musculature which is crucial to structure composition and form against gravity (posture) and the coordination of the neuromuscular units of the joint to produce the resultant force necessary to perform movement (function).[11] Restoring normal biomechanical relationships to the aging oculus facilitates the ocular structures to work with gravity in the most efficient way: the *oculociliary joint* is "postured" into optimum position to allow for the maximum potential kinetic energy to perform positive work or anterior acceleration and posterior deceleration of the lens for maximum range of dynamic visual tasks.[12] Biomechanical balance and specificity allows for efficient ocular movement, whereas, biomechanical dysfunction demands compensatory movements (due to over- or inappropriate loading) which will be 'patterned' and eventually interfere with performance. The accommodative mechanism is system of levers, and static contractions are responsible for the discrete adjustments to hold these levers in optimal alignment. The 'posture' of the lens during disaccommodation is an important baseline for determining the functional capacity of the accommodative mechanism.[13] By gaining increasing control over these processes, biomechanical proficiency increases. The LaserACE™ procedure or Laser Anterior Ciliary Excision was developed based on the fundamentals of biomechanics, neurophysiology, and kinesiology of the aging eye organ.[14] This procedure effectively and naturally restores the biomechanical interrelationships of the intraocular structures providing biomechanical efficiency and alleviating biomechanical dysfunction by decreasing anterior global scleral compression load and subsequent subliminal tissue stress, strain and deformation.[15,16]

Scleral Compression Hypothesis

The *Sclera* undergoes a gradual "*sclerosclerosis*" with age which represents the normal and *gradual irreversible changes* which occur in all connective tissues as we age.[17] In addition, increased ocular rigidity has been linearly correlated with age.[18] This sclerotic process imposes staggeringly significant load, stress and strain upon underlying and related ocular and intraocular structures (Figure 23.2).[19,20] Every tissue interrelated with the sclera therefore will respond according to the SAID principle or otherwise respond by Specific Adaptation to Imposed Demands. CT of the ocular organ adapts to stress by compensation, substitution, or overload.[21]

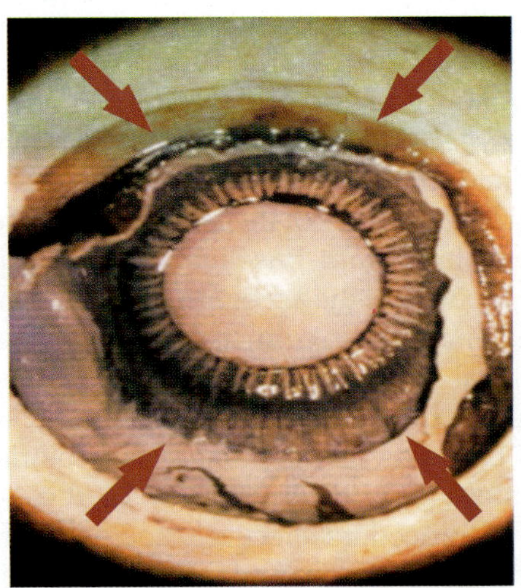

FIGURE 23.2: Scleral load vectors on underlying structures

Subsequently, all structures within the ocular organ sustain a 'gradual accumulation of microtrauma' over time. *Aging is a cyclical low grade inflammatory process ultimately resulting in irreversible changes in tissue. Unless the cycle is broken, cell death, organ death, system death and eventually organismal death occurs.* Age-related changes in connective tissue of sclera include changes in collagen composition of GAGs (glyacosaminoglycans), thickness, rigidity, tissue architecture (angle recession and changed biomechanical relationships),and changes homeostatic response.[22-24] Until now, the complex interaction of the sclera and recognition of its huge impact on the internal processing and diffusive mechanism in the eye organ has been considerably overlooked.[25] Age-related changes in the SCLERA are directly relative, indirectly relative or concomitantly relative to the impairment of the functional performance of the entire eye organ.[26] The majority of the inner anatomical and physiological areas of eye organ function lie beneath 5/6 of the outer tunic or the sclera which makes this structure a critical tissue consideration in terms of age-related changes in CT and its impact on biomechanical function of the eye organ.[27,28] One of the most critical zones is in the area of the limbus at the corneoscleral envelope (Figure 23.3).[29] A primary limiting factor in the ability to respond to near stimulus through the accommodative mechanism is the loss of mobility of the sclera. The magnitude of the response to near stimulus is also limited by the degree of "*sclerosclerosis*" or age-related fibrosis of the sclera. Muscular imbalance, which develops from biomechanical dysfunction can ultimately involve the whole ocular organ and even body function.

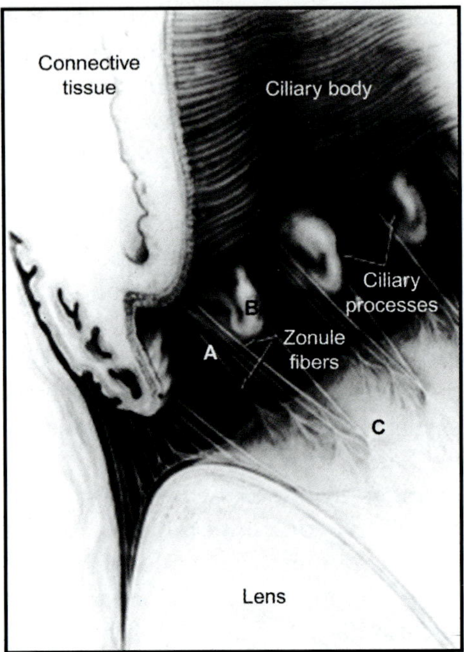

FIGURE 23.3: Physiology of the limbal structures underlying sclera at corneoscleral envelope

All of these underlying structures are impacted by the progressive scleral load either directly or indirectly creating such dysfunction as ONH atrophy, Choroid dysfunction/vascular insufficiency, decreased uveal-aqueous outflow, increased IOP, biomechanical dysfunction of EOM, and ultimately gross disturbances in ICM and ECM metabolic transport.[30-32]

In vivo, CT *Mobility* is important for the normal maintenance and turnover of PG (proteoglycans) in healthy tissue. Conversely, tissue *immobilization* or disuse results in atrophy because of a loss of PG from the matrix.[33] However, it is also noted in research that this PG loss following immobilization is *reversible* if normal tissue conditions and more importantly when mobility is restored.[34] Age-related effects of connective tissue can have enormous impact specific to overlying sclera shell thickness. "Structure = Function" is at the crux of the VisioDynamic model and is instrumental in the hypothesis and application of the LaserACE™ procedure which is based on restoring the biomechanical relationships of the ocular tunic in critical zones of physiological importance.[35] A state of equilibrium is reached and the internal stress balances the applied load (Figure 23.4). The principal goal of LaserACE™ procedure is to decrease the overall applied load stress by decompression of sclerotic CT load, to restore mobility, to rejuvenate physiological functions in the anterior globe and further retard tissue strain and deformation rates in the aging eye. The fundamental objective is to restore essential biomechanical components which are affected by age-related pathology and promote longevity of the ocular organ.

SAID PRINCIPLE: SPECIFIC ADAPTATION TO IMPOSED DEMANDS

Force and Friction play a large role in ocular functional capacity. Leonardo da Vinci has the credit to be the first who made quantitative studies on the problem of friction (1497-1493) Leonardo defined a friction coefficient as the ratio of the friction divided by the mass of the slider. Experimentally, he found a universal friction coefficient

For every Force there is an equal an opposite Force.
Isaac Newton 1668

Wt. bearing load of scleral coat to intraocular connective tissues

↓

Compression-physiologic metabolic stress

↓

Shear stress-friction caused low grade inflammatory tissue

↓

Response and change in tissue architecture

↓

Strain – deformation

↓

Hydrostatic stress- fluid and metobolic stasis

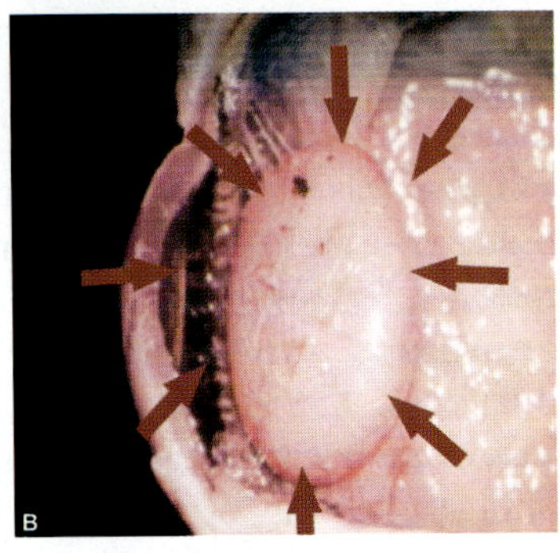

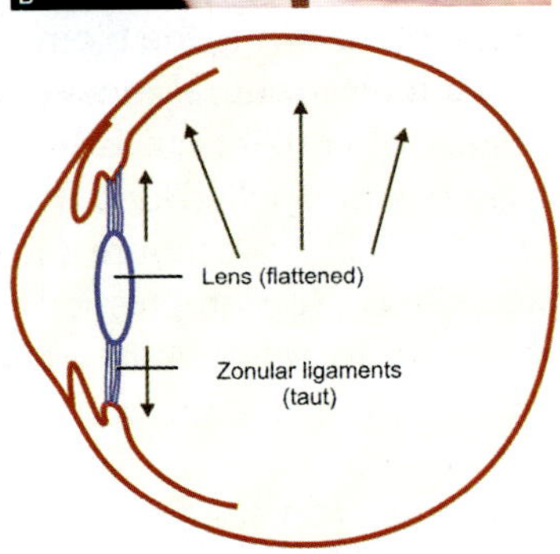

Effect of pressure exerted on sclerotic coat

FIGURE 23.4: Scleral coat load creates an internal stress response of elevated IOP to achieve equilibrium

of 0.25 independent of the material. Ocular tissues like other biological tissues like to live in a homeostatic stress/strain range. Therefore, FORCE (mass × acceleration) and FRICTION play a critical role in the ability for aging ocular tissue to function efficiently. Values of stress/strain outside of this range will lead to adaptation and changes in the tissue structure.[36] The *said principle* for Ocular aging states that: ***Age-related changes which occur in connective***

tissue increase both the static and dynamic coefficient of friction. Constant and gradual increased force and mass of the scleral load on underlying ocular tissues elicits equal and opposite force requirements resulting in intraocular physiological overload. Increased friction and load stress across tissue layers further elicits a cycle of repetitive low grade inflammatory tissue responses, changes in tissue architecture, connective tissue deformation, and biomechanical dysfunction Specific to Imposed Demands which overall decrease biomechanical efficiency of ocular organ function. Therefore, there is a constant linear deceleration of intraocular physiological processes concomitant with increased moment of inertia produced by progressive age-related scleral force (load) and friction (stress-strain).

BIOMECHANICAL SOLUTIONS FOR THE AGING OCULAR ORGAN

History of Biomechanical Surgical Solutions

During the mid-1970s in Russia, Fyodorov began treating myopia (nearsightedness) in patients using radial or spoke cuts through the cornea to biomechanically flatten its shape.[37] The biomechanics of the RK surgery evolved further to the Limbal region and to the sclera after surgeons noticed unanticipated impact on other visual functions (Fig. 23.5).

Scleral ablation was first hypothesized as a treatment for Presbyopia shortly after RK was brought to the United States (Figure 23.6). Surgeons (particularly a group led

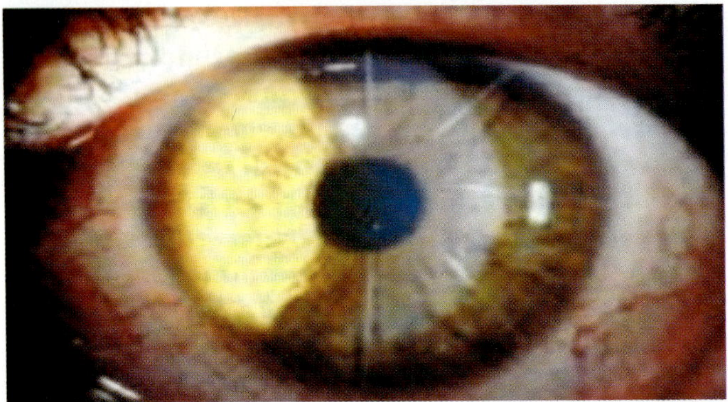

FIGURE 23.5: Early biomechanical applications in the cornea (RK)

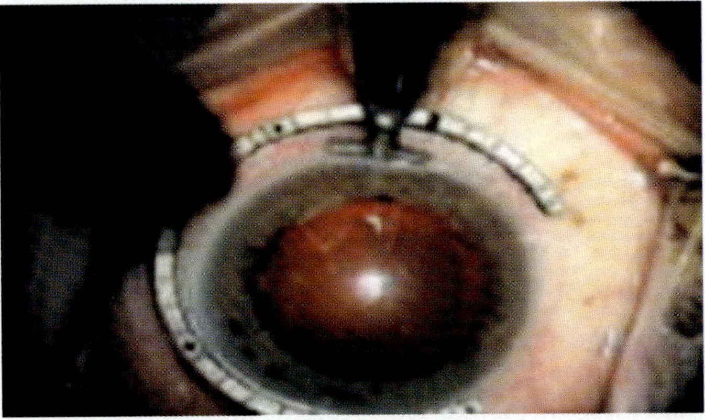

FIGURE 23.6: Thornton developed one of the first presbyopic specific procedure using scleral incisions: Anterior ciliary sclerotomy (ACS)

by Spencer Thornton, MD) began to notice that some of their patients were not developing presbyopia as expected. It appeared that this was by product of RK surgery when the radial incision went through the limbus.

Dr Thornton organized a group of leading RK surgeons worldwide to perform scleral incisions and test this theory. While the procedure held promise, the results were less dramatic mainly due to regression as the incisional sites healed. Only a small increase in the amplitude of accommodation was observed and .5 D of myopic shift was also recorded.[38] This procedure later evolved to be combined with silicone plugs having a more impressive and lasting effect. "ACS" is currently in clinical trials.

Schachar hypothesized a new model of accommodation controversial to the Hemholtz theory and performed scleral implants over the ciliary body in order to achieve an increase in accommodative power (Scleral Expansion Bands "SEB"). He hypothesized that the primary element in achieving the accommodative effect was the increase in the working distance for the ciliary muscle complex.[39]

JT Lin hypothesized that the effect of scleral incisions was not permanent due to the rapid healing response of the body and utilized an Er:YAG laser to make the incisions. Under this technique, LPC or LAPR, near full thickness ablations of the sclera are made in parallel radial orientation in the four quadrants resulting in an axial length change and anterior globe expansion.[40]

Hipsley introduced VisioDynamic Theory in 2003 based on the effects caused by the age-related changes of CT on the inner structures of critical physiological functional importance and countered that increasing scleral diameter across the globe was not ideal and in fact could superimpose even more biomechanical imbalance and possible instability to an already homeostatically challenged structure.[41] LaserACE™ procedure was developed based upon these fundamental principles of age-related changes on connective tissues and their progress load, stress/strain on subliminal tissues of the eye and imposing biomechanical dysfunction and its effects on ocular function.

LaserACE™ Biomechanical Surgical Solution

Unlike the expansion procedures, LaserACE™ is distinctly different in that it is a *decompression* procedure which emphasizes volumetric excisions in a CT matrix over critical segmental zones of fibrotic sclera in addition to creating a mechanical diaphragm pump in aponeurotic layers of the eye to rejuvenate aqueous outflow and alleviate stress from sensory receptors (Figure 23.7). Restoration of the Biomechanics of Accommodation with LaserACE™ or Laser Anterior Ciliary Excision is performed utilizing the patented VisioLite ophthalmic laser system with optical probe (Figure 23.12A).

- Since nothing can be done about lenticular hardening on must aim to increase the biomechanical efficiency of oculociliary joint complex.
- Restoration of biomechanical balance requires alleviating restrictions and maximizing intraocular structural functional performance without imposing new biomechanical challenges to the oculus.
- Resultant effects of LaserACE™ allow for a new static oculociliary joint complex resting posture which maximizes the kinetic potential of the neuromuscular system.
- Resultant effects of decompression rejuvenate ocular biotransport mechanisms both indirectly and dynamically.

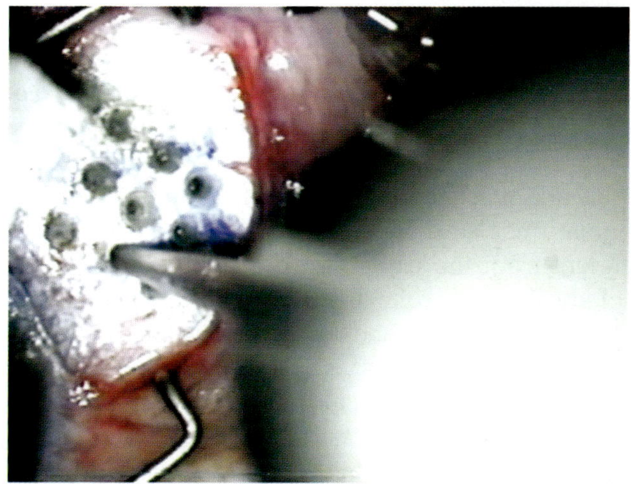

FIGURE 23.7: LaserACE™ "NeoPore" matrix decompressing fibrotic scleral mass and restoring physiological function

To distinguish LaserACE™ from scleral expansion procedures: Scleral expansion procedures have been proposed by Thornton ACS (Anterior Ciliary Sclerotomy), Fukusaku, Schachar (Scleral Expansion Bands) and LAPR procedure. Scleral expansion procedures are primarily based on the "Lens Crowding Theory" and strive to achieve improvement of the working distance of the ciliary complex or the circumlental space by inducing a 'pseudomyopic' eye shape with the polar axis longer than the equatorial diameter. Scleral implants are inserted into the superficial tunnels, causing a slight lift or 'myopic roof' in the sclera designed to reduce the crowding of the underlying muscles surrounding the crystalline lens. Alternatively, a radial ablation technique is used to create full thickness expansion of the anterior globe of the sclera producing enough substantial relaxing of the scleral tissue in the anterior globe to effectively change the stability of the anterior globe significantly enough to produce a myopic shift and axial length change. All of the expansion procedures have significant effects on eye shape of the anterior globe as a primary mechanism of action. LaserACE™ is *theoretically* different from the expansion procedures regarding the etiology of loss of ocular function as well as the mechanism and principles of restoration of ocular function. LaserACE™ procedure is based on the VisioDynamic Theory and scleral compression, biomechanical dysfunction, homeostatic, and neuromuscular hypotheses.[1] In this model, the etiology of the loss of accommodation in presbyopia is principally related to the effects of age-related changes of the eye which impact its normal biomechanical functions.[42] Scleral compression ultimately precipitates ocular biomechanical dysfunction leading to increased mechanical load, shear stress and consequential tissue strain.[43] Tissue strain and deformation has effects on micro tissue layer interactions, collagenous integral structure/remodeling and ultimately neuromuscular, physiological and extracellular matrix chemical and nutrient balance and efficiency. LaserACE™ surgical application is *fundamentally* different from these procedures in that there is *no* objective for scleral expansion or induced myopia, rather there is a zonal *decompression* of the connective tissue restriction which eliminates the compression or impingement of subliminal connective tissue, fascal tissue, and biophysiological structures of the eye organ (Figure 23.8).

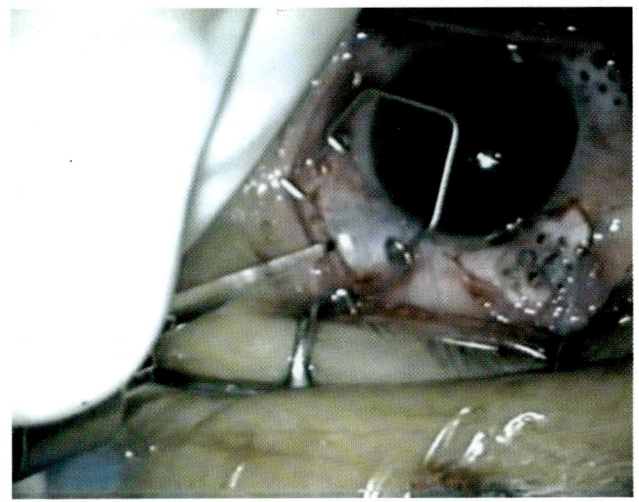

FIGURE 23.8: LaserACE™ zonal decompression decreases vertical load and creates no expansion

LaserACE™ Strategic Critical Zones of Restoration

LaserACE™ nomogram is based on mathematical calculations in anterior globe sphere specific to Three Critical zones (Figure 23.9 and 23.10). The key element in the effectiveness of the procedure lies in the ability to decompress the anterior globe with specificity to the key physiological and biomechanical areas of function. It is also critical to create the micro "NeoPores" with respect to the geometry of the sphere and the relative change in scleral thickness, CT characteristics, and rigidity across the globe (Figure 23.9). The cylindrical excisions are made in segmental zones with relativity to the natural physiological shape of the sclera and in tangential

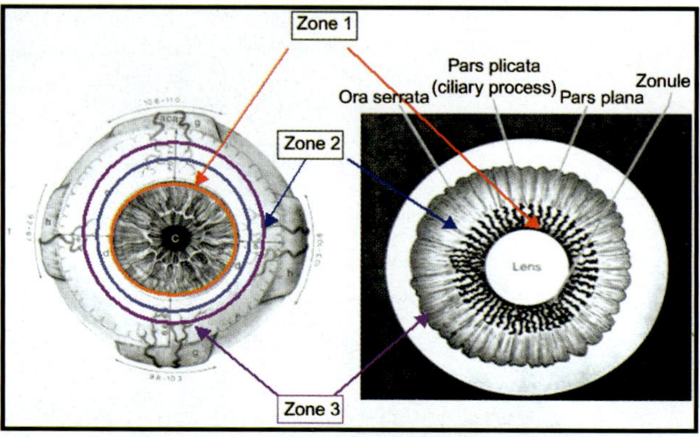

FIGURE 23.9: LaserACE™ critical zones—anatomy and geometry

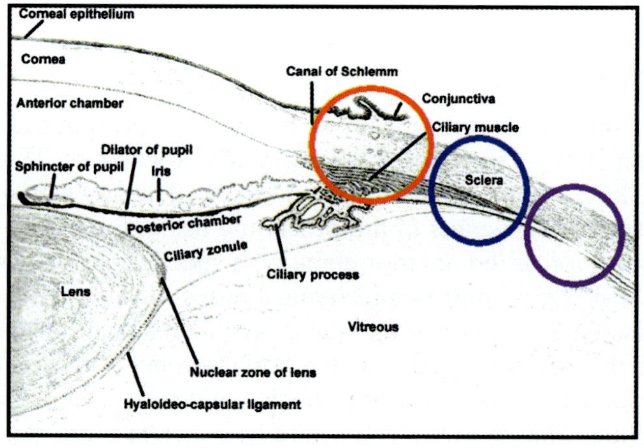

FIGURE 23.10: LaserACE™ critical zones—physiology

quadrants which allows decompression of the functional structures in the physiological planes of the spheroid of the eye globe in *three critical zones* of anatomical and physiological significance (Figure 23.10).

CRITICAL ZONES:

- Zone 1: Just distal to the corneoscleral envelope in the region of the Limbus extending to the pars plana over the girth of the ciliary body/process/complex and particularly the scleral spur 0.5 mm limbal area/tm/ scleral spur/structures of the angle.
- Zone 2: The region of the sclera which is begins just outside of pars plana and represents the largest circumferential diameter of the anterior globe sphere between the equator and the edge of the pars plana.
- Zone 3: The region of the ora serrata and the origin of the anterior radial ciliary muscles.

LASERACE™ NATURAL VISION RESTORATION SURGICAL SOLUTIONS

VisioLite™ Ophthalmic Laser System

The LaserACE™ procedure (Laser Anterior Ciliary Excision) is a revolutionary new technique which is performed with the VisioLite™ Er:YAG laser (Figure 23.11). The VisioLite™ laser's superior design and ability to control the variations of energy delivered will be the safest laser on the market for low energy soft tissue ablations for microsurgery in the eye. The laser beam of the VisioLite™ is pulsed and at a specific wavelength (2.94 um) that is very highly absorbed by water, as well as anything containing water such as CT. The laser beam causes rapid

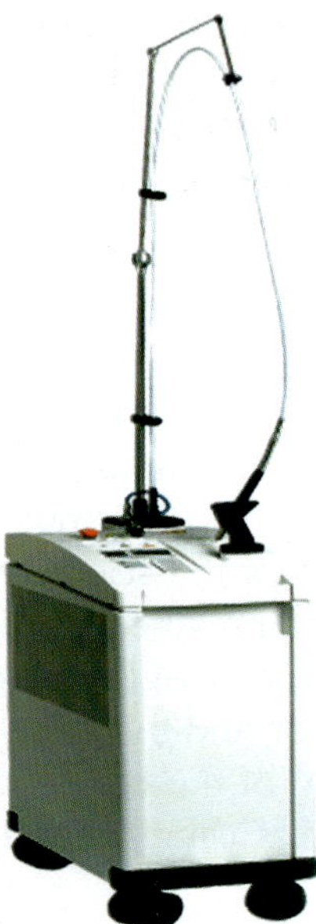

FIGURE 23.11: VisioLite™ ophthalmic laser system

vaporization, or ablation, in both hard and soft tissues. The efficiency of tissue removal varies with the available laser beam wavelength, the energy per pulse, the diameter of the pulse at the target, the pulse duration, and the repetition rate of the pulses. The optimum wavelength for energy absorption in water is 2.94 microns which is what the VisioLite™ ophthalmic laser system emits. The laser energy causes a vaporization of the water in the target tissue, causing an expansion of the water volume. The expansion causes the surrounding mineral material to be ejected. This water mediated explosive tissue removal is efficient and *transfers minimal heat to the surrounding*

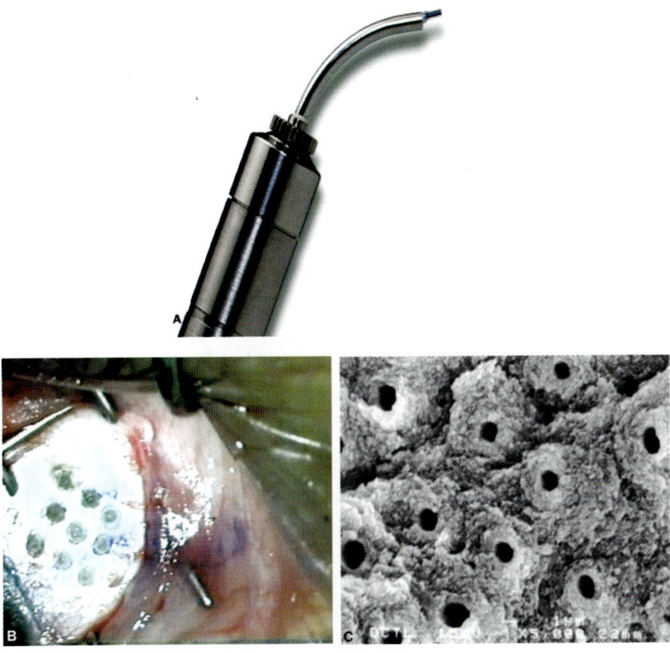

FIGURES 23.12A to C: (A) VisioLite patented optical probe and tip, (B) LaserACE™ NeoPores *in vivo* (C) LaserACE™ NeoPores (SEM 5,000 X)

tissue. The unique properties of the Er:YAG laser allow inhibition of tissue healing response therefore preserving the "NeoPores" integrity without tissue regeneration or scarring. In addition to the Er:YAG being the ideal wavelength to create efficient photoablation without significant photocoagulation[44] (Figures 23.12B and C). There are small 'desirable' thermal and mechanical effects that produce stimulation of proprioceptive and vascular tissues in the ciliary complex which facilitate accommodation. It is further proposed that the unique characteristics of the 2.94 Er: YAG laser especially contribute to the 'lasting effects' of the procedure by limiting inflammatory stress and inhibiting tissue remodeling.

How LaserACE™ Works

- *Excisions in the sclera and globe in critical zones thereby restoring the efficiency to the biomechanics of the accommodative system.*
- *Secondary impact of changing the biomechanics of the relationship of the lens/ciliary oculociliary joint complex mechanism improves mobility to achieve improved accommodative power.*
- *Improves the efficiency of the hydrodynamic system by influencing intraocular pressure and aqueous drainage. Rejuvenation of the trabecular meshwork.*

Ideal Eligibility for LaserACE™
Ideal Age: 48-65 years
Health patient with no CT diseases or ocular pathology • ±.50 spherical equivalent BCVA 20/25 or better • No more than .50 cylinder • Preferably plano or –.25 to –.50 spherical equivalent prior to LaserACE™ • PRK,RK, LASIK refractive correction can be done either before or after LaserACE™ • Ideally no more than .50 diopters of difference between manifest and cycloplegic refraction
Ideal IOP is 12-20 mmHg
Normal stereopsis
• No convergence insufficiency or eye teaming deficit, History of fusional problems (phorias and tropias – poor stereopsis) • No excessively large pupils

LaserACE™: Surgical Technique

The aim of the LaserACE™ surgical procedure is the strategic volumetric decompression of scleral tissue outside the limbus over critical zones of the anterior segment of the globe of the eye. The mathematical model for scleral decompression is based on age-related geometric and tissue characteristics. The scleral decompression is accomplished by removing strategic areas of sclera in opposing quadrants of the anterior globe segment whereby a series of zonal connective tissue partitions are created using a non-contact Er: YAG 2.94 um wavelength.

The patient is prepared with 2 percent xylocaine topical drops or subconjunctival anesthesia and draped in usual way as LASIK. One percent povidone-iodine is used to prep lashes and cul-de-sac. Mark 6 o'clock and 12 o'clock meridians with a 26 G needle dipped in gentian violet. An opaque "Hover" contact lens is used with Goniosol or other viscoelastic for corneal protection (Figure 23.13A). The Critical Zones are mapped out utilizing custom designed quadrant and matrix markers in the 4 oblique quadrants (Figures 23.13B and C).The surgeon determines method of conjunctival dissection either via flap and conjunctival spreader instrument or transconjunctival excision (Figure 23.13D).

Calipers are used to measure the total length × width parameters of the exicision zone and a gentian violet marker is used to make outer limit guidemarks for the matrix (Figures 23.14A and B).The VisioLite™ laser and patented optical probe/tip is used to create the "NeoPore" excision matrix. Depending on the protocol used, between 9-12 NeoPores are created per quadrant or between 10-12 mm cubic volume of sclerotic sclera is removed.

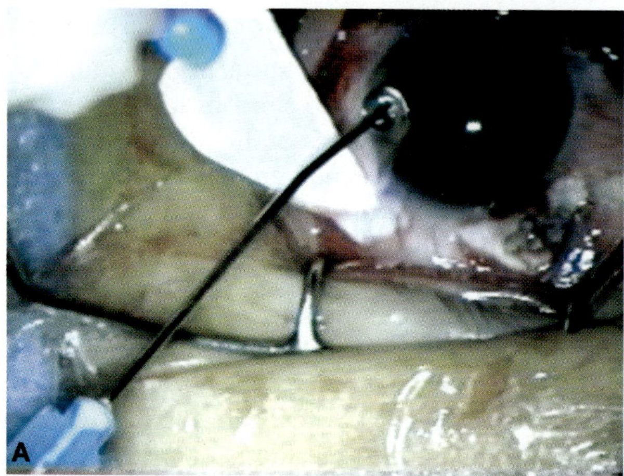

FIGURE 23.13A: Preparation for quadrant excisions: Viscoelastic and opaque corneal protector Hover lens with topical anesthetic solution

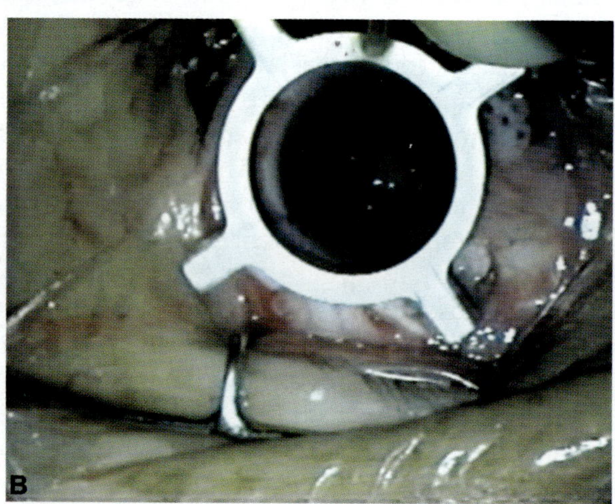

FIGURE 23.13B: Four point quadrant marker demarcates central segmental guidelines for "NeoPore" matrix

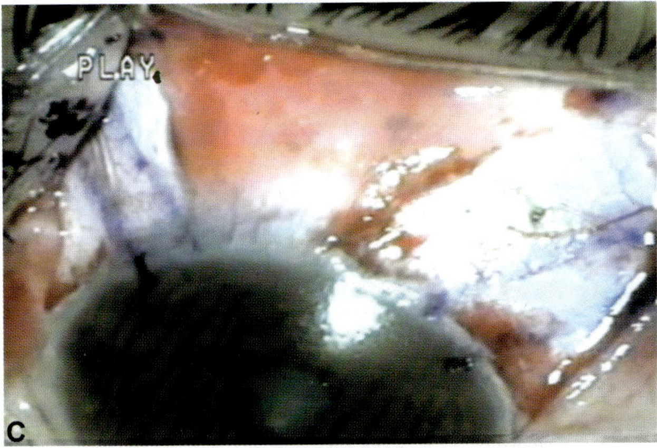

FIGURE 23.13C: Conjunctiva is opened to expose parameters of the quadrant zones. Zonal guide marks are used for excision matrix pattern

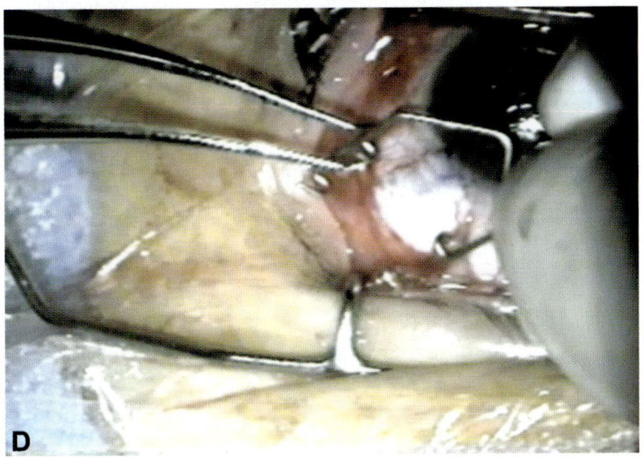

FIGURE 23.13D: Conjunctival spreader is used for optimal surgical field

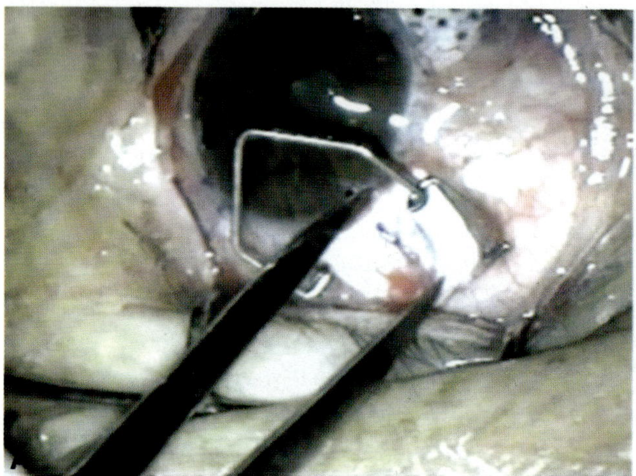

FIGURE 23.14A: Calipers are used to measure the total length of the excision zone extending from Zone 1-3

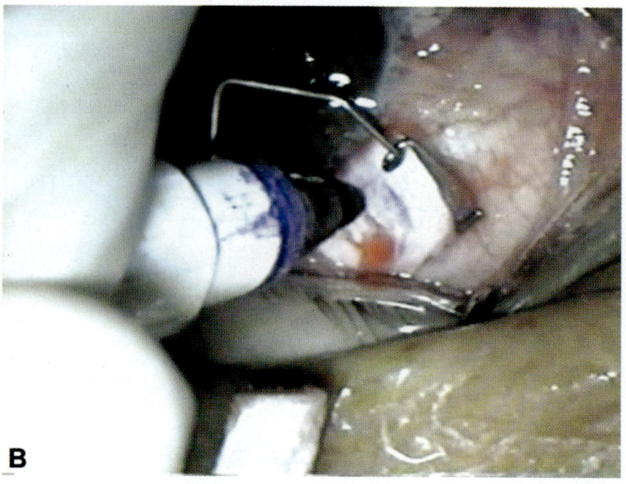

FIGURE 23.14B: Excision length and total excision surface area are marked

The NeoPore depth is approximately 90-95 percent (Figure 23.14C). The resulting "NeoPores" or 'new pores' can be created in a number of design patterns, however, they must have a critical width which is necessary to inhibit scleral residual tissue approximation thereby inhibiting normal fibroblast activity retarding the connective tissue healing cycle. Collagen reorganization and tissue healing response is further prevented by implantation of a weightless bioscaffold material having very low specific gravity and therefore adding no external loading of the structures beneath and maintaining 'NeoPore' effectiveness (Figure 23.14D). It is believed that this strategic removal of scleral tissue creates a newly formed microperforated tissue layer at the aponeurosis of the oculus or the subchoroidal lamina within the segmental zone treatment areas. These segmental regions act as biological "flexible diaphragm pumps" or extensible dividing membrane partitions which allow decompression of scleral load and shear stress, rejuvenation of intracellular /extracellular fluid exchange and restoration of biomechanical efficiency in the tissues that are internal to the scleral shell.

The conjunctival spreader is removed after each zone is completed and the conjunctiva is closed with conjunctival glue or alternatively bipolar cautery can be used. Topical anesthetic and steroid drops are placed in the eye following the procedure and are used for one week postoperatively along with biotears. Patient is instructed in VisioFlex™ accommodative exercises immediately.

LaserACE™: Kinesiology Application

The resultant effect of the LaserACE™ procedure is the immediate change in ocular mobility and indirect impact

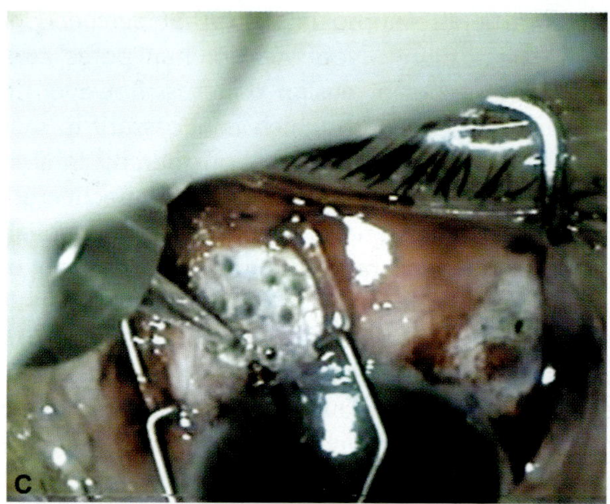

FIGURE 23.14C: LaserACE™ "NeoPore" excision matrix is made with the VisioLite patented optical probe tip

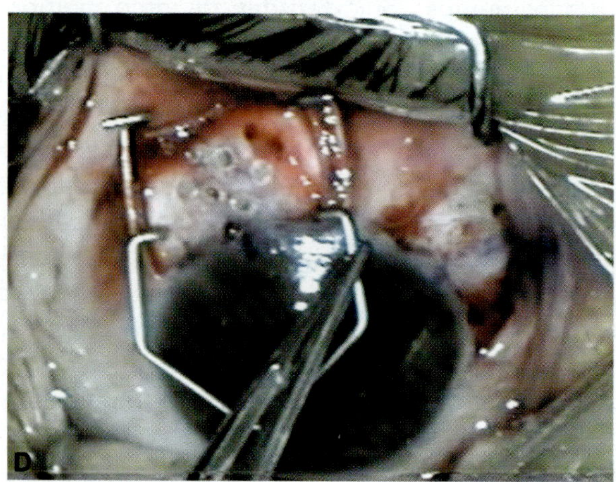

FIGURE 23.14D: Completed segmental decompression of sclera is stabilized with opaque bioscaffold fill

on viscoelastic modulus and rigidity. Enhanced mechanical efficiency of the accommodative mechanism as well as improved aqueous outflow as a result of zonal scleral excisions is demonstrated by an immediate drop in IOP (approximately 3 mmHg) and ability to respond to near visual stimulus with significant amplitude within a few hours postoperatively. Further implications regarding enhanced metabolic solute transfer in the hydrodynamic system are being studied. It is believed that the culmination of the LaserACE™ decompression results may represent an additional potential prophylactic benefit by producing an improvement of overall eye health and adding the potential effects of increasing the longevity of eye function for satisfactory performance of functional vision ADL with delay of onset of diseased states.

The neuromuscular consequences include a resetting of the oculociliary joint complex in the anterior and posterior chamber, facilitation of the inner scleral wall mobility and choroidal elastic translation of the ciliary ring forces to the lens.[45] The restored biomechanical efficiency may in fact create a positive shift in the AC/C ratio (accommodation convergence/convergence) decreasing the level of effort needed to accommodate.[46] Lens factors still contribute to the overall accommodative deficits but despite this even small changes in vector force translations to the lens produce large functional improvements biomechanical improvements and therefore large functional improvements.[47] This is due to the mass and specific gravity of the lens, compared to mass and specific gravity of the sclera in an aged eye and the postoperative resetting of the ciliary ring lens complex. Even as little as 0.25 mm of anterior translation can contribute a significant change in dioptric power for near response. In addition the increase in specific gravity and central cortex nuclear mass of the lens which accompanies age actually becomes an advantageous mechanical property to allow for an even greater fulcrum with very low requirement in overall force from the ciliary ring in order to move the lens forward to facilitate near vision acuity. Intermediate vision likewise is dramatically improved.

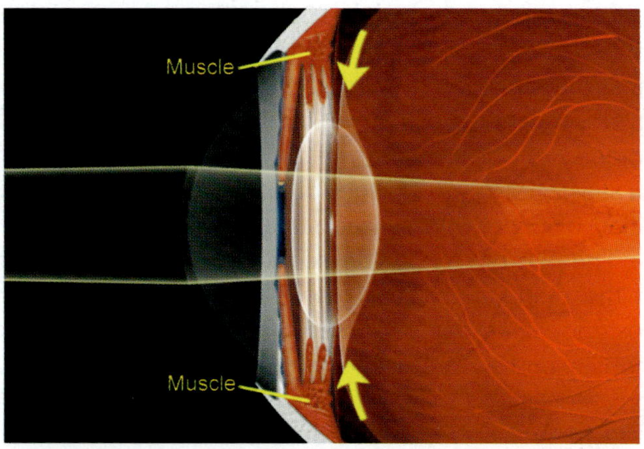

FIGURE 23.15: Improved VisioDynamic efficiency with natural restoration of accommodative function

LaserACE™ patient's also experience *"overload"* to the accommodative mechanism even at rest due to the restoration of functional capacity of the neuromuscular unit until the initial healing phase begins to stabilize and balance the globe. The "NeoPores" remain completely open for approximately 4-6 hours. A thin layer of epithelial cells begin to form in the early healing phase to close the inner fascial layer of the sphere. During this temporary initial phase, over convergence or "supervision" will occur in for a time period prior to acute stability of the healing anterior globe segment (approx. 10-14 days). This is followed by smaller variations in fluctuation, manifest stability (approx. 6-8 wks), and finally a CNS established end point resting tonus in the accommodative system (approx. 3-6 months). It is critically important during all phases, especially the initial phase for the patient to be compliant in accommodative training exercises in order to maximize potential outcomes. Patients can experience 'overload' and ciliary spasm during prolonged exercise or reading activities especially in the first one or two postoperative months. As the system becomes well trained, accommodative spasm dissipates. It is also imperative for the patient to train the newly activated neuromuscular system in both dynamic burst response and prolonged endurance modes. Accommodative insufficiency is seen more in the myopic eye and underdeveloped neuromuscular systems, whereas, Accommodative spasm is seen more frequently in hyperopic eye type and well developed accommodative systems. Semi-permanent/permanent stabilization seems to occur at about 6 months postoperative. Safety and preliminary efficacy have been determined by animal studies and *in vivo* treatment of more than 60 human eyes.

LaserACE™ Prospective Clinical Trial: Preliminary Results

In June 2003, clinical surgical validation of the LaserACE™ procedure along with diagnostic proofs for the VisioDynamic theory were initiated in Moscow Russia, with Dr Dimitrii Dementiev. A series of aberrometry and evaluative studies were performed as well as evolution of the LaserACE™ nomogram parameters and are ongoing. These early endeavors were pivotal to the efficacy of the volumetric calculations that produce the stable LaserACE™ biomechanical result without compromise of ocular stability or asymmetry. In December 2003, clinical surgical studies began in Juarez Mexico with investigator Dr Bobby Maddox. Clinical surgeries were performed during 2004 on 8 eyes or 16 patients. Results were encouraging with a mean of 3.1 diopters of improvement for accommodative amplitude for near and intermediate vision with no statistically significant change in manifest refraction.In May of 2005 clinical surgical studies began in Valencia, Venezuela with Dr Jose Manuel Vargas. LaserACE™ was performed on 3 eyes recently with similar preliminary results.

LaserACE™
Preoperative and Postoperative Exam

- Medical history
- Visual Function Questionnaire
- Complete eye examination
- Dilated fundus exam
- Video keratography
- Contrast sensitivity
- Manifest and cycloplegic refraction
- Pupillary size
- IOP
- Gonioscopy
- Amplitude of accommodation (push-up method)
- Near vision at 35 cm (14")
- Intermediate vision at 60 cm (24")
- Axial length and AC depth (Humphrey Zeiss IOL Master) pachymetry

Health Canada approved the LaserACE™ procedure for investigative study in October of 2004. Presently ongoing prospective Clinical Trials were initiated with Dr John F Blaylock in British Columbia, Canada. Clinical surgeries were performed during 2004 and 2005 on 20 eyes. The preliminary results represented herein. Patient data demonstrated a good effect in improving near vision and an excellent effect at improving intermediate or "functional" vision. Mean increase for these patients of more than 3.0 diopters. These results include 6-month data for most of the 10 patients, but a minimum of 3 month follow-up on all 10 patients. T test and linear regression analysis were performed and *accommodative amplitude* measured with a 'push-up' and 'pull up' method utilizing the K-range measurement modified prince rule showed significant increase in accommodative amplitude. Monocular increased by 1.89 ± 1.16 D; (mean ± SD, P= 0.000); Range: –0.1 to +3.8 D and Binocular increased by 3.27 ± 2.38 D;(mean ± SD, P=0.002); Range: 0.2 to +7.6 D.

LaserACE™ resulted in significant improvement of both Monocular and binocular near uncorrected visual acuity measured at 40 cm (Figure 23.16). Even greater improvements were seen for intermediate visual acuity measured at 60 cm (Figure 23.17). A majority of the patients reported on the patient questionnaire more dissatisfaction and loss of functional ADL (Activities of Daily Living) with loss of intermediate vision or 'functional-arm's length vision'. Therefore, patient satisfaction for functional ADL was over 95 percent.

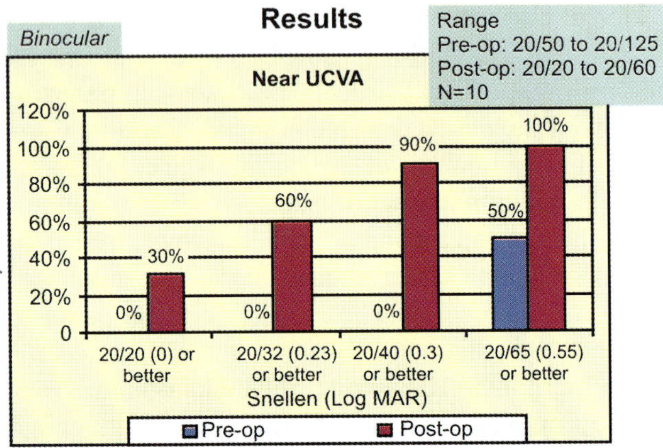

FIGURE 23.16: Binocular near uncorrected VA (40 cm) showed significant improvement by 0.47 ± 0.27 (log MAR, mean± SD) (P= 0.000); Range: 0.17 to 0.90

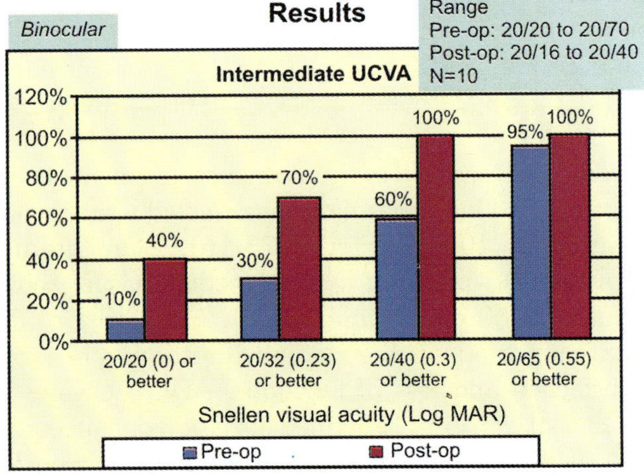

FIGURE 23.17: Binocular intermediated uncorrected VA (60 cm) showed improvements by 0.21 ± 0.18 (logMAR, mean ± SD) (P= 0.006); Range: 0.00 to 0.53

LaserACE™ results showed a statistically significant reduction for Add diopters for 20/20 of near VA (40 cm) after surgery. Monocular Add was reduced by 0.68 ± 0.45 D (mean ± SD) (P=0.000); Range: 0.00 to 1.25 D. Binocular Add was reduced by 0.73 ± 0.53 D (mean ± SD) (P=0.002); Range: 0.25 to 1.75 D (Figure 23.18).

Results

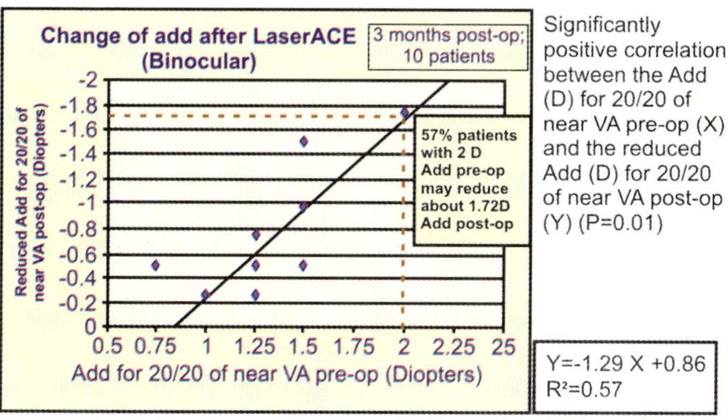

FIGURE 23.18: LaserACE™ statistical correlation between Add of near VA

There were minor changes of manifest refraction after surgery, but no statistically significant (P>0.05); Preoperative spherical refraction equivalent; 0.33 ± 0.31 D (mean ± SD); (Range: –0.25 to +0.75 D). Postoperative spherical refraction equivalent 0.31 ± 0.48 D (mean± SD);(Range: –0.50 to + 1.50 D). No statistically significant change of binocular distance uncorrected visual acuity (UCVA); Preoperative UVCA range: 20/15 to 20/25; Postoperative UCVA range: 20/15 to 20/20; N= 10 patients. There were minor changes of manifest refraction after surgery, but no statistically significant (P>0.05).

Preoperative spherical refraction equivalent 0.33 ± 0.31 D (mean ± SD);(Range: –0.25 to +0.75 D);Postoperative spherical refraction equivalent ± 0.48 D (mean± SD); (Range: –0.50 to + 1.50 D). A-Scan showed no statistically significant change of axial length (AL) after surgery (P>0.05). Preoperative AL: 23.57 ± 0.97 mm (mean ± SD).Postoperative AL: 23.56 ± 0.98 mm (mean ± SD).Topography (Humphrey) showed no statistically significant change of corneal curvature after surgery (P>0.05). Preoperative average K value: 42.92 ±1.57 D; (mean ± SD); Postoperative average K value: 43.12 ± 1.72 D (mean ± SD).

LaserACE™ Prospective Clinical Trial: Preliminary Results

Early outcomes have also shown a small statistically significant improvement in contrast sensitivity (Figure 23.19). Review of preoperative patient questionnaire shows that patient compliance with accommodative exercises gives better outcomes as well as patients who read frequently. In patients with previous LASIK or PRK, LaserACE™ appears to be preferred choice for presbyopic solution. Presbyopia with high reading Add obtain greater improvement after surgery. Overall preliminary results are promising.

LaserACE™ Complications

Very minor or low complication rate has been reported with the LaserACE™ procedure. No anterior segment ischemia has been reported and no major complications.

Contrast sensitivity

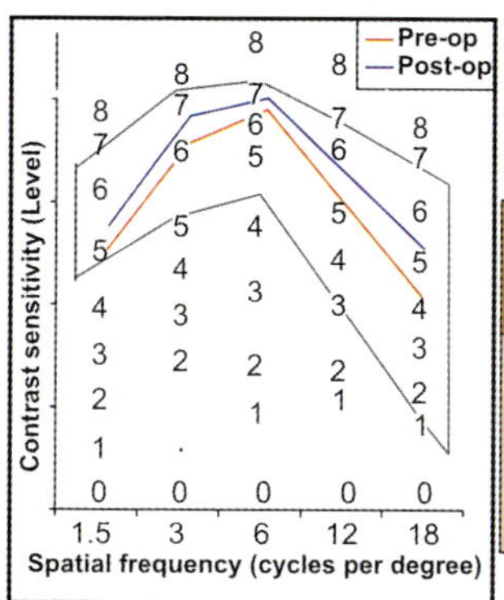

Mean contrast sensitivity level at 5 spatial frequencies before and 3 months after LaserACE

Spatial Frequency (cycles per degree)	Mean Contrast Sensitivity Level ± SD		
	Pre-op	Post-op	P Value
1.5	5.0 ± 0.6	5.4 ± 0.75	0.06
3	6.1 ± 0.8	6.6 ± 0.9	0.04
6	6.2 ± 1.1	6.8 ± 1.0	0.05
12	4.9 ± 1.0	5.5 ± 1.3	0.06
18	4.0 ± 1.2	5.1 ± 1.6	0.01

Paired samples T test

FIGURE 23.19: LaserACE™ statistical correlation between mean contrast sensitivity

LaserACE™
Complications

- 2 conjunctival cysts
- No ASI
- Subconjunctival hemorrhage
- No dry eye problem
- Temporary redness, and mild to moderate discomfort
- One patient saw shadowing at intermediate VA test in left eye 1 day and it disappeared within 1 week
- One patient had focusing problem at 20-40 feet 2 weeks postoperative and this disappeared one month post-operative

Patients experience temporary ciliary fimosis initially which can be alleviated by over the counter pain medications. Temporary redness and dryness is alleviated with biotears. Patients have improvement of near and intermediate vision within hours of the procedure.

REFERENCES

1. Hipsley AM. VisioDynamics Manuscript. VisioDynamic Theory: A Biomechanical Model for the Aging Ocular Organ, 2003.
2. Amile D, Woo SL-Y, Harwood FL, Akeson WH. The effect of immobilization on collagen turnover in connective tissue. A biochemical-biomechanical orrelation. Acta Orthop Scand 1982;53:325.
3. Viidik A, Danielsen CC, Oxluind H. Fourth International Congress of Biorheology Symposium on Mechanical Properties of Living Tissues: On fundamental and phenomenological models, structure and mechanical properties of collagen, elastic and glycosaminoglycan complexes. Biorheology, 1982;19:437.
4. Sylvie Wendling A1, Patrick CaÑadas, Christian Oddou A1, Alain Meunier A3. Interrelations Between Elastic Energy and Strain in a Tensegrity Model: Contribution to the Analysis of the Mechanical Response in Living Cells. Computer Methods in Biomechanics and Biomedical Engineering.2002;5(1): 1-6.
5. Diamant J, et al. Collagen: Ultrastructure and its relations to mechanical properties as a function of ageing. Proc R Soc Lond (Bio J) 1972;180:293.
6. Dale WC: A composite materials analysis of the structure, mechanical properties, and aging of collagenous tissues. PhD thesis, Case Wetern Reserve University, Cleveland, Ohio 1974.
7. Curtin BJ. Physiopathological Aspects of Scleral Stress-Strain". Tr Am Opht Soc 1969;67:417-61.
8. Fung YC B: Stress-strain history relations of soft tissues in simpole elongation. In: Fung YC, Perrone N, Anliker M (Eds). Biomechanics: Its Foundations and Objectives. Englewood Cliffs, Prentice-Hall 1972;1818-208.
9. Werner L, et al. Correlation between different measurements within the eye relative to phakic intraocular lens implantation. J Cataract Refract Surg 2004; 30:1982-88.
10. Fung YC. B: Biomechanics: Mechanical Properties of Living tissues, New York, Springer Verlag, 1981, 222.

11. Hutton RS. Neuromuscular physiology. In: Welsh RP, Shephard RJ (Eds). Current Therapy in Sports Medi ine 1985-1986. B. C. Decker. Philadelphia, 1985.
12. Aura O, Komi PV.Effects of prestretch intensity on mechanical efficiency of positive work and on elastic behaviour of skeletal muscle in stretch-short cycle. Int J Sports Med 1986;7:137.
13. Craik R. Biomechanics: a neural control perspective. Physical Therapy 1984;64:1810-11.
14. Hipsley AM. VisioDynamics Manuscript: Biomechanical Solutions for the Aging Ocular Organ: LaserACE™ Natural Vision Restoration.
15. Arciniegas A, Amaya LE. Mechanical behavior of the sclera. Ophthalmologica 1986;193(1-2):45-55.
16. Paul JP. Approaches to design: force actions transmitted by joints in the human body. Proc R Soc Lond B. 1976; 192,163.
17. Sigal IA, Flanagan JG, Tertinegg I, Ethier RC. Finite Element Modeling of Optic Nerve Head Biomechanics Investigative Ophthalmology and Visual Science. 2004;45:4378-87.
18. Ioannis G Pallikaris,1,2 George D. Kymionis,1,2 Harilaos S. Ginis,2 George A. Kounis,2 and Miltiadis K. Tsilimbaris1,2. Ocular Rigidity in Living Human Eyes. Investigative Ophthalmology and Visual Science. 2005;46:409-14.
20. Burgoyne CF, Downs JC, Bellezza AJ, Suh JK, Hart RT. The optic nerve head as a biomechanical structure: a new paradigm for understanding the role of IOP-related stress and strain in the pathophysiology of glaucomatous optic nerve head damage. Prog Retin Eye Res 2005 jan:24(1):39-73.
21. Battaglioli JL,Kamm RD. Measurements of the compressive properties of scleral tissue IOVS:1984.
22. Rada JA, Achen VR, Penugonda S, Schmidt RW, Mount BA. Proteoglycan composition in the human sclera during growth and aging. Invest Ophthalmol Vis Sci 2000 41(7):1639-48.
23. Rada JA, Achen VR, Rada KG. Proteoglycan turnover in the sclera of normal and experimentally myopic chick eyes. Invest Ophthalmol Vis Sci 1998;39(11):1990-2002.

24. Yamaoka A, Matsuo T, Shiraga F, Ohtsuki H. TIMP-1 production by human scleral fibroblast decreases in response to cyclic mechanical stretching. Opthalmic Res 2001;3 3(2):98-101.
25. Watson PG, Young, RD. Scleral structure, organisation and disease. A review. Exp Eye Res. 2004;78(3):609-23.
26. Julie Albona, Peter P Purslowb, Wojciech S S Karwatowskic, David L Eastyd. Age related compliance of the lamina cribrosa in human eyes. Br J Ophthalmol 2000;84:318-23.
27. Gong H, Freddo TF, Johnson M. Age-related changes of sulfated proteoglycans in the normal human trabecular meshwork. Exp Eye Res. 1992 Nov:55(5):691-709.
28. Koretz JF, Rogot A, Kaufman PL. Physiological strategies for emmetropia. Trans Am Ophthalmol Soc 1995;93:105-18; discussion 118-22.
29. Hanna KD, et al. Computer Simulation of Arcuate and Radial Incisions involving the corneoscleral Limbus", Eye, 1989;3:227-39.
30. Ross C Ethier, Mark Johnson, Jeff Rubert. Ocular Biomechanics and Biotransport. Annual Review of Biomedical Engineering. 2004;6:249-73.
31. Neacsu A, Tuchila G, Trifu M, Curea M, Boeru G. Biomechanical stress in glaucoma—cause and effect. Oftalmologia. 2004;48(4):93-8.
32. Mori F, Konno S, Hikichi T, Yamaguchi Y, Ishiko S , Yoshida A. Factors affecting Pulsatile Ocular Blood Flow. Br J Ophthalmol 2001;85:529-30.
33. Shepherd RJ. Physiology and Biochemistry of Exercise. Praeger, New York, 1982.
34. Buckwalter JA. Maintaining and restoring mobility in middle and old age: the importance of the soft tissues. Instr Course Lect 1997;46:459-69.
35. Norton TT, Siegwart JT Jr. Animal models of emmetropization: matching axial length to the focal plane. J Am Optom Assoc 1995;66(7):405-14.
36. Woo SL-Y, et al. Nonlinear Material Properties of Intact Cornea and Sclera. Exp Eye Res 1972;14:29-39.

37. Robin JB. Radial keratotomy: Procedures. Indian J Ophthalmol 1990;3 8(3):103:6.
38. Thornton S. Anterior Ciliary Sclerotomy (ACS), A Procedure to Reverse Presbyopia. Surgery for Hyperopia and Presbyopia, Neal Sher (Ed). 1997;33-37.
39. Schacar RA. Cause and treatment of presbyopia with a method for increasing the amplitude of accommodation. Ann Ophththalmol 1992;24:445-52.
40. Lin JT, Perasso A, Martinez D. A novel device for presbyopia reversal. ISRS1999; 92.
41. Hipsley AM. Influence of Biomechanics on Age-Related Changes of the Eye: Clinical Implications for Refractive Surgery. ASCRS 2005.
42. SA Strenk, JL Semmlow, LM Strenk, P Munoz, J Gronlund-Jacob, JK DeMarco. Age-related changes in human ciliary muscle and lens: a magnetic resonance imaging study. Invest Ophthalmol Vis Sci 1999;40:1162-69.
43. Battaglioli JL,Kamm RD: Measurements of the compressive properties of scleral tissue IOVS:1984.
44. Becker PC, Olsson NA, Simpson JR. Erbium-doped fiber amplifiers: Fundamentals and technology. San Diego [etc.]: 1999;Aron Rosa, Academic Press.
45. Friberg TR, Lace JW. A comparison of the elastic properties of human choroid and sclera. Exp Eye Res 1988;47(3): 429-36.
46. Mutti DO, Jones LA, Moeschberger ML, Zadnik K. AC/A ratio, age, and refractive error in children. Invest Ophthalmol Vis Sci 2000; 41(9):2469-78.
47. van Alphen GW. Choroidal stress and emmetropization. Vision Res 1986;26(5):723-34.

CHAPTER 24

LASEK (Laser Assisted Subepithelial Keratectomy)

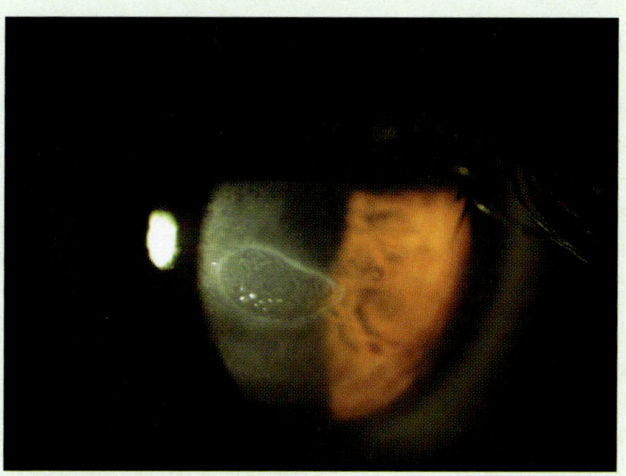

Sanjay Chaudhary (India)

WHY IS LASIK LOOSING ITS GLORY?

With the introduction of LASIK, PRK was immediately pushed to the background. Themain reasons for LASIK's popularity with the patients and the ophthalmologists were the quick recovery often termed the 'wow' factor, and the no corneal haze scenario. With the increasing numbers of LASIK, problems about this procedure started showing up. As ophthalmologists got down to correcting higher degrees of myopia and greater degrees of tissue ablation, cases of corneal ectasia began to get reported from all over the world. Initially a safe standard was set as a residual corneal bed of 300 mic. However, in a normal thickness cornea of 530 mic, and after making an allowance for a 160 mic flap, 70 mic was just sufficient tissue to correct about 5 D of refractive error. Customized LASIK and demands for prolate cornea, meant more ablation of the corneal tissue. This also meant that another one to two diopter was reduced from our capacity to correct the refractive errors. And what if the cornea was slightly thin and in the range of 500 mic. Would this mean depriving the person from the benefits of LASIK and a major loss of revenue for the ophthalmologist by increasing his rejections. Add to this the unpredictability of the flap thickness. It was demonstrated that the best of the microkeratomes, which talked of a 160 mic flap, would actually cut a flap in the range of 90 to 230 mic. Thus, with a lot of debate, the safe standard was set to 250 mic of residual corneal bed. And this gave the much-needed flexibility to the refractive surgeon to treat a mild to moderate myopia in routine clinical practice. So myopia of 1 to 8 could be handled in most of the situations. But what about the high myopes. Enterprising ophthalmologists started reducing the corneal bed further to 200 mic. As more and more cases of corneal ectasia got reported, there was a major concern for this man made complication even though the cases reported are few and far between. Doctors wanted to fell safe both for the patients and for themselves and this led to the transition to LASEK.

LASEK Gains Popularity

The more the residual stromal bed one leaves behind, the less the chances of ectasia was what makes LASEK ride the crest of popularity.

LASEK has the following advantages to offer:

1. More residual corneal bed thickness, so less chances of ectasia
2. No flap to be lifted, so
   a. No flap related complications like buttonhole, partial cut, free caps, flap wrinkling, epithelial down growth, etc.
   b. Another 90 mic of stroma available for corneal ablation thereby enhancing the limit of correction by approx. another 5D over LASIK.
   c. Less costly because the expense of a keratome and blades eliminated.
   d. In a better position to handle thin cornea. A person with a corneal thickness of 490 mic may still have an option of a 6D myopia correction.
   e. Large zone treatments for better corneal prolacity and in hyperopia are now possible. This essentially means that in LASIK the flap size was a restricting factor to the size of treatment. And it was seldom possible to go over a 9 mm treatment. The flap

size was further reduced in a flat cornea which was a catch situation in hyperopic patients who had a flat cornea, a small flap and a need for a large treatment zone. With LASEK there is no limitation to the zone of treatment.

Surgical Considerations

LASEK involves the stripping of epithelium from the Bowman's membrane in a form of a hinged flap.

An epithelial trephine of the required size in placed on the center of the cornea after anesthetizing the eye with 0.5 percent proparacaine eyedrops. A 4 mm segment of the trephine at the 12 O'clock is blunt. By placing on the cornea with pressure, the trephine cuts through the epithelium sparing the underlying stroma and the 12 O'clock epithelium. The diameter of the trephine could vary from 8.5 to 10.5 mm. A similar sized alcohol well is now centered on the cornea. Twenty percent ethyl alcohol is filled in the well and kept in position for 60 sec. It is then removed with a cellulose sponge, the well taken off the eye and the epithelium washed with BSS. After waiting another minute to allow the alcohol to weaken the epithelial Bowman's adhesions, a micro hoe is used to pick up the epithelium from the edges of the trephine marks. A hockey shaped spatula is now used to roll the epithelium slowly towards the hinge exposing a clean Bowman's to work on. Excimer laser is delivered to the cornea surface to make a correction for the refractive error. The corneal surface is washed thoroughly and scrapped to rid of the debris and the condensed plume. The epithelium is carefully rolled back with the help of an irrigating cannula. Because of the loose elasticity of the tissue, the replaced epithelium usually crosses over the natural edges to overlap some of the healthy epithelium. A bandage contact lens is now placed over the epithelium where it rests for the next five days. The patient is sent home after instilling a preservative free lubricating eyedrop, an antibiotic and a NSAID eyedrop. These are used for the next five days. Systemic antibiotic and strong pain killers are prescribed for the next three days.

LASEK with Mitomycin C

Here, all the above steps are the same. After corneal ablation the treated area of the cornea is exposed to 0.02 percent Mitomycin C for 30 seconds. The corneal surface is then thoroughly washed with BSS for a minute to remove all traces of Mitomycin and then the epithelium is reposited back. Mitomycin C is useful in containing fibroblastic activity and thereby reducing and delaying the chances of corneal haze, more so when attempting to treat high myopia.

Follow-Up

The bandage contact lens is removed when the old epithelium is replaced by the new epithelium generated from the edges of the wound. This usually coincides on the fifth postoperative day. After removing the Bandage Contact Lens, FML eyedrops are started to replace NSAID drops to contain the tissue edema and the subsequent fibroblastic reaction. In our clinical practice we use FML six times a day for a week, and then taper it off by a drop every week over the next six weeks. Antibiotic drops are used for two weeks and lubricating drops for at least two and a half month or more as per requirement.

Disadvantages of LASEK

These are similar to PRK with minor modifications:

Postoperative Pain

This is a major setback for LASEK. The pain is intense on the day of LASIK and reduces over the next 2 to 3 days. This may be accompanied with hyperemia, chemosis of the conjunctiva, and lid edema. Strong analgesics and anti-inflammatory are required over the first 2 to 3 days. The intensity of pain is definitely less than what is encountered in PRK. This is also in sharp contrast to LASIK where there is no pain and only an occasional irritation and watering on the day of the procedure.

Buttonholing

Excess exposure to alcohol does help in easily picking up the flap, but the resultant chemical trauma to the epithelium results in greater tissue reaction, more haze, pain and tissue edema. Less exposure to alcohol or less percentage of alcohol used prevents proper loosening up of the epithelium resulting in single or multiple buttonholing. Excessive breaks in the continuity of the epithelium make the flap useless and have to be discarded. The situation then mimics a PRK.

Blurred Vision

The patient encounters blurred vision for a week. This is a result of epithelial haze as the new epithelium coming in from the sides replaces the old alcohol treated epithelium. The vision clears up in a week's time. This is in stark contrast to LASIK where the patient has good vision within a few hours and has total clarity by next morning.

Corneal Haze

This has become the most feared complication in a long-standing follow-up of LASEK. The haze is similar to the one encountered in PRK and can be graded from I to IV. The use of Mitomycin C in our routine clinical practice for myopia of over 4 D seems to have helped in the following ways:

1. Haze is usually not encountered in myopia of up to 7.0 D as compared with PRK where it could be encountered after 4 D
2. Myopia of 8 to 12 usually results in Grade I haze while 12 and above may result in Grade II to III haze
3. There have been situations where even –18 D has had no haze and on the other hand, even a –5 developed a mild haze
4. Haze usually develops after 6-9 months of the procedure
5. Haze results in a regression of the refractive error and the degree of regression depends on the severity of haze
6. Haze usually regresses spontaneously over a period of 2-3 years. Low dose topical steroids could assist resolution
7. The regression of haze sometimes results in some reversal of regression of the refractive error and improvement in refractive error and vision.

The above observations are not a rule but an indication of the surgeon's experience with PRK of over 10 years and of LASEK with and without Mitomycin on over 400 eyes in 4 years.

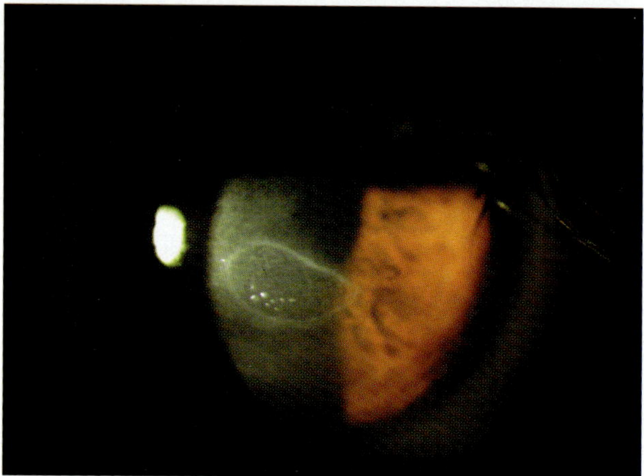

FIGURE 24.1: Delayed epithelial healing with corneal haze on 9th postoperative day after LASEK with Mitomycin C. The eye was patched with an antibiotic and lubricating ointment and the defect healed over the next 3 days

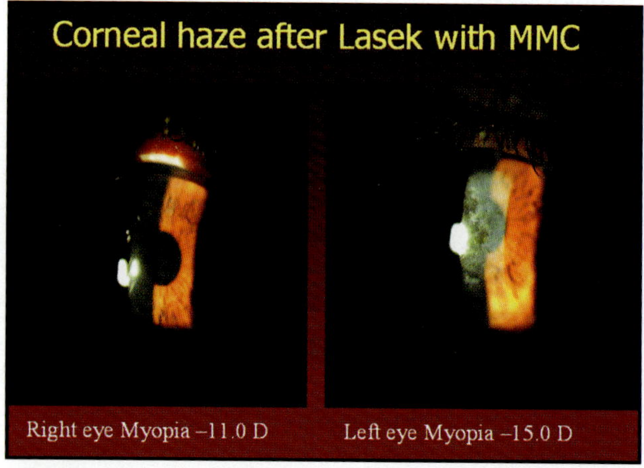

FIGURE 24.2: The patient developed a Grade I corneal haze in the right eye and a Grade II haze in the left eye after one and a half year of simultaneous LASEK with Mitomycin C in both eyes

LASEK in Relation to PRK and Epi-LASIK

PRK, LASEK and now Epi-LASIK involve the removing or stripping of the epithelium from the Bowman's membrane. In PRK, it is mechanical scrapping, in LASEK it is alcohol assisted while in Epi-LASIK, it is again separation with a blade. Since the three are essentially similar, they carry the same advantages and disadvantages with minor modifications. The postoperative pain has definitely reduced from PRK to LASEK to Epi-LASIK. This is attributed to a healthier flap over the cornea and less alcohol injury. The rate of epithelial healing has improved favoring Epi-LASIK. This has also reduced the blurring of vision to a shorter period. However, it postulates that the effect on corneal haze may be similar in LASEK and Epi-LASEK. More experience is required to understand the long-term difference between the two. Epi-LASIK is prone to buttonholing, and in such a situation, the entire epithelium has to be scrapped off to continue with the procedure, and this then becomes a PRK.

BIBLIOGRAPHY

1. Autrata R, Rehurek J. Laser-assisted subepithelial keratectomy and photorefractive keratectomy for the correction of hyperopia: Results of a 2-year follow-up. J Cataract Refract Surg 2003;29:2105-14.
2. Autrata R, Rehurek J. Laser–assisted subepithelial keratectomy for myopia: Two-year follow-up. J Cataract Refract Surg 2003;29:661-68.
3. Azar DT, Ang RT, Lee J-B, et al. Laser subepithelial keratomileusis: Electron microscopy and visual outcomes of flap photorefractive keratectomy. Curr Opin Ophthalmol 2001;12:323-28.
4. Camellin M. Laser epithelial keratomileusis for myopia. J Refract Surg 2003;19:666-70.

5. Claringbold TV II. Laser-assisted subepithelial keratectomy for the correction of myopia. J Cataract Refract Surg 2002;28:18-22.
6. Espana EM, Grueterich M, Mateo A, et al. Cleavage of corneal basement membrane components by ethanol in laser-assisted subepithelial keratectomy. J Cataract Refract Surg 2003; 29:1192-97.
7. Lee JB, Seong GJ, Lee JH, et al. Comparison of laser epithelial keratomileusis and photorefractive keratectomy for low to moderate myopia. J Cataract Refract Surg 2001;27:565-70.
8. Scerrati E. Laser in situ keratomileusis vs laser epithelial keratomileusis (LASIK vs LASEK). J Refract Surg 2001;17:S219-S221.
9. Shah S, Sebai Sarhan AR, Doyle SJ, et al. The Epithelial flap for photorefractive keratectomy. Br J Ophthalmol 2001;85:393-96.
10. Shaninian L Jr. Laser-assisted subepithelial keratectomy for low to high myopia and astigmatism. J Cataract Refract Surg 2002;28:1334-42.

Index

D

E

F

G

H

I

K

L

M

O

P

R

W

Z